Visit our website

to find out about other books from Mosby
and our sister imprints in Harcourt Health Sciences

Register free at
www.harcourt-international.com

and you will get

- the latest information on new books, journals and electronic products in your chosen subject areas

- the choice of e-mail or post alerts or both, when there are any new books in your chosen areas

- news of special offers and promotions

- information about products from all Harcourt Health Sciences imprints including Baillière Tindall, Churchill Livingstone, Mosby and W. B. Saunders

You will also find an easily searchable catalogue, online ordering, information on our extensive list of journals...and much more!

Visit the Harcourt Health Sciences website today!

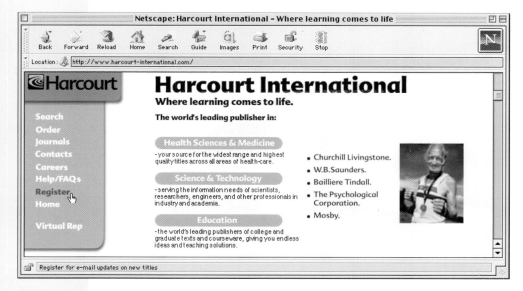

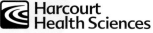

Prostate Cancer

Commissioning/Development Editor: Sue Hodgson
Project Manager: Hilary Hewitt
Production Manager: Mark Sanderson
Designer: Barrie Carr

Prostate Cancer

Second Edition

Roger S Kirby MD, FRCS
Consultant Urologist, St. George's Hospital, London, UK

Timothy J Christmas MD, FRCS
Consultant Urologist, Charing Cross Hospital, London, UK

Michael K Brawer MD
Director, Northwest Prostate Institute, Seattle, USA

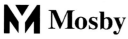 **Mosby**

London Edinburgh New York Philadelphia St Louis Sydney Toronto 2001

MOSBY
An imprint of Mosby International Limited

© Mosby International Limited 2001

M is a registered trademark of Mosby International Limited

The right of Roger S. Kirby, Timothy J. Christmas and Michael K. Brawer to be identified as authors of this work has been asserted by them in accordance with the Copyright, Designs and Patents Act 1988

First published 1996

ISBN 0 7234 3167 1

British Library Cataloguing in Publication Data
A catalogue record for this book is available from the British Library

Library of Congress Cataloging in Publication Data
A catalog record for this book is available from the Library of Congress

Note
Medical knowledge is constantly changing. As new information becomes available, changes in treatment, procedures, equipment and the use of drugs become necessary. The editors/authors/contributors and the publishers have, as far as it is possible, taken care to ensure that the information given in this text is accurate and up to date. However, readers are strongly advised to confirm that the information, especially with regard to drug usage, complies with the latest legislation and standards of practice.

The
publisher's
policy is to use
**paper manufactured
from sustainable forests**

Printed in England

Contents

Acknowledgements

'Things don't just happen, things have to be made to happen.'

We would like to acknowledge Sue Hodgson and Hilary Hewitt for their indefatigable work at Harcourt Health Sciences.

We also thank Irene Schleicher for invaluable help with proof checking and Dee McLean for enhancing the original figures and creating many new illustrations for this second edition.

We would also like to thank our wives, Jane and Patti, and our children for their unerring support and forbearance during the production of this book.

RSK and MKB

Preface to the first edition

The expression 'make it happen' seems set to become the catch-phrase of the remaining few years of this millenium, and it may certainly be aptly applied to those working in all aspects of prostate cancer. Virtually ignored for so long, this leading cause of cancer illness and death has seen an upsurge of interest over the past five years. The driving forces behind this are partly economic: it has been calculated that prostate cancer, together with benign prostatic hyperplasia (BPH), results in 4.4 million physician visits, 836 000 hospital admissions and 39 215 deaths annually at a health care cost of more than US$3 billion in the USA alone.

Moreover the ranks of those afflicted are swelling fast. Over this century in the West life expectancy has been increased by 25 years. Currently in the UK around 25% of the population is over the age of 60, and by 2031 this figure is projected to rise to 46%. The increasing numbers of men now reaching the so called Third Age (i.e. 50 to 75) hope and indeed expect to remain fit, healthy and vigorous. For them, over whom the disease hangs like the proverbial sword of Damocles, the argument that prostate cancer is a disease meriting low priority because of the relatively low number of life years lost carries little weight. Hence perhaps the increasing media fascination with the prostate over the past few years. This publicity has resulted in a rapid rise in the level of patient education relating to prostate cancer. This in turn has heightened the need for urologists and primary care physicians at every level to be conversant with the rapidly advancing knowledge in this disease area.

In this book we have tried to summarise state-of-the-art information about this very common cancer in as lucid and well illustrated a way as possible. Since in this modern world no-one, especially the busy practising urologist, has time to wade through dense and turgid text, we have tried to make the book as concise and easy to read as possible, while still covering most of the important issues in some depth. We hope that this approach will be of value, not only to health care professionals, but also to the many hundreds of thousands of men around the world in their care who face the devastating consequences of this most prevalent form of cancer.

Roger Kirby, Tim Christmas and Michael Brawer
1996

Preface to the second edition

Four years after the publication of the first edition of *Prostate Cancer* we felt that the time was right to update and expand the book. The task of extensively revising the text and refining the illustrations has only served to remind us how rapid the pace of change has been during those years. New insights into the ways that cancer develops and spreads are now poised to translate into genuine benefit to patients. Chemoprevention is now not such a distant dream and the importance of angiogenesis, for example, has become clear. New angiogenesis inhibitors, such as the once demonized thalidomide and other agents, now offer new hope to prostate cancer sufferers.

Prostate-specific antigen (PSA) testing, while still controversial, has been refined by a clearer understanding of the way that it forms complexes in the blood stream. Its widespread utilization as a screening test in the USA has certainly been responsible for a stage shift in presentation and probably contributed to the recent 7% reduction in prostate cancer mortality in that country. The chapter on this the most important tumour marker in all oncology has been extensively updated.

Once prostate cancer has been diagnosed treatment choices depend critically on the clinical stage of the tumour. Unfortunately the accuracy with which this can be accomplished is still sub-optimal. The dilemmas currently faced by clinicians and patients in this respect are covered in the chapter on staging, which has been extensively rewritten. The initial promise of PCR-PSA testing has not been fulfilled clinically, but the use of a combination of PSA, Gleason grade and information from digital rectal examination has helped to quantify the risk of extra-prostatic extension of cancer more accurately.

While radical prostatectomy remains the gold standard therapy for men with localized prostate cancer, newer treatment options such as brachytherapy are growing in popularity. An entire chapter has been devoted to this new technology. New treatment options for locally advanced prostate cancers are also considered in some depth. These include the combination of androgen ablation and external beam radiotherapy and the use of antiandrogens alone as monotherapy. The latter has now been shown to be equivalent in this situation to either orchidectomy or luteinizing hormone-releasing hormone (LHRH) analogues. New hormonal therapies such as LHRH antagonists soon will be available. Currently one of the most difficult problems that clinicians face is the management of androgen independent prostate cancer. New therapies that are safe and effective are at last beginning to emerge and these are discussed in the concluding chapters.

Quality of life is always an important consideration in cancer, especially in prostate cancer where progression is often so slow. A new chapter on sexual function and prostate cancer has been included to cover this subject which is often preeminent in the minds of our patients.

As the populations of the developed and developing worlds continue to age prostate cancer seems set to rise ever higher in both prevalence and profile. We hope that this new edition will help to bring this important disease area into sharp focus.

Roger Kirby, Tim Christmas and Michael Brawer
2000

Foreword

A generation ago, prostate cancer was relegated to a minor role in the medical curriculum and commanded little attention from primary care physicians. For the urologist of that day, understanding androgen deprivation therapy and, for the rare patient diagnosed with a small palpable nodule, how to perform a radical perineal prostatectomy constituted the core knowledge about this disease. Prostate cancer, as the educated physician knew, was a disease that elderly men died *with*, not *of*.

No more. Today, life expectancy is substantially longer. The fastest growing segment of our population is composed of those over 80 years. Prostate cancer is now recognized as the second leading cause of death from cancer in men – second in mortality only to lung cancer, which is largely preventable. No cancer increases in mortality rate so rapidly with age as prostate cancer. In those countries whose populations have the longest life span, prostate cancer has become *the* leading cause of death from cancer in men. Even limited exposure to patients with prostate cancer will convince any student of this disease that death from prostate cancer is particularly miserable. Patients rightly fear this disease and demand from their physicians a high level of knowledge about its cause, natural history, methods of detection, prognosis, and therapeutic alternatives.

The authors of this second edition of *Prostate Cancer* have performed a service to their profession and to patients by providing a lucid, concise, organized, and comprehensive review of knowledge about this disease. A particularly valuable feature of this book – evident in this edition as well as the first – is the international perspective provided by the authors, who are among the most knowledgeable and respected practitioners on both sides of the Atlantic. This is no theoretical text – it is applied science at its very best. With astute discrimination and obvious collaborative interaction, the authors selected the most relevant data and the most up-to-date studies to present. They have organized this diverse and complex field into easily digestible information by providing helpful lists, well-organized tables, and uniformly clear illustrations.

Today, when the complexity of medicine leads most editors to produce multi-authored texts, these editors have turned author and have managed to write accurate chapters on topics ranging from epidemiology to therapy with consistent style in written word, tabular presentation, and drawings. The advantage is a balanced yet comprehensive approach. There is little of importance to the field that is not mentioned here.

Prostate Cancer, second edition, will serve as an excellent starting point for the urologist-in-training who seeks greater depth of knowledge about this all-too-common disease. For the seasoned practitioner, it represents a ready reference source to keep abreast of the state-of-the-art in this disease. Few other sources can boast of such timeliness and contain such relevant data about prostate cancer.

Peter T Scardino MD
Chairman, Department of Urology,
Alfred P. Sloan Chair
Head, Prostate Cancer Program,
Memorial Sloan-Kettering Cancer Center
New York

June 2000

To all our patients with prostate cancer

Chapter **1**

The problem

As we embark on the new millenium carcinoma of the prostate constitutes a major and escalating international health problem. In many developed countries prostate cancer is the most commonly diagnosed life-threatening malignancy in men, and seems poised to overtake lung cancer as *the* major cause of cancer death[1]. It has been calculated that the current lifetime risk for a man in a Western society of developing microscopic prostate cancer is roughly 30%; the risk of developing clinical disease is about 10%, and the chances of dying from the disorder is around 3%. Risk factors for the disease include Western-type lifestyle; worldwide trends in lifestyles make exposure to these risk factors increasingly widespread. These, added to the well known demographic shifts towards an increasingly aged society (**1.1**), have led epidemiologists to predict a dramatic increase in both the incidence of and death rate from prostate cancer by the year 2020 unless effective improvements in prevention, early diagnosis and treatment are forthcoming (**1.2**)[2].

Unlike most other forms of cancer, however, not every prostate tumour constitutes a serious threat to life of the individual affected, and consequently does not automatically warrant treatment. Some elderly men in fact die *with* rather than *of* prostate cancer, leading historically to some urologists adopting a stance of therapeutic nihilism for this malignancy. However, in the era of increasingly widespread prostate-specific antigen (PSA) testing, such a position is becoming ever more difficult to maintain, at least in patients with a natural life expectancy of more than 10 years. In fact, the challenge now is to

The 'greying' of society

% of population aged 65 +

Germany — Japan - - USA — Italy — France — UK

Year

1.1 Populations will age in all countries (OECD predictions).

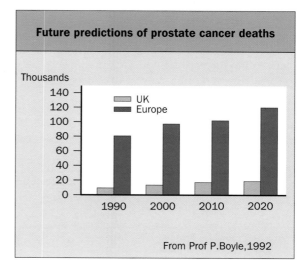

Future predictions of prostate cancer deaths

Thousands

UK
Europe

1990 2000 2010 2020

From Prof P.Boyle,1992

1.2 Predictions for prostate cancer deaths in Europe up to the year 2020.

accurately distinguish those potentially dangerous lesions from the very small, slow-growing, well differentiated cancers that are unlikely to progress to present clinically within that individual's natural lifespan.

In this respect, current progress and future prospects are encouraging. Tumour grade and stage, in terms of volume of the primary cancer, have been shown to be important prognostic indicators. Molecular markers of tumour aggressiveness and metastatic potential, such as PCNA[3], Ki-67[4] and E-cadherin[5] expression, may hold the key to distinguishing those clinically significant and dangerous tumours that have been described as the 'tigers', from the 'pussy cats', which may best be managed simply by watchful waiting.

Currently, much debate centres around the lengths to which we should go to identify prostatic cancer early, i.e. at a stage when it is still curable. Few dispute that steps should be taken to diagnose prostate cancer in those with life expectancy exceeding 10 years who present to urologists with lower urinary tract symptoms. 'Case-finding' by digital rectal examination (DRE) and PSA determination in asymptomatic individuals, particularly those at risk because of family history, is also considered legitimate. Less consensus surrounds the issue of screening for prostate cancer – i.e. the formal invitation of all men to attend for a prostate check – since there is no evidence yet that screening effects a reduction in disease-specific mortality, and over-diagnosis is a possibility[6]. However, those cancers that are detected early by PSA measurement, the so-called T1c cancers, do appear to be of clinically significant volume and grade in more than 95% of cases[7], and are specimen-confined in around three quarters of patients[8]. Long-term, randomized trials to evaluate screening and early diagnosis are currently underway in Europe and the USA.

Once prostate cancer has been diagnosed in a patient, histologically graded, and staged as accurately as possible, clinicians are duty bound to offer the best advice about treatment options, even though the risks and benefits of competing therapies have often not been formally compared in randomized trials. For the patient and his family, the decision concerning which treatment modality should be employed is often seen as a life or death scenario – perhaps one of the most important in their lives. Random assignment to a pre-judged treatment arm of a randomized clinical trial is obviously difficult in such situations, especially if one of the study arms contains a no-treatment option. In such circumstances, it is incumbent upon every urologist to be informed about all of the latest data related to risks and benefits of therapy, and to discuss these freely and frankly, not only with the patient, but also with his immediate family. In this way, patient-focused truly informed decisions can be made about various competing treatment options available with due repect to patient preferences.

Numerous new therapies for prostate cancer are now emerging for which some extravagant claims have been made, but their long-term efficacy in terms of cancer eradication and incidence of side-effects are still largely unknown. Interest of the general public in these new modalities, often fired by uncritical features in the popular press, is understandably intense.

Androgen deprivation therapy continues to be the mainstay for metastatic disease and significant advances have come with newer luteinising hormone-releasing hormone (LHRH) analogues, pure LHRH (*gonadotropin-releasing hormone (GnRH)*) antagonists[9] and antiandrogens. Alternative approaches utilizing, for example, retinoid derivatives, microtubule inhibitors and gene therapy also hold exciting promise[10]. These complex issues will be discussed and illustrated in greater depth in the following chapters; although we do not even pretend to have all of the answers in this most perplexing of diseases, we have tried to set out the facts and controversies as clearly and concisely as possible.

REFERENCES

1 Parker SL, Tong T, Bolden S, *et al.* Cancer statistics 1997. *CA Cancer J Clin* 1997;**47**:5–27.

2 Carter HB, Coffey DS. The prostate: an increasing medical problem. *Prostate* 1990;**16**:39–48.

3 Harper ME, Glynne-Jones E, Goddard L, *et al.* Relationship of proliferating cell nuclear antigen (PCNA) in prostatic carcinomas to various clinical parameters. *Prostate* 1992;**20**:243–253.

4 Harper ME, Goddard L, Wilson DW, *et al.* Pathological and clinical associations of Ki-67 defined growth factors in human prostate carcinoma. *Prostate* 1992;**21**:75–84.

5 Umbas R, Schalken JA, Adders TW, *et al.* Expression of cellular adhesion molecule E-cadherin is reduced or absent in high grade prostate cancer. *Canc Res* 1992;**52**:5104–5109.

6 Schroder FH. Prostate cancer: to screen or not to screen. *BMJ* 1993;**306**:407–408.

7 Epstein JI, Walsh PC, Carmichael M, *et al.* Pathologic and clinical findings to predict tumour extent in non-palpable (T1c) prostate cancer. *JAMA* 1994;**271**(5):368–374.

8 Scaletsky R, Koch MO, Eckstein CW, *et al.* Tumour volume and stage in carcinomas of the prostate detected by elevations of prostate-specific antigen. *J Urol* 1994;**152**:129–131.

9 Molineaux CJ, Sluss PM, Bree BS, Gefter ML, Sullivan BS, Garnick MB. Suppression of plasma gonadotrophins by abarelix: a potent new LHRH antagonist. *Molecular Urology* 1998;**2**:265–268.

10 Crawford ED, Rosenbloom M, Ziada AM, Large PH. Overview: hormone refractory prostate cancer. *Urology* 1999;**54**:1–7.

Chapter 2

Anatomical and pathological considerations

INTRODUCTION

The term 'prostate' was originally derived from the Greek word 'prohistani', meaning 'to stand in front of', and has been attributed to Herophilus of Alexandria who used the term in 335 B.C. to describe the organ located 'in front of' the urinary bladder; detailed anatomical depictions did not appear until the Renaissance (**2.1**). However, while the existence of the prostate has been recognized for over 2300 years, accurate descriptions of the gland's internal structure, physiology and pathology have occurred only relatively recently.

Over the past decade there has been a flurry of interest in relation to the major prostatic diseases, i.e. benign prostatic hyperplasia (BPH) and carcinoma of the prostate. This is partly the result of the demographic changes (alluded to in Chapter 1) which have led to an increasing proportion of the male

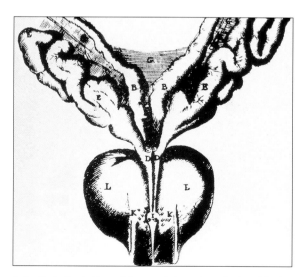

2.1 Early illustration of the prostate and seminal vesicles by Regnier de Graaf (circa 1660).

population attaining an age after which they are especially susceptible to these disorders, and is also due in part to the introduction of a number of new diagnostic and treatment options in both of these disease areas.

Central to the understanding of prostatic pathology is a comprehension of the zonal anatomy. In addition, a knowledge of the capsule and the adjacent neurovascular bundles is paramount. These will be considered in relation to an illustrated review of the pathology of premalignancy and cancer of the prostate.

ZONAL ANATOMY

The anatomy of the prostate has been a subject surrounded by controversy for many years. The early descriptions of the embryology of the prostate by Lowsley suggested that the human prostate followed a lobar pattern of development similar to that of other mammals[1]. In humans, however, the dorsal, ventral and lateral lobes of the foetal prostate coalesce in the adult to form a rather homogeneous structure.

Subsequent studies by McNeal revealed that the lack of anatomically distinct lobes in the human gland was actually the result of an alternative form of architecture[2]. His studies used sagittal, parasagittal and coronal sections of the prostate instead of simply the conventional transverse plane. McNeal described three anatomical zones: the peripheral zone, the transition zone and the central zone (**2.2**). The peripheral zone in the normal gland comprises the majority (approximately 65%) of the prostatic volume. As its name implies, it extends around the posterolateral peripheral aspects of the gland from its apex to its base, and its histological appearance is characterized by small, simple, acinar spaces lined by tall columnar secretory epithelial cells. As is true of the entire gland, prostatic acini are embedded in smooth muscle stroma whose function may be to enhance the emptying of prostatic secretions into the urethra at the time of ejaculation, thereby allowing them to intermingle and liquefy with seminal fluid from the seminal vesicles.

The second largest component of the normal prostate is the central zone; this is a cone-shaped region that comprises approximately 25% of normal prostatic volume (**2.2**). The ducts of the central zone join the urethra at the verumontanum, and the direction in which these ducts run may render them relatively immune to intraprostatic urinary reflux, in contradistinction to those of the peripheral zone (**2.3**)[3].

The prostatic ducts branch towards the base of the prostate to join their acinar lobules, and recent studies have suggested different functions and longevities of epithelial cells in the ductal system when compared to those within the acini (see **4.3**).

The central zone surrounds the ejaculatory ducts and makes up the majority of the prostatic base. Histologically, the central zone is identified by the presence of relatively large acini with irregular contours, that are lined by low columnar cuboidal epithelium. The smooth-muscle stroma of the central zone appears rather more compact than that of the peripheral zone.

The smallest, but by no means least important,

zone of the normal prostate has been termed the transition zone. This comprises only 5–10% of the prostate in young adults and is composed of two bilaterally symmetrical lobules found on the two sides of the prostatic urethra. The transition zone is separated from the two other zones by a narrow band of fibromuscular stroma which extends in an arc from the posterior urethra in the mid-prostate to the most anterior aspect of the gland. The ducts of the transition zone empty bilaterally into the urethra at the base of the verumontanum. Histologically, transition zone acini resemble those of the peripheral zone; the surrounding stroma is more compact, however, and is similar to that of the central zone.

The histological distinctions between the transition, central and peripheral zones of the prostate in man are usually difficult to perceive (either macroscopically or microscopically), because, in the absence of disease, their anatomical boundaries are relatively subtle. All of the mature, functioning, prostatic acinar and ductal epithelial cells elaborate both prostate-specific antigen (PSA) and prostatic acid phosphatase (PAP). To date, few biochemical differences between the epithelial cells of the three zones have been demonstrated. The central zone *does* differ, however, in containing a relatively large proportion of epithelial cells containing a gastric

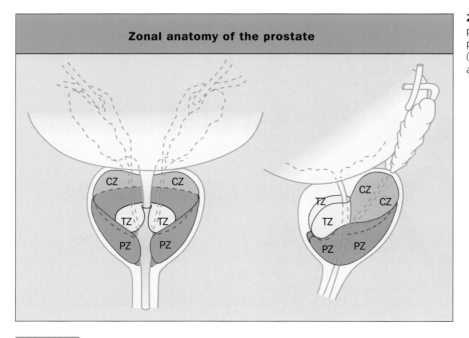

Zonal anatomy of the prostate

2.2 Zonal anatomy of the prostate in AP and sagittal planes showing central zone (CZ), peripheral zone (PZ) and transition zone (TZ).

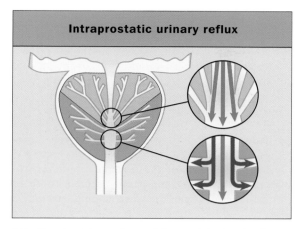

Intraprostatic urinary reflux

2.3 The glandular anatomy of the prostate showing the tendency of peripheral zone ducts to permit urinary reflux.

proenzyme called pepsinogen $2^{4,5}$. Tissue-type plasminogen activator is also found exclusively in the central zone's epithelial cells. Epidermal growth factor (EGF) receptors also seem to be present in a greater concentration in the central and transition zones than in the peripheral zone (**2.4**), but the reverse seems to be the case with androgen receptors.

The clinical significance of zonal anatomy is important in terms of the development of both BPH and prostate cancer. Nodules of benign prostatic tissue usually originate within, and then expand, the transition zone; this expansion frequently distorts and compresses the adjacent peripheral zone. In contrast, although malignancy may affect any, or all three of the zones, the majority of cancers (more

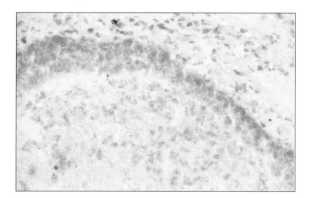

2.4 Epidermal growth factor (EGF) receptors in prostatic epithelial cells using immunoperoxidase stain and monoclonal antibody to EGF (×60).

than 70%) are believed to originate in the glands of the peripheral zone. However, it is usually difficult to pinpoint the precise origin of an individual prostatic tumour as this is obscured by the extent of its involvement as it invades across zonal boundaries.

It is still unclear whether there are distinct differences between those carcinomas that originate in the peripheral zone and those that form in the central or transition zones. Although it has been suggested that carcinomas in the transition zone demonstrate a lower malignant potential than those of the peripheral zone, recent studies have suggested that, grade for grade, tumours of the transition zone are little different from those that arise in the peripheral prostate[6]. However, the proximity of peripheral zone cancers to the neurovascular bundles may facilitate their spread along perineural and lymphatic channels (**2.5**), thereby enhancing their metastatic potential[7].

THE PROSTATIC CAPSULE

Long-standing confusion has surrounded not only the structure of the prostatic parenchyma, but also the existence of a prostatic 'capsule'. Historically, the term 'capsule' has had two very different meanings. First, in glands that have been distorted by benign prostatic hyperplasia, the term 'surgical capsule' has been used to describe the residual peripheral zone that has undergone compression by the expanding transition zone; in this situation, the peripheral zone becomes atrophic and consists mainly of stromal elements. Second, and more pertinent to the study of prostatic cancer, is the question of whether or not the prostatic parenchyma is delimited by fibroconnective tissue similar to the capsule of the kidney.

The prostate develops by a form of branching morphogenesis in which the outpouchings of the urogenital sinus invade a bed of splanchnic mesoderm. The stroma organizes itself around the epithelial buds as they penetrate through the primitive mesenchymal cells. By the 16th week of gestation, the undifferentiated mesenchymal cells take on the differentiated phenotype of smooth muscle. It is this stromal–epithelium interaction which determines the ultimate borders of the prostate. When epithelial invasion ends, those mesenchymal cells within the range of their inductive factors become the outer border of the prostate proper. Mesenchymal cells

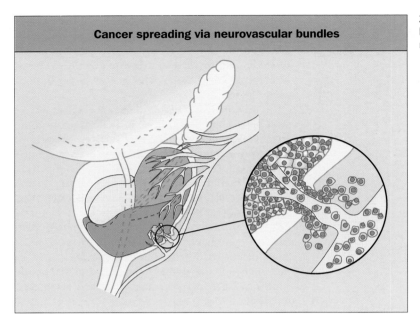

Cancer spreading via neurovascular bundles

2.5 Prostate tumour cells spreading by perineural invasion down the neurovascular bundle.

beyond this boundary remain fibroblastic and establish the zone of loose connective tissue through which supportive blood vessels and nerves travel to the gland. The capsule of the prostate is therefore more akin to the adventitia of major arteries than it is to the distinct fibroconnective capsule that encapsulates the liver and the kidney[8]. As one would expect, extensive penetration of prostatic cancer cells through this flimsy capsule (**2.6**) appears to correlate with a risk of the subsequent development of metastatic disease; this will clearly affect prognosis and survival (**2.7**) (see Chapter 9). Interestingly, microscopic capsular penetration provides very little prognostic information.

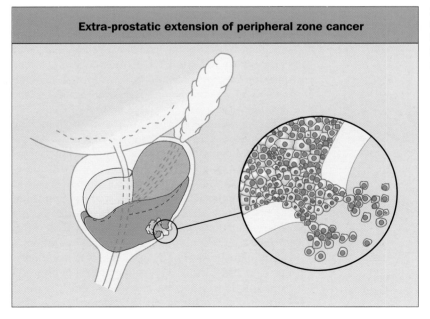

Extra-prostatic extension of peripheral zone cancer

2.6 Extensive extra-prostatic extension of prostate cancer is strongly associated with the subsequent development of distant metastases.

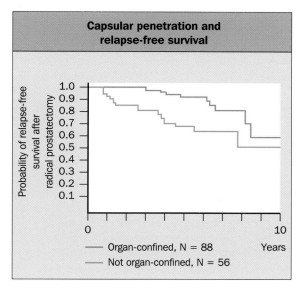

Capsular penetration and relapse-free survival

2.7 Capsular penetration by prostate cancer cells correlates with risk of tumour recurrence after radical prostatectomy. (Data supplied by Dr DF Paulson.)

THE NEUROVASCULAR BUNDLES

The neurovascular bundles lying dorsolaterally and adjacent to the prostate carry nerve fibres and blood to the corpora cavernosa, and are critical to the development of normal erectile responses[9] (**2.8**). Their division in the original radical prostatectomy procedure undoubtedly resulted in an incidence of post-operative impotence that approached 100%. The observation that these neurovascular bundles lie *outside* Denonvillier's fascia led to the development of the nerve-sparing radical retropubic prostatectomy described by Walsh[10], a procedure that leaves these bundles intact (see Chapter 9). Fortunately, this manoeuvre appears to enhance the prospects for post-operative potency, at least in younger men, even when only one of the two bundles can be spared[11].

THE SECONDARY EFFECTS OF PROSTATIC OBSTRUCTION

Prostatic enlargement from either benign or malignant disease generally results in a reduced compliance of the prostatic urethra and increasing outflow obstruction; secondary changes often occur in the bladder as a result. In anatomical terms, these consist of hypertrophy of the bladder wall, and the formation of trabeculae as well as diverticula. Upper tract dilatation may occur, rather less frequently in benign than in malignant disease. The secondary changes in the detrusor muscle may be largely responsible for the most troublesome symptoms associated with prostatic obstruction: nocturia, frequency and urgency. The underlying cause of these symptoms remains controversial, but is probably, in part, related to the development of detrusor

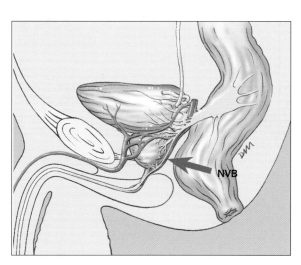

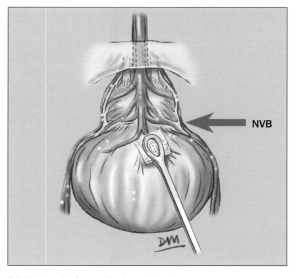

2.8 The neurovascular bundles (NVB) described by Walsh, innervating and supplying blood to the corpora cavernosa. (**a**) Lateral view.

(**b**) AP view before radical prostatectomy.

instability in the obstructed bladder. In animal models, obstruction to the bladder outlet results in detrusor muscle hypertrophy, collagen infiltration, and the development of involuntary detrusor contractions or 'instability'. A number of explanations for these unstable detrusor contractions have been suggested, the most plausible of which is an obstruction-related denervation, with the development of post-junctional supersensitivity to agonist transmitters. This is almost certainly only part of a complex overall picture, with other factors including altered adrenoceptor function, afferent nerve dysfunction, an imbalance of peptide neurotransmitters, as well as acquired myogenic deficit also playing an important role[12]. Whatever the explanations for the secondary effects of obstruction in the bladder are, it is clear that operative relief of either benign or malignant outflow obstruction can result in a reversal of the secondary changes in the bladder, provided that they are not too advanced and chronic over-distension of the detrusor muscle has not developed.

PROSTATE PATHOLOGY AND MARKERS OF PROGRESSION

The definitive diagnosis of any cancer demands cytological and/or histological confirmation of the established diagnostic criteria of malignancy. The prostate presents an exceedingly complex organ in this regard. A number of factors contribute to the difficult interpretation of pathological specimens from the prostate, including the large variations in normal histology, the changes associated with the frequent findings of inflammation and infarction, and the effects of changing the hormonal milieu. For example, follicle-stimulating hormone (FSH) is absent in young males, present in moderate amounts in benign prostatic hypertrophy, and present in abundance in prostate cancer[13]. Testosterone levels are known to increase with age. This has led to the suggestion that prostate cancer is a multihormonal disease and that progression should be monitored through measurement of several humoral factors, including FSH. These are compounded by the myriad appearances that the most common malignancy, adenocarcinoma, may exhibit, not only between patients, but even within a given individual's neoplasm.

Despite these significant constraints, major progress has been made in the realm of diagnostic accuracy. Probably the most significant factor enabling this progress is the unprecedented increase in the clinical material that pathologists are confronted with (owing to the increased prevalence and interest in prostate cancer in general). Moreover, there has been a significant improvement in the technique of biopsy, which is the most common method of making the diagnosis of cancer; the use of spring-loaded biopsy devices (which afford excellent cores for histological interpretation) in conjunction with ultrasound guidance and a systematic sector approach, lessens sampling errors. The application of immunohistochemical techniques (which may help to establish a diagnosis of malignancy in equivocal cases, and may confirm or refute the prostate as the site of origin for tumours of unknown aetiology) has greatly assisted the pathologist in more accurate tissue interpretation.

As already mentioned, the most challenging frontier in prostate cancer today is the ability to differentiate between those men whose prostate cancer is likely to lie quiescent (without significantly affecting his longevity or quality of life), and those who harbour more potentially aggressive neoplasms that justify radical treatment. A multitude of so-called 'markers of malignant potential' are currently being investigated for application in men with prostate cancer, in order to help distinguish between these two groups.

Methods of obtaining specimens for pathological interpretation of the prostate include core-needle biopsies, aspiration for cytology, transurethral resection, or simple open prostatectomy, as well as the sampling of lesions thought to represent metastatic deposits. In the US and now in the majority of other countries, the most common diagnostic specimen is the core-needle biopsy, which may be obtained by a variety of instruments. The spring-loaded biopsy devices, which are in widespread use, afford excellent tissue core, generally 12–15 mm in length and approximately 1 mm in diameter (**2.9a–c**). Owing to the low morbidity and minimal discomfort associated with obtaining biopsies with this instrument[14], multiple specimens are generally obtained (under sonographic guidance to improve the likelihood of sampling significant lesions), which, when cancer is encountered, effects a more representative assessment of the grade and extent of the neoplasm[15].

In a number of countries, but primarily in Scandinavia, aspiration cytology is still used. This technique, with its associated minimal morbidity and

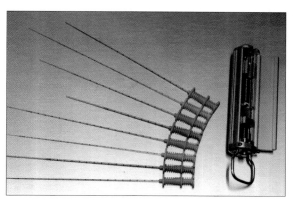

2.9(a) Transrectal ultrasound-guided prostate biopsy using an automatic biopsy device.

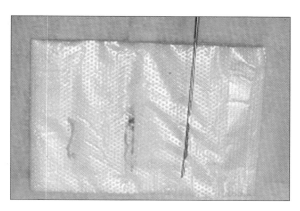

(b) Prostatic needle-biopsy specimens.

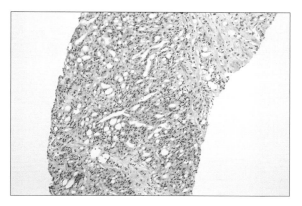

(c) Histology of a needle biopsy showing invasion by cancer.

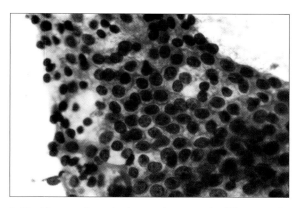

2.10 Fine-needle aspiration cytology: poorly differentiated adenocarcinoma. (Reproduced with permission from Weiss MA, Mills SE. *Atlas of Genitourinary Tract Disorders*. London: Gower; 1988.)

the opportunity it presents to sample a large volume of the gland, has a number of advocates (**2.10**). Excellent correlation with core-needle biopsy has been reported[16,17] in centres with a dedicated cyto-pathologist, but there exists considerable variability between different institutions in the accuracy of cytologic diagnosis. This, coupled with difficulty in correlating aspiration-cytology grade with the more commonly used histological grading systems and the advances of the spring-loaded biopsy devices, has led to a reduced use of this method.

The normal prostate consists of an admixture of luminal spaces, stroma comprised of smooth muscle and fibroblasts, with interposing collagen, blood vessels, as well as lymphatic and epithelial tissue. In the benign prostate, the epithelium consists of two cellular layers, one being of basal cells (flat

cells with a horizontal orientation), and the other of luminal cells (which lie perpendicularly to the basal cells but have basally oriented nuclei) (**2.11**). The basal cells, whose function remains unknown, can be difficult to identify on standard histological preparations; however, one can readily identify this layer with high-molecular-weight cytokeratin staining, which identifies only the basal cells[18]. This is an important feature, as carcinoma of the prostate is always devoid of the basal-cell layer, offering an excellent immunohistochemical confirmation of the presence of benign or malignant tissue (**2.12**).

Owing to the ubiquitous nature of benign prostatic hyperplasia, most men who undergo examination for prostate cancer will harbour histological BPH. A thorough discussion of this entity is beyond the scope of this chapter, but may be found else-

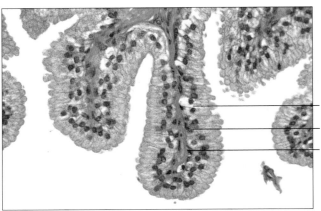

2.11 Benign prostatic epithelium as seen in BPH.
(Reproduced with permission from Weiss MA, Mills SE. *Atlas of Genitourinary Tract Disorders.* London: Gower; 1988.)

Uniform columnar cell nuclei

Basal cell nuclei

Fibrovascular stalk

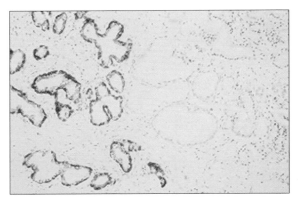

2.12 High-molecular-weight cytokeratin: normal (left-hand side) and prostate cancer (right-hand side).

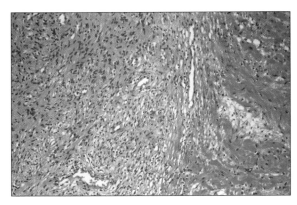

2.14 BPH – stromal nodule of the fibromuscular variant.

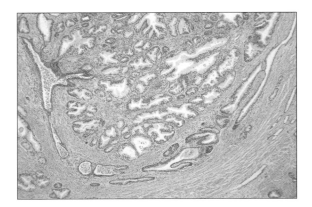

2.13 BPH hyperplastic nodule of the highly epithelial variant.

where[19]. Histologically, BPH is an extremely variable entity, ranging from a highly epithelial variant (**2.13**) to a fibromuscular type that is largely devoid of epithelial components (**2.14**).

PREMALIGNANCY IN THE PROSTATE

The early detection and cure of cancer has often depended on the ability to recognize premalignant change. The definitive identification of the precursors of invasive carcinomata of the prostate has lagged many years behind equivalent organ sites, such as the uterine cervix. This is partly due to the technical difficulties in performing repeated biopsies on the same exact location of the prostate, e.g. when compared to repeating a PAP cervical smear or undertaking cervical colposcopy. Even with trans-rectal ultrasound-guided (TRUS-guided) biopsy, it is impossible to be sure that a given rebiopsy is taken from an identical microscopic field. For this reason, the interpretation of transformations within the prostate from dysplastic to frankly malignant states is handicapped by the lack of data concerning the progression of specific lesions over time.

Prostatic Intraepithelial Neoplasia

Progress in the area of identifying precursors was made in the mid 1980s, however, when McNeal and Bostwick[20] reported the existence of a lesion that they termed 'intraductal dysplasia'. This entity was proposed as a precursor of malignancy on the grounds of cytological atypia, exhibiting nuclear pleomorphism and nucleolar prominence similar to that seen in prostate cancer (**Table 2.1**). Following a consensus conference in 1989 the term 'prostatic intraepithelial neoplasia' (PIN) was adopted as the most appropriate nomenclature for this lesion (**Table 2.2**), bringing it into line with other pre-malignant lesions elsewhere in the body, such as cervical intraepithelial neoplasia (CIN).

In general, our understanding of PIN is based on its association with other areas of unequivocal malignancy. Transition-zone cancers are not usually associated with PIN but, in peripheral-zone tumours, PIN is frequently found adjacent to carcinomas[21,22]. Severe PIN is often more extensive in multifocal cancers[21]. Apart from the nuclear pleomorphism already mentioned, PIN lesions also share other

Table 2.2 Prostatic premalignant lesion synonyms
Atypical epithelial hyperplasia
Atypical glandular hyperplasia
Atypical hyperplasia
Cytologic atypia
Cellular atypia
Duct-acinar dysplasia
Glandular atypia
Intraductal dysplasia
Intraepithelial neoplasia
Intraglandular dysplasia
Large acinar atypical hyperplasia

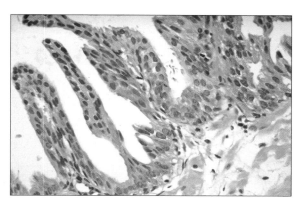

2.15 Low-grade prostatic intraepithelial neoplasia (PIN).

Table 2.1 Evidence that PIN is premalignant
Morphologic similarity to invasive cancer
Phenotypic similarity to cancer
Incidence is greater in organs harbouring invasive cancer
Severity is increased with cancer
Extent is greater with concomitant cancer
Spatial relationship to invasive cancer
Microinvasion present from the premalignant change
Progression to invasive cancer identified on serial biopsy*

* Not proven in PIN owing to 3-dimensional arborization of prostate epithelium

characteristics of malignancy such as the loss of basal layer continuity[23], the production of acid mucin[24], altered lectin binding[25], evidence of differentiation as evidenced by decreased PSA immuno-staining[26,27] and abnormalities of ploidy. **2.15** is an example of low-grade PIN.

The diagnosis of high-grade PIN (**2.16**) is established by increasing proliferation and cytological changes. PIN is commonly associated with prostate cancer (**2.17**) and disruption of the basal-cell layer, as identified by high-molecular-weight cytokeratin immunohistochemistry. This has led to development of a model for prostate carcinogenesis, which has become increasingly accepted (**2.18**).

Another lesion which has been suggested to represent a premalignant change is atypical adenomatous hyperplasia (**2.19**). This entity, which is similar in appearance to low-grade carcinoma, may also be focally associated with disruption of the

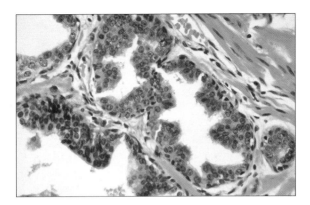

2.16   High-grade PIN.

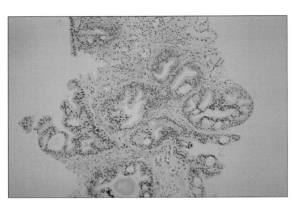

2.17b   PIN shown with an H and E stain.

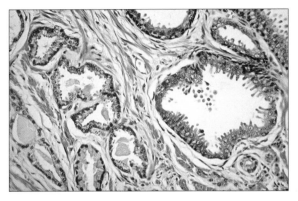

2.17a   Slide showing high-grade PIN on the right and a focus of adenocarcinoma on the left.

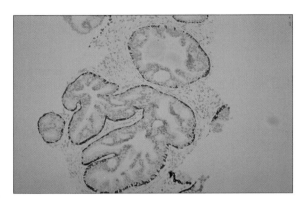

2.17c   PIN using LP34 staining.

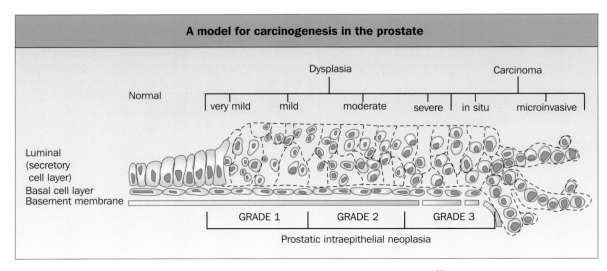

2.18   Model for PIN – carcinogenesis in the prostate. (Reproduced from Bostwick and Brawer[23] © 1987 American Cancer Society. Reprinted by permission of Wiley-Liss, Inc., a subsidiary of John Wiley & Sons., Inc.)

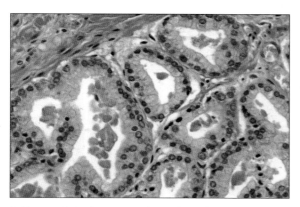

2.19 Atypical adenomatous hyperplasia. (Reproduced with permission from Weiss MA, Mills SE. *Atlas of Genitourinary Tract Disorders.* London: Gower; 1988.)

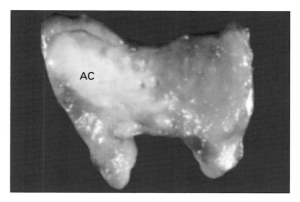

2.20 Gross pathological specimen showing prostate cancer. The site of origin is difficult to determine. AC, adenocarcinoma. (Reproduced with permission from Weiss MA, Mills SE. *Atlas of Genitourinary Tract Disorders.* London: Gower; 1988.)

basal-cell layer. However, current evidence suggests that this is not a premalignant change.

Pathology of Prostate Cancer

Microscopically, most carcinomas of the prostate are classical adenocarcinomata, being made up of epithelial cells with varying degrees of glandular architecture. As noted, there is a departure from the normal two layers of cells (with absence of the basal-cell layer) which may be confirmed immunohistochemically. Additionally, there is an infiltrative growth pattern that often results in difficulty delineating the actual edge of the tumour. As mentioned, this makes the definitive site of origin difficult to identify in many cases (**2.20**).

One of the hallmarks of prostate cancer is the frequent finding of glands growing 'back-to-back' with no intervening stroma. Cytologically, prostate cancer is extremely variable but, in general, enlarged pleomorphic nuclei and prominence of nucleoli are found.

Histological Grading

Just as in other organ systems, the grade of a malignancy or its degree of departure from normal has been established as an important prognostic marker in the prostate. A number of grading systems have been advocated, the most widely applied of which is that of Gleason[28]. The Gleason grading system uses low-power architectural findings on microscopy to define the pattern of the tumour.

A 5-step grading system is used, and the two most prominent grades are added together to afford the so-called 'Gleason score', which ranges from 2–10. **2.21** illustrates the architectural changes for each

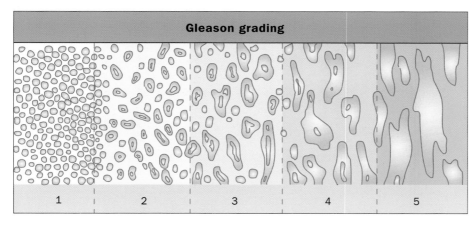

Gleason grading

1 2 3 4 5

2.21 Gleason grading system shown diagrammatically. The system grades the cancer according to its ability to form gland-like structures. Poorly differentiated tumours (grade 4–5) lose this ability.

grade as described by Gleason. The Gleason system has been shown not only to offer significant prognostic information but also to be reasonably reproducible between pathologists[29,30].

Histological grading offers valuable prognostic information. Evidence of this comes from many settings, including a meta-analysis of a watchful-waiting series by Chodak and associates[31]. They noted that grade 1 (Gleason score 2–4) had a 2.1% annualized rate of developing metastases; grade 2 (Gleason score 5–7) had a 5.4% rate and grade 3 (Gleason score 7–10) had a rate of 13.5%.

2.22 shows a Gleason grade 1 tumour comprised of small, uniform glands exhibiting minimal nuclear changes. This low-grade neoplasm, which frequently consists of nodules with well-defined borders, has been shown to be of low biological potential. The most common grade is Gleason grade 3 (**2.23**). This lesion exhibits the largest degree of variation in architecture, glandular size, shape and regularity; infiltrative borders are generally found. Gleason grades 4 and 5 (**2.24**, **2.25**) represent more aggressive neoplasms with marked cytologic atypia, extensive infiltrative borders (most likely associated with capsular penetration), positive surgical margins, seminal-vesicle extension, and/or metastatic spread.

Marked heterogeneity of the histological appearance of the high-grade carcinoma may be present and, at times, it may be difficult to establish the prostate as the site of origin, particularly in lesions extending beyond the prostate, either locally in the pelvis, or in metastatic deposits. The specificity of prostate-specific antigen (PSA) as described in Chapter 6 on tumour markers, affords an excellent immunohistochemical test for the diagnosis of prostate cancer in such clinical scenarios (**2.26**).

THE ENIGMA OF 'LATENT' PROSTATE CANCER

In 1954, Franks was the first to point out the extraordinarily high prevalence of microfoci of 'latent'

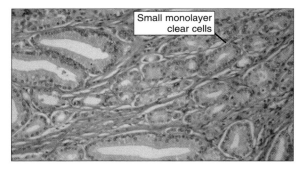

2.22 Gleason grade 1.

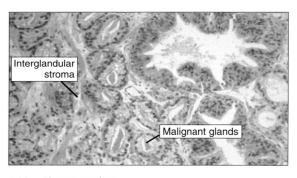

2.23 Gleason grade 3.

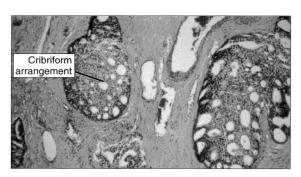

2.24 Gleason grade 4.

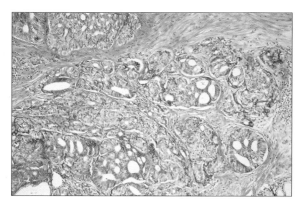

2.25 Gleason grade 5 infiltrating stroma.

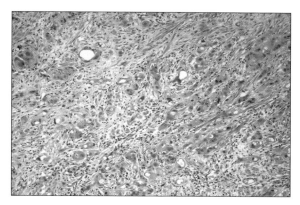

2.26 PSA immunohistochemistry from involved lymph nodes.

prostate cancer in the post-mortem examination of men dying from other diseases[32]. Since then, numerous other investigators have confirmed this observation and noted that the incidence of these tiny cancers appears to increase with age; overall around 30% of men over 50 are apparently affected[33] and this figure does not seem to vary markedly between countries. Recently, a study of younger men dying of diseases other than prostate cancer has highlighted the surprisingly early age of onset of these pathological changes[34]. The low growth rate of these microscopic tumours (some prostate cancers have a cell-doubling time of more than 4 years) is probably the reason that they often carry little danger for the individual. A proportion, though, *will* enlarge (and also dedifferentiate), to a point where they become both clinically significant and identifiable by modern screening methods within the natural lifespan of the patient. The threshold of 'clinically significant' volume is currently regarded as 0.5 cm^3; by the time a volume of 3.5 cm^3 is reached, a high proportion of prostate cancers will have penetrated through the capsule[35].

The sobering statistics of the rising morbidity and mortality associated with prostate cancer must be balanced against the fact that the histological incidence of prostate cancer far exceeds the prevalence of clinically manifest disease. While perhaps 30% of men over age 50 harbour tiny foci of well-differentiated prostate cancer, it is estimated that only 10% of men will have a diagnosis of prostate cancer during their lifetime, and that only 3% will succumb to the disease[36]. The progression to malignant disease may be related to FSH exposure and increased numbers of FSH receptors in these cells. For example, the presence of FSH has been found in benign prostatic hyperplasia and prostatic adenocarcinoma (Gleason score of 5–9[37]). Further research will determine the importance of tissue-specific FSH and its receptors. Of the three methods for reducing cancer-related mortality – decreasing the incidence, improving therapy, and providing early detection – only the latter is currently at hand. However, an obvious problem exists with the widespread application of early detection or screening for this common malignancy: we may identify malignancies in some men who have little likelihood of a clinical manifestation of this disease, and who would actually be better off were their cancer to remain undetected. The overdetection of these malignancies, and the few methods of identifying those with a high propensity of causing patient morbidity or mortality, may lead to overtreatment. Several randomized studies of screening are now underway to determine whether screening results in a reduction in the disease-specific mortality rate from prostate cancer. What are clearly needed in prostate cancer management today are reliable methods to stratify those malignancies that may well give rise to patient disease from those likely to lie quiescent. Considerable effort is currently directed towards the development of potential markers of future biological behaviour (**Table 2.3**).

Table 2.3 Potential markers of malignant potential for prostate cancer
Histological grade
Clinical stage
Pathological stage
Tumour volume
Prostatic acid phosphatase
Prostate specific membrane antigen
Prostate specific antigen
DNA ploidy
Nuclear morphometry
Neovascularity
Oncogenes
Tumour-suppressor genes
Invasion markers (e.g. cathepsin, collagenase)
Cell adhesion factors
Basement membrane (collagen)
FSH and FSH receptors

STAGE MIGRATION OF PROSTATE CANCER

The increasing application of early detection programmes has created what appears to be a 'stage migration'. That is, more men are identified with malignancies of lower stage and are thus perhaps more likely to be cured with conventional therapy. Recently, Ohori et al.[38] examined a series of men undergoing radical prostatectomy at Baylor School of Medicine. They classified the neoplasms into three categories (latent, clinically important, or curable), and compared these tumours to incidental cancers found in 90 cystoprostatectomy specimens. A total of 78% of the patients undergoing cystoprostatectomy had what were described as latent cancers (cancers smaller than 0.5 cm^3 with Gleason grade of 1, 2, or 3) which were pathologically confined. In 22% of patients, cancers were found that were deemed curable with significant malignant potential; that is to say, they had either a Gleason grade 1, 2, or 3 tumour with a volume greater than 0.5 cm^3 that was confined to the prostate, a grade 4 or 5 tumour of any volume that was confined, or demonstrated microscopic extracapsular extension in cancers of any grade and any volume. Advanced neoplasms, defined as those that have extensive extracapsular extension, seminal-vesicle extension or pelvic lymph-node metastases, were not found in the cystoprostatectomy specimens.

Of 360 men undergoing radical prostatectomy, latent carcinoma was found in 9%, curable malignancy in 62%, and in 29% of patients it was thought that advanced cancer was present and was not likely to have been cured. Among the 246 men who had palpable tumours, 8% were deemed latent, 58% curable, and 34% advanced. Of the 55% of patients who had nonpalpable carcinoma (stage T1c), identified by elevation of serum PSA, 13% were felt to be latent, 76% curable, and 11% advanced.

TUMOUR VOLUME AND GLEASON GRADE

McNeal has reported that tumour volume and Gleason grade are closely correlated[39]. His data indicate that extraprostatic extension only begins when tumours have exceeded a volume of 0.5 cm^3, and occurs frequently when tumour volume is greater than 1.4 cm^3 (**2.27**). Oesterling[40] has also found that the Gleason grade is correlated with capsular penetration, seminal-vesicle invasion (**2.28**)

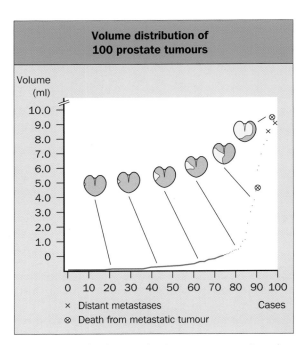

2.27 Volume distribution of 100 prostate cancers in rank order. Only those with volume >1.5 cm^3 had metastasized. (Modified with permission from McNeal et al.[35] © by The Lancet Ltd, 1986.)

and lymph-node metastases in Stage B (T2) disease. Unfortunately, at present it is usually not possible to make an accurate determination of tumour volume pre-operatively. In practical terms, therefore, in patients with high-grade tumours (Gleason grade >7), additional staging procedures such as computed tomography (CT) and magnetic resonance imaging (MRI) scanning and pelvic lymph-node dissection should be considered before radical surgery, to decrease the likelihood of operating inappropriately on patients with locally advanced or metastatic disease.

PSA AND PATHOLOGICAL STAGE

Serum prostate-specific antigen (PSA) is discussed in detail in Chapter 6. Its utility as a staging tool and, by extrapolation, as a method of assessing malignant potential, was initially felt to be of low utility owing to the considerable overlap of pathological stage in patients with pre-operative PSA value. **2.29** demonstrates one initial experience, and this was reflected by the observations of many other authorities[41,42]. However, in these reports, care was not taken to ensure that significant prostate

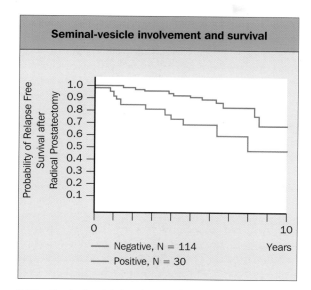

2.28 Seminal-vesicle involvement by prostate cancer carries a high risk of tumour recurrence and a poor prognosis. (Data from Dr DF Paulson.)

perturbation (which we now know can influence the serum PSA levels for a long period of time) did not contaminate these findings. In a recent radical prostatectomy series, in which preoperative PSA was obtained prior to significant prostatic perturbation (i.e. biopsy), the potential prognostic yield for elevated PSA (greater than 10.0 ng/ml) was not inconsiderable (**2.30**). In the individual patient, however, PSA is a rather poor predictor of stage.

Tumour volume, as well as serum PSA, offer objective methods of assessing the malignant potential of prostate cancer. Goto and associates[43] examined 105 men and attempted to use these parameters (**Table 2.4**) to identify 19 patients with clinically insignificant cancers from those with cancer that was more likely to impact on their life.

Bluestein and associates[44] have conducted clinical studies of primary Gleason grade on biopsy and serum PSA to quantitate the risk of pelvic lymph-node metastasis in men who are subjected to a radical prostatectomy. As can be seen in **Table 2.5** for clinically localized prostate cancer, Gleason

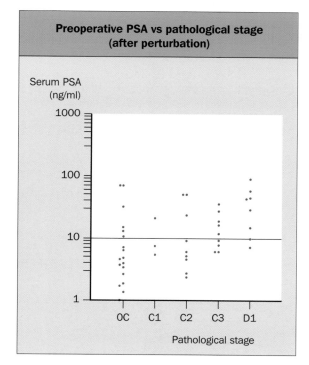

2.29 PSA and tumour stage without regard to perturbation. (Reproduced with permission from Ellis WJ, Brawer MK. Management decisions in the patient with an elevated PSA. *AUA Update Series* 1993;**XII(34)**:265–272.)

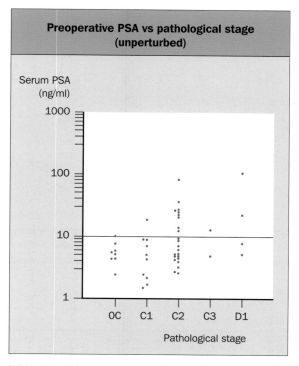

2.30 PSA and tumour stage (prebiopsy). (Reproduced with permission from Ellis WJ, Brawer MK. Management decisions in the patient with an elevated PSA. *AUA Update Series* 1993;**XII(34)**:265–272.)

Table 2.4 Distinguishing clinically unimportant (CU) prostate cancers (N = 105, 19 CU)	
PSA and tumour volume	**C.U. (%)**
PSA < 4.0 ng/ml and < 1 mm	86
PSA < 4.0 and 1–5 mm	45
PSA 4–20 < 1 mm	50
PSA 4–20	14
PSA > 20 and 5 mm	0

Table 2.5 Combinations of local clinical stage, primary Gleason grade and serum PSA to yield a false negative rate of 3% for positive lymph nodes		
Local Clinical Stage	**Primary Gleason Grade**	**Serum PSA (ng/ml)**
T1a–T1b (A1–B1)	1 and 2	17.1
	3	8.0
	4 and 5	4.2
T2c (B2)	1 and 2	4.1
	3	2.0
	4 and 5	1.0
T3a (C1)	1 and 2	1.4
	3	0.7
	4 and 5	0.3

grade 1–2 and PSA less than 17.1 would afford this performance. In contrast, if the grade was Gleason 4–5, then the PSA had to be less than 4.2. These authors argued that this would mitigate against the presence of pelvic lymph-node metastasis in a very high percentage of patients.

DNA PLOIDY

DNA ploidy has been extensively investigated as a prognostic marker. While several authors have felt that this modality offers significant stratification of patients' prostate cancer risk[45–47], significant problems surround this approach. O'Malley and asso-

ciates[48] recently reported significant heterogeneity in the DNA ploidy. In nine radical prostatectomy specimens, they performed biopsies of the tumour and compared the DNA ploidy by flow cytometry in different aliquots. Marked ploidy differences (diploid versus tetraploid or aneuploid) were seen in five of the nine cases. Greene et al.[49] recently confirmed these findings by utilizing static image-analysis ploidy determinations. This degree of variability of ploidy within a given tumour markedly constrains the potential utility of this approach.

It has long been recognized[50,51] that once a neoplasm exceeds 1 mm in diameter it has to induce a blood supply and develop an angiogenic phenotype. Weidner and associates[52] were able to stratify women with breast cancer as to the likelihood of metastasis based on the microvessel quantification. Utilizing factor VIII immunohistochemical correlations of prostate cancer, Brawer et al. were able to develop a computerized image-analysis system which afforded excellent correlation to manual counting of microvessels in human prostate[53]. It has recently been demonstrated that neovascularity is a reasonable predictor of pathological stage[54] (**2.31**). Moreover, it has been shown recently that in men who underwent radical prostatectomy and were shown to have pathological stage C (T_3)

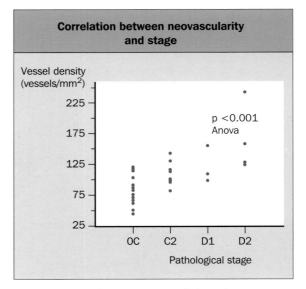

2.31 Correlation between neovascularity and tumour stage. (From Brawer et al.[54] © 1994 American Cancer Society. Reprinted by permission of Wiley-Liss, Inc., a subsidiary of John Wiley & Sons, Inc.)

disease with a minimum of 10 years follow-up, neovascularity was able to stratify those patients who did not progress, whereas tumour grade was not discriminatory[53]. In addition, it has been demonstrated that there is a good correlation between microvessel density as obtained on needle biopsy, and in that found by radical prostatectomy (**2.32**). The clinical significance of neovascularity in prostate cancer has been confirmed by Weidner and associates[55] (see **4.13**).

Berges *et al.*[56] studied proliferation and apoptosis in normal prostate, in high-grade prostatic intraepithelial neoplasia, and in prostatic carcinoma. They noted no difference in the percentage of proliferating cells between high-grade PIN and carcinoma, but there was more than a two-fold increase in proliferation over normal in these two conditions. What was intriguing was their observation that, when compared to normal, apoptosis, a measure of programmed cell death, was increased in high-grade PIN associated with cancer and in carcinoma itself, but was decreased in high-grade PIN not associated with cancer (**Table 2.6**).

Another important hallmark of tumour aggressiveness is its ability to invade. The prostate cancer must transgress the basement membrane to gain access to the stroma. Basement membrane has been quantified immunohistochemically using antibodies to collagen and fibronectin[57]. A strong correlation

Table 2.6 Cell proliferation and death in the normal prostate vs high-grade PIN and prostatic cancer (CaP)

Histology	Proliferation (%)	Apoptopic (%)
Normal	1.0	1.0
High-grade PIN	2.3 ± 0.8	0.66±0.15* 4.3 ± 0.4**
CAP	2.2 ± 0.5	5.0 ± 0.4

* PIN without CaP
** PIN with CaP
(Reproduced with permission from Berges *et al.*[56])

with the Gleason grade was observed, but these studies were hampered by the use of antibodies to type IV collagen, which could also be expressed by stromal cells. This phenomenon has been examined using antibodies to type VII collagen, which is specific to epithelial-derived basement membrane. A complete absence of basement membrane was demonstrated in carcinoma, suggesting that one of the early phenotypic changes in prostate cancer is the ability to degrade the basement membrane enzymatically to facilitate local invasion.

UNUSUAL PROSTATIC TUMOURS

Adenocarcinomas arising from the epithelial lining of the secretory acini constitute by far the commonest form of malignancy of the prostate. However, other forms of tumour may occur, most of which are uncommon. These include carcinomas of other epithelial linings, such as the urethra and major prostatic ducts, as well as lymphomas, sarcomas and small-cell carcinomas. Detailed descriptions of their pathology can be found elsewhere[58] as can a discussion of their clinical manifestations[59]. Of these cancers, only a few occur with sufficient frequency to warrant description here.

Ductal Carcinomas

The glandular acini of the prostate deliver their secretions into the urethra via a complex ductal system. Tumours that arise within this system have

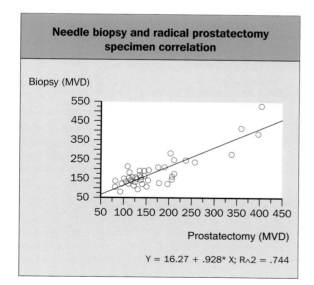

Needle biopsy and radical prostatectomy specimen correlation

Biopsy (MVD)

Prostatectomy (MVD)

$Y = 16.27 + .928* X; R^2 = .744$

2.32 Microvessel density (MVD) on needle biopsy and radical prostatectomy specimen. Note strong correlation.

been recognized as histologically distinct from the much more common acinar carcinomas.

Periurethral prostatic duct carcinomas have been described in detail by Kopelson et al.[60]. These carcinomas are characterized by their mixed transitional-cell/acinar morphology, and typically produce only minimal amounts of PSA.

Papillary tumours of the major prostatic ducts were originally referred to as 'endometrial' carcinomas of the prostate[61], and were thought not to be derived from prostatic duct linings. Subsequently, 'endometrial' carcinomas were shown to produce acid phosphatase[62] and PSA[63] and are now recognized as a variant of ductal carcinoma. It has been suggested, but not proven, that ductal carcinomas are more clinically aggressive than acinar tumours[64-66].

Mucinous Carcinomas

The production of mucus is not usually thought of as a characteristic of prostatic cancers, but it has been estimated that up to 20% of prostatic adenocarcinomas contain areas of mucin production[67]. However, if the suggested criterion of requiring at least 40% of the tumour demonstrating mucinous elements is applied, then the incidence of this tumour falls to less than 4%[68]. Fortunately, these tumours continue to secrete both acid phosphatase

and PSA, and immunohistochemical stains can therefore be used to differentiate them from other mucinous carcinomas arising from either the lung or gastrointestinal tract[69] (**2.26**).

CONCLUSIONS

The anatomy of the prostate in the adult is largely a reflection of its embryological development. The various anatomical zones are prone to different pathological processes: BPH in the transition zone and adenocarcinoma in the peripheral zone. The underlying mechanisms for the stepwise development of these most prevalent diseases are now beginning to be unfolded by molecular biological techniques.

Although detailed pathological analysis and grading can yield some insight into the aggressiveness or otherwise of prostatic tumours, more sophisticated multivariant analysis of molecular markers will be necessary to predict more precisely the metastatic potential of a cancer in a given individual. Much research is currently directed towards identifying such markers; this work, together with an insight into the molecular mechanisms of induction of prostate cancer, are the subject of the following chapters.

REFERENCES

1 Lowsley OS. The development of the human prostate gland with reference to the development of other structures of the neck of the urinary bladder. *Am J Anat* 1912;**13**:299.

2 McNeal JE. Regional morphology and pathology of the prostate. *Am J Clin Pathol* 1968;**49**:347–357.

3 Kirby RS, Lowe D, Bultitude MJ. Intraprostatic urinary reflux: an aetiological factor in abacterial prostatitis. *Br J Urol* 1982;**54**:729–731.

4 Reese JH, McNeal JE, Redwine EA, *et al*. Differential distribution of pepsinogen II between the zones of the human prostate and the seminal vesicle. *J Urol* 1986;**136**:1148.

5 Reese JH, McNeal JE, Redwine EA, *et al*. Tissue type plasminogen activator as a marker for functional zones, within the human prostate gland. *Prostate* 1988;**12**:47.

6 Villers AA, McNeal JE, Freiha FS, *et al*. Development of prostatic carcinoma: morphometric and pathological features of early stages. *Acta Oncol* 1991;**30**:145–149.

7 Villers A, McNeal JE, Redwine EA, Freiha FS, Stamey TA. The role of perineural space invasion in the local spread of prostatic adenocarcinoma. *J Urol* 1989;**142**:763.

8 Ayala AG, Ro JY, Babian R, Troncoso P, Grignon DJ. The prostatic capsule: does it exist? *Am J Surg Pathol* 1989;**13**:21.

9 Lepor H, Gregerman M, Crosby R, Mostofi FK, Walsh PC. Precise localization of the autonomic nerves from the pelvic plexus to the corpora cavernosa: a detailed anatomical study of the adult male pelvis. *J Urol* 1985;**133**:207–212.

10 Walsh PC, Epstein JI. Radical prostatectomy with preservation of sexual function. Impact on cancer control. *Problems in Urology* 1987;**1**(1):42–52.

11 Walsh PC, Epstein JI, Lowe FC. Potency following radical prostatectomy with wide unilateral excision of the neurovascular bundle. *J Urol* 1987;**138**:823–827.

12 Brading AF, Turner WH. The unstable bladder: towards a common mechanism. *Br J Urol* 1994;**73**:3–8.

13 Garde SV, Sheth AR, Shah MG, Kulkarni SA. Prostate – an extrapituitary source of follicle-stimulating hormone (FSH): occurence, localization, and de novo biosynthesis and its hormonal modulation in primates and rodents. *Prostate* 1991;**18**:271–287.

14 Desmond PM, Clark J, Thompson IM, Zeidman EJ, Mueller EJ. Morbidity with contemporary prostate biopsy. *J Urol* 1993;**150**:1425–1426.

15 Hodge KK, McNeal SE, Terris MK, Stamey TA. Random systematic versus directed ultrasound-guided

transrectal core biopsies of the prostate. *J Urol* 1989;**142**:71.

16 Ekman H, Hedberg K, Persson PS. Cytological versus histological examination of needle biopsy specimens in the diagnosis of prostatic cancer. *Br J Urol* 1967;**39**:544–548.

17 Esposti PL. Cytologic malignancy grading of prostatic carcinoma by transrectal aspiration biopsy. *Scand J Urol Nephrol* 1971;**5**:199–209.

18 Brawer MK, Bostwick DM, Peehl DM, Stamey TA. Keratin immunoreactivity in the benign and neoplastic human prostate. *Canc Res* 1985;**45**(8):3663–3667.

19 Kirby RS, Christmas TJ. *Benign Prostatic Hyperplasia.* London: Gower Medical Publishing, 1993; 1–109.

20 Gleason DF. Histologic grading and clinical staging of prostatic carcinoma. In: Tannenbaum M, ed. *Urologic Pathology: The Prostate*. Philadelphia: Lea & Febiger, 1977;171–198.

21 Epstein JI, Cho KR, Quinn BD. Relationship of severe dysplasia to Stage A (incidental) adenocarcinoma of the prostate. *Cancer* 1990;**65**:2321–2327.

22 Quinn BD, Cho KR, Epstein JI. Relationship of severe dysplasia to stage B adenocarcinoma of the prostate. *Cancer* 1990;**65**:2321–2327.

23 Bostwick DG, Brawer MK. Prostatic intraepithelial neoplasia and early invasion in prostate cancer. *Cancer* 1987;**59**:778–794.

24 Humphrey PA. Mucin in severe dysplasia in the prostate. *Surg Pathol* 1991;**4**:137–143.

25 Perlman E, Epstein JI. Blood group antigen expression in dysplasia and adenocarcinoma of the prostate. *Am J Surg Pathol* 1990;**14**:810–818.

26 McNeal JE, Alroy J, Leau I, Redwine EA, Freiha FS, Stamey TA. Immunohistochemical evidence for impaired cell differentiation in the premalignant phase of prostate carcinogenesis. *Am J Clin Pathol* 1988;**90**:23–32.

27 Nagle RB, Brewer MK, Kittelson J, Clark V. Phenotypic relationship of prostatic intraepithelial neoplasia to invasive prostatic carcinoma. *Am J Pathol* 1991;**138**:119–128.

28 Gleason DF. Histologic grading and clinical staging of prostatic carcinoma. In: Tannenbaum M, ed. *Urologic Pathology: The Prostate*. Philadelphia: Lea & Febiger, 1977.

29 Miller GJ. New developments in grading prostate cancer. *Semin Urol* 1990;**8**:9–18.

30 Gleason DF. Histologic grading of prostate cancer: a perspective. *Hum Pathol* 1992;**23**:273–279.

31 Chodak GW, Thisted RA, Gerber GS, *et al.* Results of conservative management of clinically localized prostate cancer. *New Eng J Med* 1994;**330**(4):242–248.

32 Franks LM. Latent carcinoma of the prostate. *J Pathol Bacteriol* 1954;**68**:603–616.

33 Breslow N, Chan CW, Dhom G, *et al.* Latent carcinoma of the prostate at autopsy in seven areas. *Int J Cancer* 1977;**20**:680–688.

34 Sakr WA, Haas GP, Cassin BF, *et al.* The frequency of carcinoma of the prostate and intraepithelial neoplasia of the prostate in young male patients. *J Urol* 1993;**150**:379–385.

35 McNeal JE, Bostwick DG, Kindrachuk RA, *et al.* Patterns of progression in prostate cancer. *Lancet* 1986;**1**:60–63.

36 Scardino PT, Weaver R, Hudson MA. Early detection of prostate cancer. *Hum Pathol* 1992;**23**(3):211.

37 Dirnhofer S, Berger C, Steiner G, Maderbacher S, Berger P. Co expression of gonadotrophic hormones and their corresponding FSH- and LH/CG-receptors in the human prostate. *Prostate* 1998;**35**:212–220.

38 Ohori M, Wheeler TM, Dunn JK, *et al.* Pathologic features and prognosis of prostate cancers detectable with current diagnostic tests. *J Urol* 1994;**151** (**Suppl**):451A No.894.

39 McNeal JE. Cancer volume and site of origin of adenocarcinoma in the prostate: relationship to local and distant spread. *Hum Pathol* 1992;**23**:258–266.

40 Oesterling JE, Brendler CB, Epstein JI, *et al.* Correlation of clinical stage, serum prostatic acid phosphatase and preoperative Gleason grade with final pathological stage in 275 patients with clinically localized adenocarcinoma of the prostate. *J Urol* 1987;**138**:92–98.

41 Oesterling JE, Chan DW, Epstein JI, *et al.* Prostate specific antigen in the preoperative and postoperative evaluation of localized prostatic cancer treated with radical prostatectomy. *J Urol* 1988;**139**:766–772.

42 Stamey TA, Yang N, Hay AR, *et al.* Prostate-specific antigen as a serum marker for adenocarcinoma of the prostate. *New Engl J Med* 1987;**317**:909–916.

43 Goto Y, Ohori M, Arakawa A, Wheeler TM, Scardino PT. Distinguishing clinically important from unimportant prostate cancers before treatment: preliminary report. *J Urol* 1994;**151**(**Suppl**):289A No.248.

44 Bluestein DL, Bostwick DG, Bergstralb EJ, *et al.* Eliminating the need for bilateral pelvic lymphadenectomy in select patients with prostate cancer. *J Urol* 1994;**151**:1315–1320.

45 Lee SE, Currin SM, Paulson DF, *et al.* Flow cytometric determination of ploidy in prostatic adenocarcinoma: A comparison with seminal vesicle involvement and histopathologic grading as a predictor of clinical recurrence. *J Urol* 1988;**140**:769–774.

46 Stephenson RA, James BCHG, Fair WR, *et al.* Flow cytometry of prostate cancer: Relationship of DNA content to survival. *Canc Res* 1987;**47**:2504–2507.

47 Zetterberg A, Eposti PL. Prostatic significance of nuclear DNA levels in prostatic carcinoma. *Scand J Urol Nephrol* 1980;**55**:53–56.

48 O'Malley FP, Grignon DJ, Keeney M, *et al.* DNA heterogeneity in prostatic adenocarcinoma: A DNA flow cytometric mapping study with whole organ section of prostate. *Cancer* 1993;**71**(9):2797.

49 Greene DR, Taylor SR, Wheeler TM *et al.* DNA ploidy by image analysis of individual foci of prostate cancer: A preliminary report. *Canc Res* 1991;**51**:4084.

50 Folkman J, Cole P, Zimmerman S. Tumour behaviour in isolated perfused organs: in vitro growth and metastasis of biopsy material in rabbit thyroid and canine intestinal segment. *Ann Surg* 1966;**164**:491.

51 Folkman J. Tumour angiogenesis: therapeutic implications. *N Engl J Med* 1971;**285**:1182.

52 Weidner N, Semple J, Welch W, *et al.* Tumor angiogenesis and metastasis – correlation in invasive breast carcinoma. *New Engl J Med* 1971;**285**:1182.

53 Brawer MK, Jonsson E, Gibbons RP, *et al.* Extent of prostate neovascularity predicts progression in patients with pathologic stage C adenocarcinoma treated with radical prostatectomy. *J Urol* 1994;**151**(Suppl):289A No.246.

54 Brawer MK, Deering RE, Brown M, *et al.* Predictors of pathologic stage in prostatic carcinoma. The role of neovascularity. *Cancer* 1994;**73**(3):678–687.

55 Weidner N, Carrol PR, Flax J, *et al.* Tumour angiogenesis correlates with metastasis in invasive prostate carcinoma. *Am J Pathol* 1993;**143**(2):401–409.

56 Berges R, Carmichael M, Epstein JI, *et al.* Cell proliferation and death in the normal prostate vs. high grade PIN and prostatic cancer. *J Urol* 1994;**151** (**Suppl**):No.196.

57 Fuchs MF, Brawer MK, Rennels MA, *et al.* The relationship of basement membrane to histologic grade of human prostatic carcinoma. *Modern Path* 1989;**2**(2):105–111.

58 Miller GJ. An atlas of prostatic biopsies: dilemmas of morphologic variance. In: Fenoglio-Preiser CM, Wolff M, Rilke F, eds. *Progress in Surgical Pathology VIII.* Philadelphia: Field and Wood, 1988;81–112.

59 Efros MD, Fischer J, Mallouh C, *et al.* Unusual primary prostatic malignancies. *Urology* 1992;**39**:407–410.

60 Kopelson G, Harisiadis L, Romos NA, *et al.* Periurethral prostatic duct carcinoma: clinical features and treatment results. *Cancer* 1978;**42**:2894–2902.

61 Melicow MM, Pachter MR. Endometrial carcinoma of prostatic utricle (uterus masculinus). *Cancer* 1967;**20**:1715–1722.

62 Nadji M, Tabei SZ, Castro A, *et al.* Prostatic origin of tumours: an immunohistochemical study. *Am J Clin Pathol* 1980;**73**:735–739.

63 Walker AN, Mills SE, Fechner RE, *et al.* 'Endometrial' adenocarcinoma of the prostatic urethra arising in a villous polyp: a light microscopic and immunoperoxidase study. *Arch Pathol Lab Med* 1982;**106**:624–627.

64 Dube VE, Farrow GM, Greene LF. Prostatic adenocarcinoma of ductal origin. *Cancer* 1973;**32**:402–409.

65 Greene LF, Farrow GM, Ravits JM, *et al.* Prostatic adenocarcinoma of duct origin. *J Urol* 1979;**121**:303–305.

66 Lemberger RJ, Bishop MC, Bates CP, *et al.* Carcinoma of the prostate of ductal origin. *Br J Urol* 1984;**56**:706–709.

67 Elbadawi A, Craig W, Linke CA, *et al.* Prostatic mucinous carcinoma. *Urology* 1979;**13**:658–666.

68 Epstein JI, Lieberman PH. Mucinous adenocarcinoma of the prostate gland. *Am J Surg Pathol* 1985;**9**:299–308.

69 Odom DG, Donatucci CF, Deshon GE. Mucinous adenocarcinoma of the prostate. *Hum Pathol* 1990;**21**:593–600.

Chapter 3

Epidemiology and natural history of prostate cancer

INTRODUCTION

Although prostate cancer seems set to become the most common life-threatening malignant disease to affect males in both the developed and developing world, the high prevalence of other concurrent diseases that can also be fatal in elderly males means that this neoplasm is not always the primary cause of death. As most patients with prostate cancer are beyond middle age, the average number of life-years lost – around 9 – is lower than that for other tumours (**Table 3.1**). However, since the disease is so common, the *cumulative* potential years of life lost make it third among all cancers (**Table 3.2**). Also, as noted in the previous chapter, although the prevalence of clinical prostate cancer is very high, it has become apparent that there are far larger numbers of males who have a so-called 'latent', well-differentiated microscopic form of the disease that may never progress to invasive clinical disease with metastatic potential; the natural history of these 'incidental' cancers is currently not well understood.

INCIDENCE

It is difficult to estimate the worldwide prevalence of clinical prostate cancer due to insufficient data from developing countries. Of course, the shorter life-expectancy in these countries means that prostate cancer is less likely to be a clinical problem or cause of death. The most complete epidemiological data derive mainly from the USA, where the incidence of clinical prostate cancer has been fairly accurately documented. In the USA, the incidence of newly diagnosed cases of prostate cancer was 100 000 in 1988, and this had risen incrementally to 132 000 in 1992[1]; the incidence for 1994 was only a little less than 200 000 (**3.1**). Although this rise in new cases of prostate cancer may result, at least in part, from an increased awareness of

Table 3.1 Average life-years lost by premature death from several cancers in the USA			
	Prostate (men)	**Breast (women)**	**Lung (both sexes)**
Average years of life lost	9.0	19.2	13.5 (men) 14.8 (women)

Table 3.2 Potential life-years lost by premature death from several cancers in the USA			
	Prostate (men)	**Breast (women)**	**Lung (both sexes)**
Potential years of life lost	228 547	763 511	2 870 113

and search for the condition by screening programmes utilizing prostate-specific antigen (PSA), it is becoming clear that clinically significant prostate cancer is also on the increase. Autopsy studies have identified foci of prostate cancer in approximately 20% of men in their 20s, 30% of men in their 50s and 70% of the over 80s[2]. However, as mentioned, the lifetime chance of a man developing clinically apparent prostate cancer is less than 10%[3]; hence, the large majority of the small prostate cancers detected at autopsy are clinically insignificant, or 'latent' cancers. Although the majority of these tiny, well-differentiated prostate cancers apparently grow only very slowly within the natural lifespan of the individual, a proportion dedifferentiate, grow rapidly and usually metastasize, often leading to a fatal outcome. Mortality attributable to prostate cancer was 28 000 in the USA in 1988 and has risen steadily since then to around 36 000 in 1994 (3.2). Recently this seems to have peaked and may actually be falling[4]. A similar time trend in both incidence and mortality of prostate cancer is also apparent in England and Wales (3.3). The rise in incidence and mortality attributable to prostate cancer in the Netherlands has been shown to be due to a 'birth-cohort' effect in which males born in consecutive years have an increasing risk of developing prostate

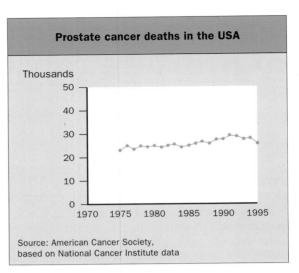

Source: American Cancer Society, based on National Cancer Institute data

3.2 Increased mortality rate from prostate cancer in the USA showing recent 7% decline.

cancer[5]. This increase in prostate cancer-related death is more than one would expect from demographic changes in the age of the population alone. More recently, however, a 7% decline in mortality rate has occurred in the USA. This has been attributed by some to the efforts of early detection and the active treatment of localized disease by radiation and radical prostatectomy.

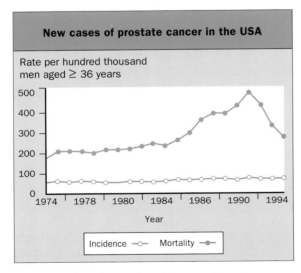

3.1 Age-adjusted rates of prostate cancer in western Washington state, 1974–1994. (Reproduced with permission from Newcomer LM, et al. Temporal trends in rates of prostate cancer: declining incidence of advanced stage disease, 1974 to 1994. *J Urol* 1997;**158**:1427–1430.)

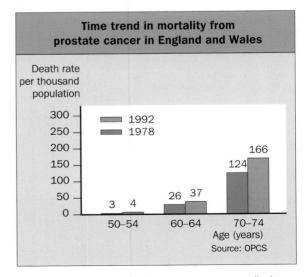

3.3 Time trend in increased prostate cancer mortality by age in England and Wales, 1978 and 1992.

Clinically significant prostate cancer is rare in men under the age of 50 years. As with latent prostate cancer, however, the incidence increases more rapidly with age than that of any other tumour. In addition to this, the mortality attributable to prostate cancer increases steadily with increasing age from 50 years upwards (**3.4**). However, a significant number of those dying are younger than 75 years of age (**Table 3.3**). The impact of age as a risk factor will make prostate cancer an even more important disease owing to the increasing longevity (**3.5**; **Table 3.4**).

Familial Prostate Cancer

It has recently become apparent that there is a greater-than-expected incidence of prostate cancer in the male relatives of men who have died from the disease. A study of 228 men dying of prostate cancer revealed a relative risk of prostate cancer in fathers and siblings that was nearly three times higher than that of a control group[6]. A genealogical study of cancer in Mormons living in Utah examined the occurrence of 2 821 cases of prostate cancer occurring between 1958 and 1961. This demonstrated that prostate cancer had the fourth highest familial association of all cancers studied, with a stronger familial link than both colonic and breast cancer, which are generally regarded as having a

Table 3.3 Deaths in 1990 from several cancers in individuals under age 75 years

Cancer	Deaths
Prostate	12 423
Lung	100 253
Breast	29 931
Colon/rectum	29 805

Table 3.4 New cases of prostate cancer in Europe

Country	1990	2000	2010	2020
Belgium	2796	3156	3248	3939
Denmark	1120	1120	1307	1596
France	16 444	19 507	20 497	26 157
FR Germany	17 658	21 727	27 416	28 927
Greece	1207	1511	1621	1752
Ireland	549	546	621	814
Italy	11 321	11 510	14 836	16 313
Luxembourg	63	76	86	106
The Netherlands	3559	4087	4861	6512
Portugal	1753	1993	2068	2347
Spain	8056	9938	10 454	11 933
UK	14 125	14 421	15 352	18 099

(Data with permission from Boyle P. Evolution of an epidemic of unknown origin. In: Denis L, ed. *Prostate Cancer 2000*. Heidelberg: Springer-Verlag; 1994.)

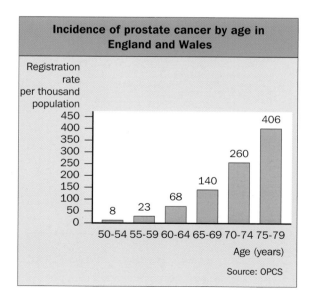

Incidence of prostate cancer by age in England and Wales

3.4 Mortality from prostate cancer in England and Wales by age cohort, 1987.

significant genetic component[7]. A study of 691 men with prostate cancer revealed twice the expected incidence of prostate cancer in those with first-degree relatives with the disease. Also, those men with two or three affected first-degree relatives had a 5-fold and 11-fold increased lifetime risk of developing prostate cancer respectively[8]. Currently, about 9% of all cases of prostatic cancer are thought to have a genetic basis – this is about twice the percentage of the familial tumours seen in breast cancer.

Clearly the increased incidence of prostate cancer among members of the same family could result from environmental factors rather than a genetic predisposition. Recently, however, some evidence

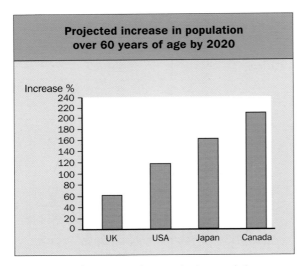

3.5 Projected percentage increase in the population over 60 years of age by the year 2020. (Adapted with permission from Kirby R, Fitzpatrick J, Kirby M, Fitzpatrick A. *A Shared Care for Prostatic Diseases*. Oxford: ISIS Medical Media; 1994, p. 2.)

Geographical and Ethnic Variations

The worldwide prevalence of clinical prostate cancer varies remarkably from one country to another. The highest reported incidence is from the Scandinavian countries (60 per 100 000 per year), with intermediate incidence in the USA (50 per 100 000) and the UK (20 per 100 000). The lowest incidence is in the Far East, especially in mainland China and Japan (4 per 100 000). The difference between the highest and lowest is almost 100 fold. Unfortunately, accurate figures are not available from many countries of the world, although high-risk, medium-risk and low-risk zones can be identified (**3.6**). Although overreporting may be an issue, it is estimated that of the approximately 1 million men worldwide who have diagnosed prostate cancer, 90% reside in developed nations[12].

The rate of mortality attributable to prostate cancer is also highly variable worldwide. The highest rate of mortality from prostate cancer occurs in the West Indies and Bermuda, at 28–29 per

has emerged to suggest that a genuinely hereditary form of prostate cancer may exist. Hereditary prostate cancer is characterized by Mendelian autosomal dominant inheritance, and an early onset of the disease[9]. Based on the familial clustering of prostate cancer, a number of groups have worked to identify the genes involved. Generally, they have used linkage analysis of large families affected by prostatic carcinoma. The exact location and determinants of the gene or genes that might be responsible for hereditary prostate cancer have not been elucidated, but loss of one or more tumour suppressor gene loci seems the most likely explanation and the 24–25 positions on the long arm of chromosome 1q is one candidate location[10], a second resides on the X chromosome, suggesting an X-linked mode of inheritance[11] (see Chapter 4).

Mass screening by specific invitation of asymptomatic men for prostate cancer is at present controversial (see Chapter 7). However, there is now some evidence to support the value of screening of first-degree male relatives of men with prostate cancer, particularly male relatives of those developing the disease at a young age and those with a strong positive family history of the disease. Since congenital prostate cancer has an early onset, this screening process should start around the age of 40.

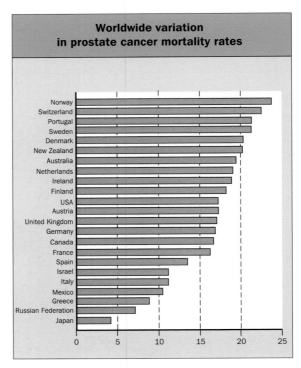

3.6 Age-adjusted prostate cancer mortality rates per 100 000 males by country. (Reproduced from Parker SL, Tong T, Bolden S, Wingo PA. Cancer Statistics, 1996. *CA Cancer J Clin* 1996;**46**:5–27.)

100 000. The mortality rates from the USA and the UK are 15 per 100 000 and 12 per 100 000 respectively. It is interesting to note the disparity between the incidence:mortality ratio between the USA and the UK: 50:20 per 100 000 and 15:12 per 100 000 respectively. It has been suggested that this might result from aggressive therapy for early disease in the form of radical prostatectomy that is common practice in the USA, but less commonly performed in the UK. However, until recently in the USA, the death rate from prostate cancer has increased together with the incidence rates, in spite of an increase in the number of radical prostatectomies performed. It is therefore possible that the increasing incidence of prostate cancer in the USA, over and above that seen in the UK, to some extent reflects an increase in the early diagnosis by PSA driven screening programmes. This raises the question of whether at least a proportion of the early prostate cancers diagnosed in the USA might not progress to clinically significant disease if left untreated. This bias may be even more skewed owing to racial differences in participation in screening programmes in the USA (**Table 3.5**).

This issue will be further addressed in subsequent chapters.

Further analysis of the statistics for the incidence of prostate cancer in multiracial communities has shown wide differences between races. The highest incidence is found in blacks, and the lowest in Chinese and Japanese races. This finding also explains, at least in part, the enormous geographical variation in the incidence of prostate cancer. The highest worldwide incidence of prostate cancer is in blacks living in Atlanta, Georgia (91.2 per 100 000), while the lowest is in Chinese residents of Shanghai (1.3 per 100 000). However, blacks living in Africa appear to have a lower rate of prostate cancer, although this may simply result from the shorter life expectancy in Africa and the limited facilities for diagnosis. Epidemiological data have also shown a disparity between the incidence of prostate cancer in racial groups in their native countries and migrants of the same group living in countries with a higher endemic rate of prostate cancer[13]. In particular, Japanese migrants to San Francisco have an incidence of prostate cancer of 16.5 per 100 000, while their counterparts remaining in Osaka, Japan, have an incidence of only 6.1 per 100 000). A similar difference has been described in Japanese migrants to Hawaii[14]. However, the incidence of prostate cancer in such Japanese migrants does not rise anywhere near as high as that for endemic whites in San Francisco (50 per 100 000). Similar differences are found in migrant Chinese, Jews and Indians. It is interesting to note that the incidence of latent or incidental prostate cancer appears to affect all groups equally. These data suggest an in-born genetic predisposition for the development of clinical prostate cancer associated with specific racial groups, with superadded promotion of disease progression by environmental factors, including diet.

AETIOLOGICAL AND PREDISPOSING FACTORS FOR PROSTATE CANCER

Apart from the 9% or so of men with hereditary prostate cancer, the strongest predetermining factor for the development of prostate cancer is age (**Tables 3.6 and 3.7**). As already mentioned, prostate cancer is rarely found in the under 50s but is increasingly common with rising age (**3.4**). The racial characteristics outlined above are also quite strong predisposing factors with North American blacks, having roughly twice the lifetime risk of the disease compared with their white counterparts[15].

Hormones

Circulating androgens are an essential prerequisite for the growth of normal prostate, and for the development of benign prostatic hyperplasia and prostate-cancer change. The precise role of androgens in terms of carcinogenesis within the prostate is not entirely clear, but they seem to act by promoting

Table 3.5 African–Americans in screening programmes	
Investigator	**Proportion of African–Americans (%)**
Mettlin	7
Brawer	5
Catalona	2–3
Crawford	5

(Data with permission from Brawer MK. Prostate cancer: epidemiology and screening. *Prostate Cancer and Prostatic Diseases* 1999;**2(Suppl)**:2–6.)

Table 3.6	Predisposing factors for clinical prostate cancer
Genetic	Familial autosomal dominant in some
Racial	Commoner in blacks, Scandinavians, US whites and Western Europeans
Age	Commoner with increasing age
Hormones	Testosterone and dihydrotestosterone apparently essential
Sexual history	Commoner in men with early sexual experience and multiple sexual partners
Diet	Animal fats
	Low intake of yellow/green vegetables
Pollution	Urban dwelling
	Cadmium exposure
	Exposure to radioactive agents: Tritium, ^{51}Cr, ^{59}Fe, ^{60}Co, ^{65}Zn
Infection	Gonococcal infection?
	Herpes simplex type 2?
	RNA viruses?
Vasectomy	Increases risk?

? = possible risk factors

Table 3.7	Protective factors for clinical prostate cancer
Racial	Rare in Asians
Age	Rare in young men
Hormones	Absent in pseudo-hermaphrodites and eunuchs
Diet	High intake of yellow/green vegetables
	Low fat intake, especially red meat
Environment	Less common in rural dwellings
Hepatic cirrhosis	Due to increased oestrogen

cell growth and division. Although the amount of circulating testosterone is variable from one individual to another, there is apparently no direct correlation between the serum testosterone level and the risk of developing prostate cancer[16]. It is interesting to note that although serum testosterone levels gradually decline with advancing age, the incidence of prostate cancer steadily increases. This apparent anomaly might be explained by the lengthy lag period between initial early neoplastic change and the appearance of clinically apparent prostate cancer, as well as by changes in androgen receptor levels.

Testosterone is metabolized within the prostate to dihydrotestosterone (DHT) by the enzyme 5 alpha-reductase. It is now known that it is DHT rather than testosterone which is the major intracellular androgen that promotes growth within the prostate[17]. The role of DHT in the promotion of prostate cancer is as yet unclear. However, prostate cancer does not appear to occur in a cohort of pseudohermaphrodite men in whom 5 alpha-reductase is absent. It is also possible that the variable geographical incidence of prostate cancer might be related in some way to different levels of DHT in ethnic groups. In particular a reduced activity of 5 alpha-reductase has been reported in Japanese men – this could perhaps account for the lower, but currently rising, prevalence of prostate cancer in Japan[18].

Cirrhosis of the liver can lead to a decrease in the level of circulating testosterone as well as an increase in circulating oestrogens; both of these changes could account for the reduced risk of developing prostate cancer in this condition[19].

The precise role of androgens in the induction and promotion or progression of prostate cancer is not yet fully understood. However, once malignant transformation has become established, androgens almost certainly have a role in stimulating malignant cell division and invasion.

Diet

There has been considerable interest in the role of dietary components in the aetiology of prostate cancer. The high incidence of prostate cancer in the USA appears to correlate with an increase in fat consumption. Regions within the USA where dairy product and red-meat ingestion is greatest also have a higher age-adjusted incidence of prostate cancer[20].

The US health professionals' follow-up study[21] evaluated over 4700 men with respect to, among other things, diet and the risk of the development of cancer. During the course of this study 300 men had a diagnosis of prostate cancer. Food fat consumption was directly related to the risk of prostate cancer and the risk was primarily associated with saturated fat. The authors went on to demonstrate that red meat consumption had the greatest correlation with cancer risk. The original studies supporting the relationship of dietary fat have shown similar results[22,23]. The effect of dietary fat in different racial groups was reported by Whittemore as well as the World Health Organization[24,25]. The association between saturated fat and cancer was greatest in the Asian–Americans.

There are several potential modes of action of fats in prostate cancer. In some strains of genetically susceptible rats, certain fats reduce the induction time for testosterone to stimulate the development of prostate cancer[26]. Another possible mechanism whereby high levels of fat consumption increase the risk of prostate cancer is reduction in the absorption of vitamin A. An increase in the circulating level of beta-carotene, which depends upon the amount of vitamin A absorption, appears to be protective against the development of some cancers[27]. Circulating testosterone levels decrease by as much as 30% in men converted to a vegetarian low-fat diet, and could hence reduce the induction of prostate cancer by testosterone[28]. In Japan, where the traditional diet is low in fat, the incidence of prostate cancer has recently begun to rise in association with increasing 'Westernization' of lifestyle. Similar trends seem to be occurring in China[29].

The traditional diets in Japan and other Asian countries consist of large quantities of yellow and green vegetables. High levels of vitamin A in this diet may protect against the induction of prostate cancer. Phyto-oestrogens such as genistein and daidzein found in vegetables such as soya may alter the hormonal milieu and counteract the effects of testerone upon the prostate. They also have antioxidant activity and act as free radical scavengers. Other possible mechanisms of anticarcinogenic activity include inhibition of angiogenesis and inhibition of tyrosine-specific protein kinase of the growth factor receptors.

The substantial worldwide variation in the incidence of prostate cancer appears to depend to some extent upon genetic factors, but dietary differences could account for the changes in incidence in migration studies. It seems likely that the Western diet, which is high in animal fats and relatively low in vegetables, confers a higher risk for the development of prostate cancer.

Vitamins and Prostate Cancer

Dietary supplements of vitamin E and selenium may possibly afford some protection against the development of prostate cancer.

In a recent case control study higher levels of selenium in the toenail clippings of men in the health professionals follow-up study were associated with lower risks of advanced prostate cancer[30]. In a recent intervention trial the risk of prostate cancer was reduced by one third in men taking 200 mcg of selenium.

A link between the levels of alpha-tocopherol and beta-carotene in the diet has been suggested. Long-term supplementation with alpha-tocopherol has been shown to reduce the incidence of prostate cancer in male smokers; by contrast, beta-carotene seems to increase the incidence[31]. Although there are considerable data in the literature, a recent Finnish study of male smokers showed an increased rate of prostate cancer in a group receiving beta-carotene. This supports previous observations of an increased risk of prostate cancer in men receiving this substance[32]. A very intriguing finding from the study[32] was a negative association between prostate cancer and intake of vitamin E. Among those men receiving alpha-tocopherol there was a significant decreased rate of prostate cancer. Caution must be noted, however, in that the study was not specifically designed to demonstrate a change in prostate cancer incidence and therefore the findings must be considered preliminary.

Schwartz and Hulka[33] noted an increase in prostate cancer with distance from the equator. On the basis of this, vitamin D deficiency is a potential contributing cause and has been investigated. Vitamin D has been shown to have an antiproliferative and differentiating effect on human prostate cancer cell lines[34]. Epidemiological studies, however, have shown conflicting results.

Sexual Activity

It has been suggested that frequent sexual activity initiated early in life, multiple sexual partners and a history of sexually transmitted diseases may all increase the risk of prostate cancer[35]. Correlation between a history of gonococcal infection and prostate cancer, with a 45-year delay period, has been reported[36]. However, there are also conflicting data suggesting an increase in prostate cancer in men with low levels of sexual activity[37], and a study has shown that prostate cancer mortality in 1400 reputedly celibate Catholic priests was comparable to that within the general male population[38]. At present, the influence of sexual activity on the development of prostate cancer should be considered uncertain, but the changes in sexual mores occurring since the 1960s may well manifest themselves in a greater prevalence of prostate cancer in years to come. The median age at first intercourse for men in the UK, for example, has fallen from 20 to 17 over the last 25 years. The number of sexual partners during the lifetime of the average man has also increased considerably[39].

Vasectomy

Considerable controversy has surrounded a study suggesting a causal link between vasectomy and the subsequent development of prostate cancer[40]. However, this case-control surveillance can be criticized since it was not a prospective analysis, did not take account of other potential variable influences (such as sexual history and testosterone level) and did not exclude the presence of occult cancer in case controls. Two recent studies by Giovannucci[41,42] suggested a relative risk for vasectomy patients for prostate cancer of 1.85 and 1.56. Other studies of larger numbers of men who had undergone vasectomy failed to demonstrate conclusively an increased risk of prostate cancer[43,44]. At present, there seems no good reason to counsel against this important method of limiting world population growth, although individuals contemplating this procedure should probably be advised that the question remains open[45].

Environmental Factors

Over the last few decades, attention has increasingly been focused on the possible role of environmental pollution in promoting a number of neoplastic diseases. Exposure to a variety of chemicals that have been widely used in industry has been shown to contribute towards the development of particular malignant tumours. Prostate cancer is less likely to develop in men living in a rural environment than in their counterparts living within cities, and the latter group are also at greater risk of dying from the disease[29]. The factor, or factors, responsible for this could be environmental pollution by chemical agents, as well as exposure to substances within the workplace. Workers exposed to chemicals in the rubber, textile, chemical, drug, fertilizer and atomic energy industries have an increased risk of devel-

oping prostate cancer. The precise chemicals responsible for inducing prostate cancer are not known, although the finding of increased levels of cadmium in patients with prostate cancer has led to the suggestion that this might induce the condition[46]. There is also evidence to suggest that exposure to tritium, ^{51}Cr, ^{59}Fe, ^{60}Co, and ^{65}Zn may increase the risk of prostate cancer in employees of the United Kingdom Atomic Energy Authority[47]. Car salesmen, caretakers, personnel managers and shipping clerks have also been suggested to be at increased risk of developing prostate cancer. It is difficult to explain these associations (at least in terms of chemical exposure), and it seems likely that there are many other, as yet unknown, environmental factors associated with twentieth century living that might act to promote microscopic foci of incidental prostate cancer to become locally invasive.

Sunlight and Vitamin D

As mentioned, prostate cancer incidence appears to correlate with latitude[33]. The disease is more common in the northern states of the USA and Europe than in more southerly locations. This observation has led to the suggestion that vitamin D (1,25 dihydrocholecalciferol) may to some extent be protective against the development of the disease[34].

Smoking

Although tobacco smoking has been implicated as an aetiological factor in malignant tumours of the lung and bladder and many other neoplasms, no such association has yet been found in prostate cancer[48].

Viruses

Infectious agents, particularly viruses, are known to be the cause of carcinogenesis in some forms of genital malignancy such as cervical cancer. Viruses are certainly a potential environmental trigger for prostate cancer, but this is difficult to prove since many viruses are ubiquitous and others are impossible to isolate from tumour cells.

A possible candidate for the aetiology of prostate cancer is herpes simplex virus type 2. Antibodies to this virus were detected within the serum of 71% of prostate cancer cases, but in only 66% of controls with benign prostatic hyperplasia[49]. The virus has also been demonstrated within prostate cancer cells by electron microscopy[50]. It is intriguing to note also that wives of men with prostate cancer were reported to have an increased incidence of cervical carcinoma in one study[51].

RNA viral particles have also been identified within prostate cancer cells[52]. Further support for an aetiological role for RNA viruses is the presence of the H-*ras* oncogene p21 within prostate cancer cells. This seems to be associated with less well-differentiated prostate cancers[53].

PROSTATE CANCER AND BENIGN PROSTATIC HYPERPLASIA

The possibility of a causal association between prostate cancer and benign prostatic hyperplasia (BPH) is still controversial. Prostate cancer most commonly arises within the peripheral part of the prostate, while BPH predominantly develops within the transition zone[54]. However, Armenian *et al.*[55] reported that patients with BPH have a risk of developing prostate cancer that is several times greater than that of men without BPH. It was also suggested that prostatectomy reduces the chance of the subsequent development of prostate cancer. This study, however, can be criticized since the diagnosis of BPH in some of the cases was made on clinical rather than precise histological grounds.

A conflicting conclusion was reached by Greenwald and colleagues in a prospective study of men undergoing sub-total prostatectomy and a control group. The relative risk for the development of prostate cancer in the BPH group was found to be 0.88[56].

Both BPH and prostate cancer are very common in elderly males, and both are neoplastic conditions characterized by disturbances of the control of growth of prostatic epithelium. As will be discussed in the next chapter, the stepwise accumulation of genetic changes could underlie the pathogenesis of both conditions, although it currently seems unlikely that BPH is a direct precursor of adenocarcinoma.

NATURAL HISTORY OF PROSTATE CANCER

Attempts to study the natural history of prostate cancer have often been confounded by the addition of surgical, radiotherapeutic and endocrine therapies, which undoubtedly alter the long-term outcome of the disease. In the majority of circumstances, ethical and humanitarian reasons usually make it impossible to observe the natural course of this malignant disease without therapeutic intervention. However, a recent, pooled multicentre analysis of 828 men with clinically localized prostate cancer that was treated conservatively has revealed a disease-specific 10-year survival of 94% for men with a well-differentiated tumour. By contrast, there was only a 58% 10-year survival for men with a less well-differentiated tumour[57] (3.7).

This, and other studies, have supported the concept that some well-differentiated prostate cancers may not require active treatment, especially in older patients. Any therapeutic intervention, radical prostatectomy, radiotherapy or endocrine treatment, it has been argued, may be of no greater benefit than watchful waiting in such cases. Small foci of well-differentiated prostate cancer appear much earlier than had previously been appreciated. Recent autopsy studies have demonstrated small foci of intra-epithelial neoplasia and adenocarcinoma within the prostate in men in their 20s[58]. It seems, therefore, that the natural history of prostate cancer in at least some individuals is much more prolonged than had been appreciated.

There are probably three important steps in the natural history of prostate cancer. First, the development of microfoci of 'incidental' prostate cancer. Second, the progression from occult to clinically

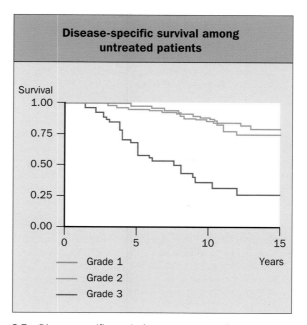

3.7 Disease-specific survival among untreated patients with prostate cancer according to tumour grade. (Reproduced with permission from Chodak *et al.*[57] © 1994 Massachusetts Medical Society. All rights reserved.)

significant localized prostate cancer and, third, metastasis of the cancer to lymph nodes, bones or other organs. The factors influencing each of these steps are discussed in the next chapter. There are two basic explanations for the progression of prostate cancer from occult disease to clinically significant disease. The first, championed by Stamey, suggests that the development of prostate cancer is a slow but unrelenting progression. The doubling time for prostate cancer has been shown to be much slower than in other tumours (up to 4 years in some cases) so that the progression time from initial malignant transformation until the appearance of a

1 ml volume tumour may be as long as 10 years[59]. The second proposition is that multiple genetic hits are necessary for transformation into clinically significant prostate cancer and subsequent de-differentiation, and that in some men occult prostate cancer will never in fact progress. This could also explain the fact that, although the prevalence of histological prostate cancer is evenly distributed worldwide, clinical disease develops to a variable extent in different countries dependent upon environmental factors[60] that act as promoters of progression. These issues are considered in greater depth in the next chapter.

REFERENCES

1 Boring CC, Squires TS, Tong T. Cancer statistics 1993. *CA Cancer Clin J* 1993;**43**:7–26.

2 Sheldon CA, Williams RD, Fraley EE. Incidental carcinoma of the prostate; a review of the literature and critical reappraisal of classification. J Urol 1980;**124**:626–631.

3 Silverberg E, Lubera JA. Cancer statistics. *CA* 1989;**39**:3–20.

4 Mettlin CJ, Murphy GP. Why is the prostate cancer death rate declining in the United States? *Cancer* 1998;**82**:249–251.

5 van der Gulden JWJ, Kiemeney LALM, Verbeek ALM, *et al.* Mortality trend from prostate cancer in the Netherlands (1950–1989). *Prostate* 1994;**24**:33–38.

6 Woolf CM. An investigation of the familial aspects of carcinoma of the prostate. *Cancer* 1960;**13**:739–743.

7 Cannon L, Bishop DT, Skolnick M, *et al.* Genetic epidemiology of prostate cancer in the Utah Mormon genealogy. *Cancer Survey* 1982;**1**:47.

8 Steinberg GS, Carter BS, Beaty TH, *et al.* Family history and the risk of prostate cancer. *Prostate* 1990;**17**:337–340.

9 Carter BS, Beaty TH, Steinberg GD, *et al.* Mendelian inheritance of familial prostate cancer. *Proceedings of the National Academy of Science* 1992;**89**:3367–3370.

10 Smith JR, Freije D, Carpten JD, *et al.* Major susceptibility locus for prostate cancer on chromosome 1 suggested by a genome wide search. *Science* 1996;**274**:1371–1374.

11 Xu J, Meyers D, Freije D, *et al.* Evidence for a prostate cancer susceptibility locus on the X chromosome. *Nature Genet* 1998;**20**:175–178.

12 Boyle P. Evolution of an epidemic of unkown origin. In: Denis L, ed. *Prostate Cancer 2000.* Heidelberg: Springer-Verlag; 1994:5–11.

13 Cook LS, Goldoft M, Schwartz SM, *et al.* Incidence of adenocarcinoma of the prostate in Asian immigrants in the United States and their descendants. *J Urol* 1999;**161**:152–155.

14 Akazaki K, Stemmermann GN. Comparative study of

15 Pienta KJ, Esper PS. Risk factors for prostate cancer. *Ann Intern Med* 1993;**118**:793–803.

16 Ghanadian R, Pugh CM, O'Donoghue EPN. Serum testosterone and dihydrotestosterone in carcinoma of the prostate. *Br J Cancer* 1979;**9**:696.

17 Bruchovsky N, Wilson JD The conversion of testosterone to 5-alpha-androstan-17-beta-ol-3-one by rat prostate *in vivo* and *in vitro. J Biol Chem* 1968; **243**:2012–2021.

18 Ross RK, Bernstein L, Loba RA, *et al.* 5-alpha-reductase activity and risk of prostate cancer among Japanese and US white and black males. *Lancet* 1992;**9**:887–889.

19 Glantz GM. Cirrhosis and carcinoma of the prostate gland. *J Urol* 1964;**91**:291.

20 Blair A, Fraumeni JF. Geographic patterns of prostate cancer in the United States. *J Natl Cancer Inst* 1978;**61**:1379.

21 Giovannucci E, Rimm EB, Colditz GA, *et al.* A prospective study of dietary fat and risk of prostate cancer. *J Natl Cancer Inst* 1993;**85**:1571–1579.

22 Mills P, Beeson L, Philips R, Fraser G. Dietary habits and breast cancer incidence among Seventh Day Adventists. *Cancer* 1989;**64**:582–590.

23 LeMarchand L, Kolonel L, Wilkens LR, Myers BC, Hirohata T. Animal fat consumption and prostate cancer: a prospective study in Hawaii. *Epidemiology* 1994;**5**:276–282.

24 Whittemore AS, Wu AH, Kolonel LN, *et al.* Family history and prostate cancer risk in black, white and Asian men in the United States and Canada. *Am J Epidemiol* 1995;**141**:732–740.

25 WHO. Trends in prostate cancer 1980–1988. *WHO Weekly Epidemiol Rec* 1992;**67**:281–288.

26 Pollard M, Luckert PH. Promotional effects of testosterone and dietary fat on prostate carcinogenesis in genetically susceptible rats. *Prostate* 1985;**6**:1.

27 Peto R, Doll R, Buckley JD, *et al.* Can beta-carotene materially reduce human cancer rates? *Nature* 1981;**290**:201.

latent carcinoma of the prostate among Japanese in Japan and Hawaii. *JNCI* 1973;**50**:1137.

28 Hill PB, Wynder EL. Effect of a vegetarian diet and dexamethasone on plasma prolactin, testosterone and dehydroepiandrosterone in men and women. *Cancer Lett* 1979;7:273–282.

29 Gu FL, Xia TL, Kong XT. Preliminary study of the frequency of benign prostatic hyperplasia and prostatic cancer in China. *Urology* 1994;44:688–691.

30 Yoshizawa Y, Willett WC, Morris SJ, *et al.* Study of the prediagnostic selenium level in toenails and the risk of advanced prostate cancer. *JNCI* 1998;90:1184–1185.

31 Heinonen OP, Albanes D, Virtamo J, *et al.* Prostate cancer and supplementation with alpha-tocopherol and beta-carotene: incidence and mortality in a controlled trial. *JNCI* 1998;90:440–446.

32 Tretli S, Engeland A, Haldorsen T, *et al.* Prostate cancer – look to Denmark? *JNCI* 1996;88:128.

33 Schwartz GG, Hulka BS. Is vitamin D a risk factor for prostate cancer? [Hypothesis]. *Anticancer Res* 1990;10:1307–1312.

34 Feldman D, Skowronski RJ, Peehl DM. Vitamin D and prostate cancer. *Adv Exp Med Biol* 1996;375:53–63.

35 Steele R, Lees RE, Kraus AJ, *et al.* Sexual factors in the epidemiology of cancer of the prostate. *J Chron Dis* 1971;24:29–37.

36 Heshmat MY, Kovi J, Herson J. Epidemiologic association between gonorrhoea and prostatic carcinoma. *Urology* 1975;6:457.

37 Rotkin ID. Studies in the epidemiology of prostate cancer: expanded sampling. *Cancer Treatment Rep* 1977;61:173.

38 Ross RK, Deapen D, Casagrade J, *et al.* A cohort study of mortality from cancer of the prostate in Catholic priests. *British Journal of Cancer* 1981;43:223–235.

39 Editorial. Sex education in schools: peers to the rescue? *Lancet* 1994;344:899–900.

40 Rosenberg L, Palmer JR, Zauber AG, *et al.* Vasectomy and the risk of prostate cancer. *Am J Epidemiol* 1990;132: 1051–1055.

41 Giovannucci E, Tosteson D, Speizer FE, *et al.* A retrospective cohort study of vasectomy and prostate cancer in US men. *JAMA* 1993;269:878–914.

42 Giovannucci E, Ascherio A, Rimm EB, *et al.* A prospective cohort study of vasectomy and prostate cancer in US men. *JAMA* 1993;269:873–877.

43 Sidney S. Vasectomy and the risk of prostate cancer and benign prostatic hypertrophy. *J Urol* 1987;138:795–797.

44 Stanford JL, Wicklund KG, McKnight B, Daling JR, Brawer MK. Vasectomy and risk of prostate cancer.

JNCI 1999;8:881–886.

45 Howards SS, Peterson HB. Vasectomy and prostate cancer, chance bias, or a causal relationship? *JAMA* 1993;269: 913–914.

46 Kipling MD, Waterhouse JAH. Cadmium and prostatic carcinoma. *Lancet* 1967;1:730.

47 Rooney C, Beral V, Maconochie N, *et al.* Case-control study of prostate cancer in employees of the United Kingdom Atomic Energy Authority. *BMJ* 1993;307:1391–1397.

48 Wynder EL, Mabuchi K, Whitmore WF. Epidemiology of cancer of the prostate. *Cancer* 1971;28:344–360.

49 Herbert JT, Birkhoff JD, Feorino PM, *et al.* Herpes simplex virus type 2 and cancer of the prostate. *J Urol* 1976;116:1608–1611.

50 Centifano YM, Kaufman HE, Zam ZS *et al.* Herpes virus particles in prostate cancer cells. *J Virol* 1973;12:1608.

51 Feminella JJ, Lattimer JK. An apparent increase in genital carcinomas among wives of men with prostatic carcinoma: an epidemiologic survey. *Pirquet Bulletin of Clinical Medicine* 1974;20:3–9.

52 McCombs RM. Role of oncornaviruses in carcinoma of the prostate. *Cancer Treatment Rep* 1977;61:131.

53 Viola MV, Fromowitz F, Oravez S, *et al.* Expression of ras oncogene p21 in prostate cancer. *New Engl J Med* 1986;314:133–136.

54 Breslow N, Chan CE, Dhom G, *et al.* Latent carcinoma of the prostate at autopsy in seven areas. *Int J Cancer* 1977;20:680–688.

55 Armenian NK, Lilienfeld AM, Diamond EL, *et al.* Relation between benign prostatic hyperplasia and cancer of the prostate: a prospective and retrospective study. *Lancet* 1974;2:115–117.

56 Greenwald P, Kirmss V, Polan AK, *et al.* Cancer of the prostate among men with benign prostatic hyperplasia. *J Natl Cancer Inst* 1974;5:35–40.

57 Chodak GW, Thisted RA, Gerber GS, *et al.* Results of conservative management of clinically localised prostate cancer. *New Engl J Med* 1994;330:242–248.

58 Sakr WA, Haas GP, Cassin BF, *et al.* The frequency of carcinoma and intra-epithelial neoplasia of the prostate in young male patients. *J Urol* 1993;150:379–385.

59 Stamey TA. Cancer of the prostate: An analysis of some important contributions and dilemmas. *Monographs in Urology* 1982;3:67–74.

60 Carter HB, Piantadosi S, Isaacs JT. Clinical evidence for and implications of the multistep development of prostate cancer. *J Urol* 1990;143:742–746.

Chapter 4

The molecular basis of prostate cancer

The molecular basis of prostate cancer has been an enigma for decades. However, progress has been made in leaps and bounds recently. This is due to the exponential growth in our understanding of cell biology that has mainly stemmed from recombinant DNA technology. Perhaps because prostate cancer is a disease affecting men mainly beyond middle-age, it has received only a fraction of the research endeavour dedicated to other common forms of cancer such as that of the colon or lung. This situation is at last changing; more funds are being devoted to the study of a disease that is now perceived as an ever-increasing menace. Moreover, much of the new information gained about the basic science of other cancers (such as cancer of the colon and hormone-dependent breast cancer) is also applicable to malignant disease of the prostate.

HORMONAL INFLUENCES ON PROSTATE GROWTH

The normal prostate, although present structurally from around the 12th week of intrauterine life, remains rudimentary throughout childhood and develops only after puberty under the influence of increased levels of circulating androgens.

Testosterone (T) is the hormone that is mainly responsible, and is synthesized by the Leydig cells of the testis under the influence of luteinizing hormone (LH) of pituitary origin. The secretion of this decapeptide is itself regulated by luteinizing hormone-releasing hormone (LHRH) from the hypothalamus. It is at this location that testosterone has a negative feedback effect which enables levels of circulating testosterone to be maintained within the normal limits (10–35 μg/l). Diurnal variation in testosterone levels (within this range) is usual, with peak plasma concentrations being recorded in the early morning. Ninety five percent of circulating testosterone is bound to a number of plasma proteins, the predominant form of which is sex-hormone binding globulin (SHBG). This leaves only a small proportion of the residual free androgen to enter cells by simple diffusion. A further, much smaller source of androgens is the adrenal cortex. Under the influence of adrenocorticotropic hormone (ACTH), androstene and androstenedione are released into the circulation from the adrenal glands. When testicular function is intact, this minor additional androgen activity has little impact; after chemical or physical castration, however, their residual androgenic effect may result in the survival of some clones of androgen-dependent cancer cells, possibly to the detriment of the patient[1] (**4.1**).

Recent research has gone beyond the concept of prostate cancer as a 'testosterone-centric' disease as first described by Huggins. As it became clear that mortality and incidence rates continued to climb after orchidectomy or oestrogen ablation therapy, other hormonal pathways came under scrutiny. For example, the identification of follicle-stimulating hormone (FSH) and its receptor in prostate cancer cells, and the ability of FSH to stimulate proliferation of prostate cancer cells in-vitro has suggested an autocrine–paracrine regulatory mechanism of growth[2]. These and other interactions of FSH with the prostate are shown in detail in **4.2**.

Once within the prostate, both testosterone and the adrenal androgens are rapidly metabolized by 5 alpha-reductase (5 alpha-R; an enzyme which is located mainly on the nuclear membrane), to dihydrotestosterone (DHT). The 5 alpha-reduced hormone, DHT, is three to five times more potent as an androgen than testosterone itself. Its androgenic action is accomplished in the nucleus by a physical association with androgen receptors which are located mainly on the nuclear membrane. The binding of DHT to the androgen receptor liberates heat-shock protein (hsp90), and unmasks the DNA-binding domain of the receptor, allowing it to

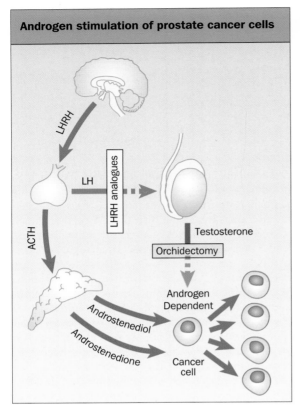

Androgen stimulation of prostate cancer cells

4.1 The pituitary–gonadal axis interrupted by castration. 5% of residual androgens are derived from the adrenals.

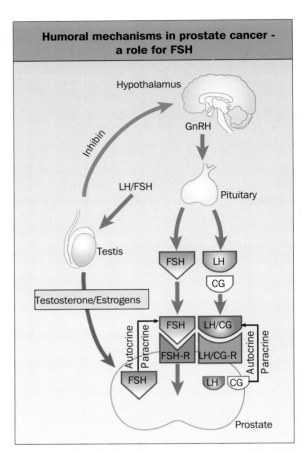

Humoral mechanisms in prostate cancer – a role for FSH

4.2 Humoral mechanisms in prostate cancer – a role for FSH. CG, chorionic gonadotropin, GnRH, gonadotropin-releasing hormone (Adapted from Porrer A, Ben-Josef E, Garde SV. *Humoral mechanisms in prostate cancer – a role for FSH*. The Institute for Medical Studies; 2000.)

dimerize and bind to the specific regulatory sequences, the so-called 'hormone response element' (HRE) of the target genes on the genome. This binding occurs upstream of the transcription start sites of the various androgen-sensitive genes, and thereby stimulates DNA transcription. The messenger RNA molecules (mRNA) thus produced encode a number of proteins, including several important growth factors, such as epidermal growth factor (EGF) and platelet-derived growth factor (PdGF) which modulate and promote prostatic cell growth (**4.3**).

Normal prostate development and maintenance is dependent upon a delicate homeostasis between cell death and cell replacement. Androgens are necessary for this homeostasis, since either medical or surgical castration results in rapid onset of epithelial 'apoptosis' or 'programmed cell death', as well as stromal depletion. The DNA content of androgen-deprived prostatic cells is reduced to 10% within 10 days[3]. Stem cells survive, however, as subsequent replacement of circulating androgens

appears capable of restoring both prostatic architecture and function to normal by rapidly switching on the processes concerned with cell proliferation[4].

MOLECULAR CONTROL OF THE CELL CYCLE

Normal prostatic growth and development depends upon a particular pattern of cell division, with some cell types dividing much more often than others, and all divisions occurring in a timely and appropriate fashion.

Prostate epithelial cells divide regularly to maintain the structural integrity of the glandular and ductal epithelial surfaces. The most active epithelial division occurs at the distal tips of the prostate glands; those in the intermediate portion are main-

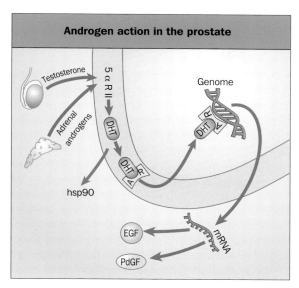

4.3 Androgen activation of androgen-response elements on the genome stimulates transcription and the production of growth factors.

tained in a differentiated state undergoing active secretion, and those in the proximal ducts nearest to the urethra undergo programmed cell death (**4.4**).

This active process of apoptosis which counter-

balances new cell formation is also seen after androgen deprivation; it is currently the subject of much research. Two genes that appear to be pivotal in apoptosis are the *bax* and *bcl*-2 genes. The principal morphological feature of apoptosis is the condensation of chromatin caused by production of 180–200 base pair DNA fragments, resulting from the activation of endonucleases[5]. Phosphatase inhibitors appear to synergize with tumour necrosis factor (TNF) to activate DNA fragmentation[6] in this in-built 'cell suicide' system. It is this system that comes into play when androgen support to the prostate is withdrawn.

CELL DIVISION

The cell-division cycle is traditionally divided into four phases: G1, S, G2 and M (**4.5**). Most differentiated prostatic cells are in G1, which stands for 'gap 1' – when no activity is visible. The S phase denotes the 'synthesis' of DNA, with the cell's chromosomal DNA replicating itself during this phase; this replication process is extremely accurate in that the sequence of the new strands is exactly complementary to the template, and in that every portion of the chromosomal DNA is copied exactly once – no more and no less. The expression of certain genes whose products are needed for DNA replication, such as the histone proteins, is limited exclusively to S phase.

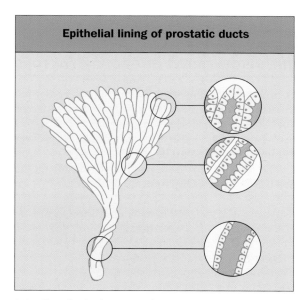

4.4 The arborized prostatic duct system. Cells are produced in the apices of the glands, and migrate down the ductal system undergoing programmed cell death (apoptosis) in the proximal ducts nearest the urethra.

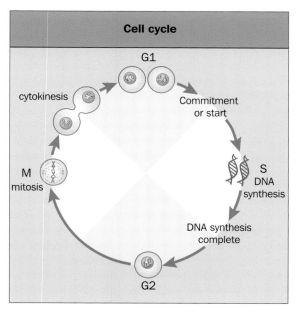

4.5 The cell cycle illustrated diagramatically.

G2 stands for 'gap 2', the second break in visible intracellular activity. At the boundary of S and G2, the replication machinery somehow signals that DNA synthesis is complete; the nature of this signal is unknown, but the cell then enters G2 and prepares itself for mitosis.

The M phase is 'mitosis' – chromosomes condense and become visible as discrete bodies. The two microtubule organizers (or spindle-pole bodies), move apart to opposite sides of the nucleus, and arrays of microtubules grow from the two spindle-pole bodies to form the mitotic spindle. Some of these microtubules become attached to so-called 'kinetochores' on the chromosomes, with the attached chromosomes becoming aligned on the 'metaphase plate' (the plane that lies halfway between the spindle-pole bodies). When all of the kinetochores are attached to microtubules and aligned on the metaphase plate, a biochemical signal is sent, and anaphase begins. The chromosomes start moving towards the poles, and the poles move apart from each other. Finally, the cell pinches in two (cytokinesis), producing two G1-phase daughter cells (**4.6**).

Normal Controls on Cell Division

Controls on the growth of cells within the prostate fall into two categories. First, there are those controls whose regulatory mechanisms influence cell metabolism and enlargement; the normal prostate smooth-muscle cell should neither enlarge nor divide, and should make only enough protein to replace what is lost. The second form of controls influence cell division itself. Epithelial cells within the prostate have a fairly high turnover, but are normally under strict regulation that coordinates both enlargement and cell division.

The nature of both of these controls is currently being elucidated. Molecular biologists have identified and cloned several genes, known collectively as the *Cdc2* family, whose normal function is necessary for cell division to proceed. *Cdc2* genes appear to encode proteins which are members of the protein kinase family. (A protein kinase is an enzyme that can transfer a phosphate group from adenosine triphosphate (ATP) onto another protein; phosphorylation either increases or decreases the activity of the protein in question, and is a widely used method of regulating protein activity in biological systems[7].)

Another protein that is also intimately involved in the control of the cell cycle has been named 'cyclin'[8]; the gene encoding it has also been cloned[9]. This polypeptide appears to form a stable complex with Cdc2 protein, with the binding of cyclin appearing to activate the protein such that Cdc2 has protein-kinase activity only when cyclin is present. Removal of cyclin from the Cdc2 molecule by intracellular proteases inactivates Cdc2 and may be the key event in completing mitosis (**4.7**).

THE INVOLVEMENT OF GROWTH FACTORS

A number of polypeptides, including epidermal growth factor (EGF), basic fibroblast growth factor (bFGF) and platelet-derived growth factor (PdGF) – see **Table 4.1**, have been identified as potent stimulators of prostate growth.

The receptors for these polypeptides reside on the

Chromosomal activity during cell division

Daughter cells · Interphase · Prophase · Prometaphase · Cytokinesis · Metaphase · Telephase · Anaphase

4.6 Chromosomal behaviour during mitosis.

Table 4.1 Growth factors identified in the prostate
Epidermal growth factor (EGF)
Insulin-like growth factors I and II (IGF I, II)
Keratinocyte growth factor (KGF)
Transforming growth factor alpha (TGF α)
Transforming growth factor beta (TGF β)
Basic fibroblast growth factor (bFGF)

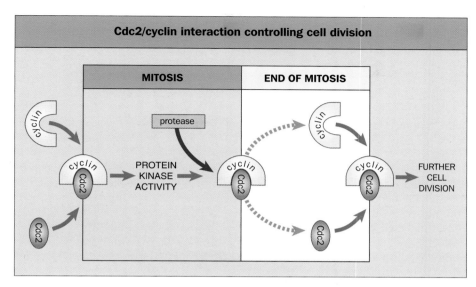

4.7 The control of cell division by Cdc2 and cyclin interaction. The combination of these two proteins results in protein kinase activity.

surfaces of both epithelial and stromal cells, and all seem to possess a large extracellular ligand-binding domain, a single membrane-spanning helix, and a sizable cytoplasmic domain. The cytoplasmic domain is usually an enzyme in the form of a ligand-stimulated protein kinase; these important enzymes are capable of transferring phosphate to tyrosine residues of other proteins. EGF receptors are linked to protein-kinase enzymes and appear to work in pairs or so-called 'dimers', which are produced by EGF binding that induces the receptors to pair off ('dimerize') and to phosphorylate each other. This, in turn, appears to result in the recruitment of several cellular enzymes to the cytoplasmic domain of the receptor. These recruits include enzymes that are involved in the production of phospholipid second messengers, and perhaps of other protein kinases, thus amplifying and distributing the signal within the cell. By these means, the genes controlling growth (such as the *Cdc2* and cyclin families) are turned on, various key proteins are synthesized, and prostatic cell division occurs (**4.8**).

PUTATIVE EVENTS LEADING TO PROSTATE CANCER

Invasive prostate cancer develops when a mutation (or a series of mutations) occurs within a single cell, and gives it a growth advantage over its neighbours. As the number of descendants of the original mutant increases, so does the likelihood that one

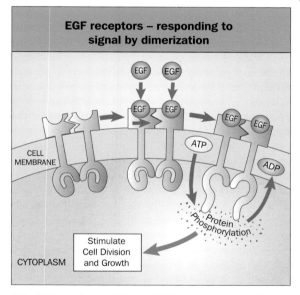

4.8 Epidermal growth factor (EGF) receptors respond to EGF signal by dimerization and autophosphorylation. This process results in the production of phospholipid second messengers which amplify the signal within the cell.

of these will sustain a further mutation that in turn allows its descendants to grow even faster. This deadly cycle of dedifferentiation continues as cells accumulate additional mutations that allow them to accelerate their growth further and to start invading surrounding tissues. Further mutations then permit metastasis – the dangerous propensity of certain prostate cancers to escape and seed new tumours elsewhere in the body, especially in bone.

Although the individual events on the road to prostate cancer are rare, men in developed countries now have an increasingly long lifespan and chance dictates that from time to time this lethal stepwise combination of events will unfold. Overall it is predicted that about 9% of all men will develop prostate cancer in their lifetime.

ACTIVATION OF ONCOGENES

The discovery that DNA tumour viruses are capable of transforming cells by inserting their own genes (which are capable of inducing cell growth and division) into the host genome, and the knowledge that this genetic material is stably transferred to daughter cells, led to the search for so-called 'viral oncogenes'. It subsequently became apparent that inactive forms of similar genes – proto-oncogenes – were in fact present in almost all mammalian cells. These proto-oncogenes encode the proteins involved with various forms of intercellular and intracellular signal transduction, including those of growth factors. But how do these proto-oncogenes become activated to produce virulent oncogenes? The answer to this question came from the study of the *c-ras* gene in bladder cancer, rather than prostate cancer. Comparison of the normal, cloned *c-ras* gene and the activated oncogene revealed only the subtlest of differences: a guanidine nucleotide had been substituted by a thymidine in the oncogene. This mutation changed the twelfth codon of the *ras* gene from a codon encoding glycine to one encoding another amino acid, valine (**4.9**). It soon became clear that it was this single base-pair change that was the driving force that induced these cells to form bladder tumours.

The Mechanisms of Action of Oncogenes

Oncogenes have diverse mechanisms of action. The *ras* gene for example is part of a larger family of genes encoding guanidine nucleotide-binding proteins, the so-called 'G proteins'. The G proteins are molecular switches that regulate a number of signal transduction pathways, including incidentally the alpha-1 adrenoceptor smooth-muscle response within the prostate. They are in their active conformation when bound to a molecule of high-energy guanosine trinucleotide (GTP), and possess an

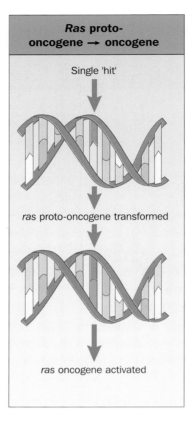

4.9 A single base-pair alteration in the *ras* oncogene bestows carcinogenic properties.

Ras proto-oncogene → oncogene

Single 'hit'

ras proto-oncogene transformed

ras oncogene activated

intrinsic enzyme activity that hydrolyses bound GTP to its lower-energy form, guanosine dinucleotide (GDP), returning the G proteins to their ground state. The mutation in the activated *ras* oncogene (**4.9**) destroys this GTP hydrolysis activity, thereby locking the protein in its active conformation (**4.10**).

Other proto-oncogenes act as growth factors. For example, the *sis* oncogene encodes a form of PdGF, the potent mitogen for mesenchymal cells to which prostate cells respond. In tissue culture, cells infected with a *sis*-carrying virus become transformed via autocrine stimulation. That is, they secrete a growth factor to which they can also respond. Thus, the cells bathe themselves continually in a factor that makes them grow and divide. Other oncogenes encode altered receptors that trigger growth signals even in the absence of ligand. The viral *c-erb*B gene, for example, encodes a truncated form of EGF receptor that is reduced at each end. In particular, its entire extracellular binding domain has been lopped off. This decapitated receptor acts as if it is constantly responding to

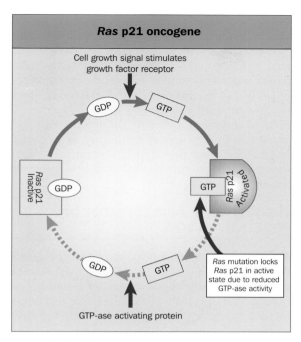

4.10 The 'locked on' *ras* p21 oncogene continually stimulates cell proliferation.

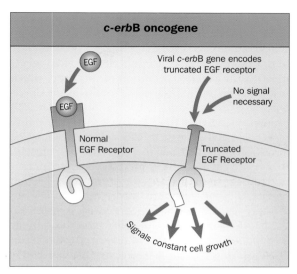

4.11 The c-*erb*B oncogene, when mutated, has a truncated cell-surface receptor. This abnormal receptor continually stimulates cell growth without the requirement of an EGF signal being present.

ligand EGF, and therefore sends constant growth promoting signals to the interior of the cell in spite of an absence of signal (**4.11**). A subset of human prostate cancers has been shown to express the c-*erb*B oncogene in immunohistochemical assays[10].

The largest class of oncogenes is still the least well understood. These encode proteins that occupy a strategic location just inside the plasma membrane. As mentioned before, protein-tyrosine kinases are intimately involved in the control mechanisms of cell division. The very large number of oncogenic protein-tyrosine kinases confirms that tyrosine phosphorylation is a critical event in growth control. Their individual functions are being elucidated and specific inhibitors of them have important therapeutic possibilities.

The proto-oncogenes *c-myc*, *c-fos* and *c-jun* all encode proteins concerned with the regulation of gene transcription[11]. They represent some of the earliest genes to be expressed in the prostate of castrated rats after administration of androgens[12]. These proto-oncogenes transduce the extranuclear mitogenic signals into the expression of genes that then encode the transcription factors – the fos, jun, and myc proteins, which regulate the secondary

genes concerned with growth. The fos and jun proteins bind to activating protein (AP-1), which is intimately involved in the regulatory processes controlling cell growth and differentiation. Epidermal growth factor (EGF) and fibroblast growth factor (FGF) both induce *c-fos* and *c-jun* genes, which have stimulatory effects unless the inhibitory influence of factors such as TGF-beta prevails. In this finely tuned and complex regulatory process, the fos and jun proteins autoregulate the expression of their own genes.

Many oncogenes have been identified and cloned, and some have been implicated in prostatic cancer[13,14]. In virtually every case, oncogene proteins lie on the strategic signalling pathways by which cells receive and execute cell growth and division instructions. The mutations that activate these genes are either structural mutations that lead to the stimulatory activity of a protein without an incoming signal, or regulatory mutations that lead to the production of the protein at the wrong place or time. Damage to oncogenes thus gives the cell a persistent internal growth signal – the so-called 'autocrine signal' – in the absence of any external stimuli.

Tumour-Suppressor Genes (Anti-Oncogenes)

As oncogene research has progressed, it has become apparent that there exist naturally genes that have the ability to overpower oncogenes and thereby keep them in check. These have been termed anti-onco-genes, or 'tumour-suppressor genes'; probably the best example is the retinoblastoma (*RB*) gene. Inherited or acquired mutation of this gene, which is located on chromosome 13, results in the development of retinal tumours in childhood. The *RB* protein, encoded by the *RB* gene, has the capability of keeping cell growth in check; certain oncogene viruses act by negating the effect of this protein, thus removing the 'brakes' on cell growth. A mutant protein, expressed as a result of an exon deletion of the *RB* gene, has been reported in the DU145 prostatic cancer cell line[15]. Moreover, transfection of the cloned, normal *RB* gene into the tumour cells in nude mice suppressed tumorigenicity. There is evidence that the *RB* protein may regulate *c-myc* expression, such that levels of myc protein are controlled. Loss of the *RB* gene and its suppressor protein would consequently lead to *myc* activation and enhanced cell proliferation. Allelic deletions on chromosome 13, the location of the *RB* gene, have been reported in some patients with prostate cancer[16,17].

Another important example of a tumour-suppressor gene is the *p53* gene, the absence of which leads to a dramatically increased incidence of various forms of cancer[18] (**4.12**). The relatively small size of the *p53* gene when compared to the *RB* gene means that it is a gene with which molecular biologists can work more easily. Various reports have described *p53* alterations in prostate-cancer tissue, with most studies suggesting an incidence in 6–20% of specimens tested[19,20]. However, there are several reports describing alterations in up to 80% of specimens analysed[21]. It appears that *p53* mutations tend to appear more often in late-stage hormone-resistant tumours. This event may therefore be involved in the final stages of prostatic oncogenesis.

THE STEP-WISE DEVELOPMENT OF PROSTATE CANCER

The epidemiology of many human tumours suggests that cancer is a multistep process in which the genome is sequentially subjected to a number of random 'hits'. Statistical calculations based upon the increasing frequency of cancer with age have estimated the number of these steps or 'hits' to be between four and six. As already discussed, about 9% of prostate cancers appear to be the result of an inherited tendency[22]. Inheritance of this disease leads to a greater than two-fold increase in the risk of developing prostate cancer, and those tumours that do develop do so at an unusually young age.

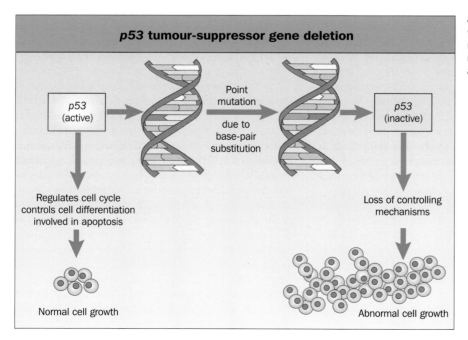

4.12 Mutation of the *p53* tumour-suppressor gene results in loss of controlling mechanisms and promotes abnormal cell growth.

p53 tumour-suppressor gene deletion

p53 (active)

Point mutation due to base-pair substitution

p53 (inactive)

Regulates cell cycle controls cell differentiation involved in apoptosis

Loss of controlling mechanisms

Normal cell growth

Abnormal cell growth

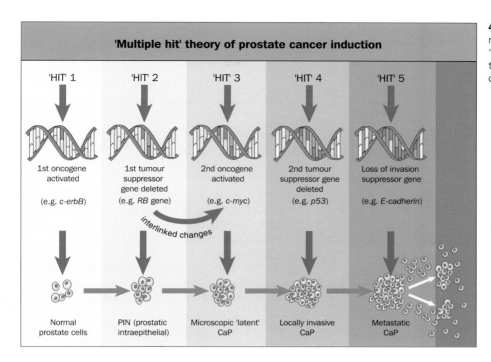

'Multiple hit' theory of prostate cancer induction

'HIT' 1	'HIT' 2	'HIT' 3	'HIT' 4	'HIT' 5
1st oncogene activated	1st tumour suppressor gene deleted	2nd oncogene activated	2nd tumour suppressor gene deleted	Loss of invasion suppressor gene
(e.g. c-erbB)	(e.g. RB gene)	(e.g. c-myc)	(e.g. p53)	(e.g. E-cadherin)

interlinked changes

Normal prostate cells	PIN (prostatic intraepithelial)	Microscopic 'latent' CaP	Locally invasive CaP	Metastatic CaP

4.13 A schematic representation of the 'multiple hit' theory of the induction of prostate cancer.

Chromosomal mapping of affected families is currently underway, and cytogenetic studies have shown chromosomal abnormalities in association with prostate cancer at 7q, 8p, 10q, 16q, and 18q loci. The 24–25 segment of chromosome 1q has also been implicated[23] as has the x chromosome[24].

The oncogene *her-2* has also been found to be associated with prostate cancer[9]. Elevated *c-myc* mRNA levels have also been demonstrated in prostate cancer, with suggestions that higher concentrations relate to higher-grade cancer. A proposed order of events in the development of prostate cancer is illustrated in **4.13**. These are certainly not the sole or specific events involved, and the order of their occurrence is probably not critical. It is the accumulation of events resulting in what has been described as 'a complementary misbehaviour of genes', rather than their order, that counts in terms of prostatic tumour development[25].

MOLECULAR FACTORS INFLUENCING THE DEVELOPMENT OF METASTASES

For a prostate cancer cell to metastasize (usually to bone or, less commonly, soft tissue), it has to acquire the ability to migrate from its original site and to grow and divide in a new environment. The molecular events involved in producing this often lethal tendency are currently under intense scutiny[26]. One factor may be the loss of cell-adhesion molecules such as E-cadherin, which normally binds cells together. The gene for E-cadherin, which has been termed an 'invasion suppressor gene', is located on chromosome 16q. In human cancer specimens, a correlation was found between E-cadherin expession and the Gleason grade of the tumour[27]. A correlation of E-cadherin expression and survival of patients with prostate cancer is also apparent.

Other features relating to the metastatic potential of a given prostatic tumour include the ability of cells to invade tissues by local secretion of collagenase enzymes. In addition, as mentioned in Chapter 2, prostate cancer metastases require a local blood supply to sustain themselves[28,29] (**4.14**). The release of peptides that stimulate the growth of new blood vessels (angiogenesis factors) may be important in this respect, and these themselves possibly act in synergy with local growth factors such as bFGF[30,31]. Recent studies also suggest the presence of an antimetastatic nm23 protein, encoded by the *nm23* gene, located on chromosome 17[32,33]. Loss of this restraining influence may be one of several further factors in determining the presence of the lethal tendency of a given tumour to spread.

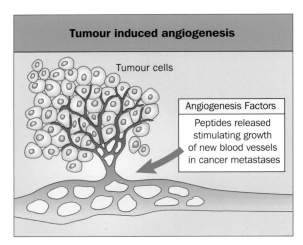

Tumour induced angiogenesis

Tumour cells

Angiogenesis Factors

Peptides released stimulating growth of new blood vessels in cancer metastases

4.14 The ability of tumour cells to metastasize is dependent upon their capacity to induce their own blood supply; this process is known as angiogenesis, and may develop in response to secreted angiogenesis factors[27,28].

FACTORS INFLUENCING THE DEVELOPMENT OF ANDROGEN INDEPENDENCE

Androgen-dependent cells undergo apoptosis and die in the absence of hormone, whereas androgen-sensitive cells can survive in the absence of androgen stimulus, but grow more quickly in its presence. In addition, some cells may be indirectly dependent upon androgens, requiring paracrine growth-promoting factors from neighbouring androgen-sensitive cells. It is presumed that the automatous growth of androgen-independent cells occurs by clonal selection and results in cancer progression. But it is not inconceivable that androgen-sensitive cells adapt to lower levels of androgen by means of the constitutive expression of growth-related oncogenes, a factor we shall consider later in relation to the use of maximum androgen blockade versus monotherapy (see Chapter 13). Genetic instability of a developing tumour could easily lead to the formation of cell variants with different degrees of sensitivity to androgen, including the production of androgen receptor mutants akin to the situation with oestrogen receptors in breast cancer[34]. Androgen receptor mutants are well recognized as a cause

of congenital androgen-insensitivity syndrome, and a mutant receptor has been identified in one variant of the so-called LNCaP prostate-cancer cell line[35]. In this case, the so-called changes in ligand specificity were such that growth responses could be elicited by the administration of antiandrogens.

TO WHAT EXTENT DOES MOLECULAR BIOLOGICAL KNOWLEDGE TRANSLATE INTO IMPROVED PATIENT CARE?

Although the recent exponential increase in our understanding of the molecular biology of cancer has yet to translate into improved patient care, the seeds of change have germinated and are now growing fast. As our knowledge improves, the possibility of preventing prostate cancer by the use of chemopreventive agents such as retinoids or 5 alpha-reductase inhibitors that block some of the molecular events on the road to cancer seems feasible. Early detection, already possible by means of prostate-specific antigen (PSA) assay, may certainly be enhanced by the development of newer, more cancer-specific, tumour markers. In addition, chromosomal mapping is likely to identify more precisely the genes responsible for familial prostate cancer, and to provide a means of confirming a need for increased cancer surveillance in defined individuals. Improved staging, utilizing polymerase chain technology (PCR) to amplify tiny amounts of metastatic tumour DNA or mRNA, may help to identify those patients whose disease is already beyond hope of purely local therapies. 'Gene therapy' for prostate cancer is still some way off, but the possibilities of replacing tumour-suppressor genes, neutralizing oncogenes, employing antisense oligonucleotides[36], and specifically enhancing the immune responses to a given prostate cancer now appear attainable (see Chapter 14). The limitations of androgen-deprivation therapy may be circumvented by the development of more specific growth factor, tyrosine kinase or angiogenesis inhibitors[37], and other new strategies which utilize apoptosis as a target for therapy[38]. Many of these latest developments and future possibilities in these exciting areas are discussed in subsequent chapters.

REFERENCES

1 Crawford ED, Eisenberger MA, McLeod DG, *et al.* A controlled trial of leuprolide with and without flutamide in prostatic cancer. *N Engl J Med* 1989;**321**:419–424.

2 Ben-Josef E, Yang SY, Ji TH *et al.* Hormone refractory prostate cancer cells express functional follicle-stimulating hormone receptor (FSHR). *J Urol* 1999;**161**:970–976.

3 Bruchovsky N, Lesser B, Van Doorn E, *et al.* Hormonal effects on cell proliferation in rat prostate. *Vitam Horm* 1975;**33**:61–102.

4 Isaacs JT. Antagonistic effect of androgen on prostatic cell death. *Prostate* 1984;**5**:545–557.

5 Oberhammer F, Wilson JW, Dive C, *et al.* Apoptotic death in epithelial cells: cleavage of DNA to 300 and/or 50 kb fragments prior to or in the absence of internucleosomal fragmentation. *The EMBO Journal* 1993;**12(9)**:3679–3684.

6 Wright SC, Zheng H, Zhong J, *et al.* Role of protein phosphorylation in TNF-induced apoptosis: phosphatase inhibitors synergize with TNF to activate DNA fragmentation in normal as well as TNF-resistant U937 variants. *J Cell Biochem* 1993;**53**:222–223.

7 Nurse P. Universal control mechanism controlling onset of M phase. *Nature* 1990;**344**:503–508.

8 Evans TE, Rosenthal J, Youngblom D, *et al.* Cyclin: a protein specified by maternal mRNA in sea urchin eggs that is destroyed at each cleavage division. *Cell* 1993;**33**:389–396.

9 Motokura T, Bloom T, Kim HG, *et al.* A novel cyclin encoded by a bcl1-linked candidate oncogene. *Nature* 1991;**350**:512–515.

10 Zhau HE, Wan DS, Zhou J, *et al.* Expression of c-erbB-2/neu proto-oncogene in human prostatic cancer tissues and cell lines. *Mol Carc* 1992;**5**:320–327.

11 Evan GL, Littlewood TD. The role of c-myc in cell growth [Review]. *Current Opinion in Genetics & Development* 1993;**3(1)**:44–49.

12 Katz AE, Benson MC, Wise GJ, *et al.* Gene activity during the early phase of androgen-stimulated rat prostate regrowth. *Canc Res* 1989;**49(21)**:5889–5894.

13 Schalken JA, Bussemakers MJG, Debruyne FMJ. Oncogene expression in prostate cancer. *Oncogenes* 1990;**7**:97–105.

14 Klotz LH, Auger M, Andrulis I, *et al.* Molecular analysis of neu, sis, c-myc, fos, and *p53* oncogenes in benign prostatic hypertrophy and prostatic carcinoma. *J Urol* 1990;**143**:401A.

15 Bookstein R, Rio P, Madreperla SA, *et al.* Promoter deletion and loss of retinoblastoma gene expression in human prostate carcinoma. *Proc Natl Acad Sci* 1990;**87**:7762–7766.

16 Brooks JD, Bova GS, Marshall FF, *et al.* Allelic losses of retinoblastoma gene in primary renal and prostate cancers. *J Urol* 1993;**149**:376A(652).

17 Sarkar FH, Sakr W, Li YW, *et al.* Analysis of retinoblastoma (*RB*) gene deletion in human prostatic carcinoma. *Prostate* 1992;**21**:145–152.

18 Hollstein M, Sidransky D, Vogelstein B, *et al.* p53 mutations in human cancers. *Science* 1991;**253**:49–53.

19 Van Veldhuizen PJ, Sadasivan R, Garcia F, *et al.* Mutant *p53* expression in prostate carcinoma. *Prostate* 1993;**22**:23–30.

20 Bookstein R, MacGrogan D, Sharkey F, *et al.* p53 mutations in human prostate cancer. *Proc Am Assoc Cancer Res* 1993;**34**:537–543.

21 de Vere White RW, Gumerlock PH, Chi SG, *et al.* p53 tumour suppression gene abnormalities are frequent in human prostate tissues. *J Urol* 1993;**149**:376A–(654).

22 Isaacs WB, Carter BS. Genetic changes associated with prostate cancer in humans. *Cancer Surveys* 1991;**11**:15–23.

23 Smith JR, Freije D, *et al.* Major susceptibility locus for prostate cancer on chromosome 1 suggested by a genome wide search. *Science* 1996;**274**:1371–1374.

24 Xu J, Meyers D, Freije D, *et al.* Evidence for a prostate cancer susceptibility locus on the X chromosome. *Nature Genet* 1998;**20**:175–178.

25 Weinberg RA. Oncogenes, antioncogenes, and the molecular basis of multistep carcinogenesis. *Canc Res* 1989;**49**:3713–3732.

26 Steeg PS, Bevaliaqua G, Kopper L, *et al.* Evidence for a novel gene associated with low tumor metastatic potential. *J Natl Cancer Inst* 1988;**80(3)**:200–204.

27 Umbas R, Schalken JA, Aalders TW, *et al.* Expression of cellular adhesion molecule E-cadherin is reduced or absent in high-grade prostate cancer. *Canc Res* 1992;**52**:5104–5109.

28 Myers C, Trepel J, Sartor O, *et al.* Predictors of pathologic stage in prostatic carcinoma. The role of neovascularity. *Cancer* 1993;**71(3)**:1172–1178.

29 Folkman J, Watson K, Ingber D, *et al.* Induction of angiogenesis during the transition from hyperplasia to neoplasia. *Nature* 1989;**339**:58–61.

30 Wakui S, Furusato M, Itoh T, *et al.* Tumour angiogenesis in prostatic carcinoma with and without bone marrow metastasis: a morphometric study. *J Pathol* 1992;**168**:257–262.

31 Weidner N, Carroll PR, Flax J, *et al.* Tumour angiogenesis correlates with metastasis in invasive prostate carcinoma. *Am J Pathol* 1993;**143**:401–409.

32 Leone A, Flatow U, Vanlloutte K, *et al.* Transfection of human nm23-H1 into the human MDA-MB-435 breast carcinoma cell line: effects on tumor metastatic potential, colonization and enzymatic activity. *Oncogene* 1993;**8(9)**:2325–2333.

33 Stahl JA, Leone A, Rosengard AM, *et al.* Identification of a second human nm23 gene, nm23-H2. *Canc Res* 1991;**51(1)**:445–449.

34 King RJ. Progression from steroid sensitive to insensitive state in breast tumours. *Cancer Surveys* 1992;**14**:131–146.

35 French FS, Lubahn DB, Brown TR, *et al.* Molecular basis of androgen insensitivity [Review]. *Recent Progress in Hormone Research* 1990;**46**:1–38; discussion 38–42.

36 Gleave ME, Miayake H, Foldie J, *et al.* Targeting bcl-2 gene to delay androgen-independent progression and enhance chemosensitivity in prostate cancer using antisense oligodeoxynucleolides. *Urology* 1999;**54**:36–46.

37 Yamoaka M, Yamamoto T, Ikeyama S, *et al.* Angiogenesis inhibitor TNP-470 (AGM-1470) potentially inhibits the tumour growth of hormone-independent human breast and prostate carcinoma cell lines. *Canc Res* 1993;**53**:5233–5236.

38 Costa-Pereira AP, Cotter TG. Molecular and cellular biology of prostate cancer – the role of apoptosis as a target for therapy. *Prost Can Pros Dis* 1999;**2**:126–139.

Chapter 5

Clinical diagnosis

INTRODUCTION

The pattern of presentation of prostate cancer changed little until a decade ago; since then there has been a pronounced 'downward' stage migration towards earlier stage disease. This change has been driven by increasing knowledge of the condition, awareness of the dangers of neglecting symptoms, and increasing attempts to detect the condition early, especially using the serum marker, prostate-specific antigen (PSA). In the first three quarters of this century, a large proportion of men with clinically significant prostate cancer presented with the symptom complex of weight loss, bone pain, lethargy (due to anaemia and uraemia) and bladder outflow symptoms, all attributable to either locally advanced or metastatic prostate cancer. Prostate cancer still does present in this way in many men beyond middle-age, but now it is increasingly being detected at an earlier asymptomatic stage (**5.1**). This earlier presentation not infrequently confronts both the urologist and primary-care physician with a dilemma concerning treatment, since it is not always clear (especially in the elderly) whether the tumour will progress within the natural lifespan of the individual in which it is found. Nor is it apparent which of the competing treatment options yields the best long-term outcome.

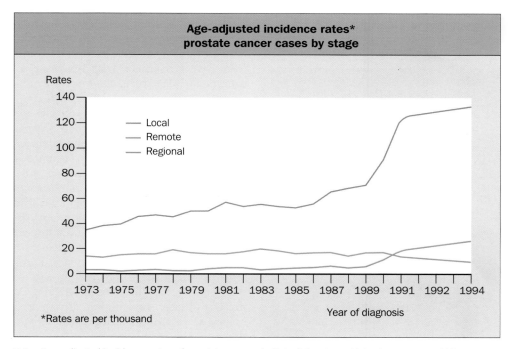

5.1 Age-adjusted incidence rates of prostate cancer in Detroit by stage. Note the recent rapid increase in localized cancers from 1990, probably resulting from the increased use of PSA testing. (SEER data.)

PRESENTING SYMPTOMS

Men with prostate cancer can present with a variety of different symptoms, and most often nowadays with no symptoms at all. Screening for prostate cancer in the asymptomatic male is such a complex and controversial issue that an entire chapter of this book is devoted to this subject (see Chapter 6). However, few would deny that an inquisitive, asymptomatic patient over the age of 45, with concerns about prostate cancer, should receive some basic investigations, if only to reassure him that there is little chance that he does in fact have prostate cancer. The investigation of asymptomatic men with a family history of prostate cancer in one or more first degree relatives seems likely eventually to become standard practice.

The presenting symptoms of men with prostate cancer can be broadly divided into:

- Bladder outflow obstruction symptoms.
- Symptoms attributable to local extension of the tumour (e.g. haematuria, ureteric obstruction causing loin pain, etc.).
- Symptoms from metastases (e.g. bone pain and weight loss).

The most frequently encountered presenting symptoms are outlined in **Tables 5.1** and **5.3**.

Table 5.1 Presenting symptoms of localized prostate cancer	
Local	Poor stream
	Hesitancy
	Sensation of incomplete emptying
	Frequency
	Urgency
	Urge incontinence
Locally invasive	Haematuria
	Dysuria
	Pain
	Impotence
	Incontinence
	Loin pain (ureteric obstruction)
	Symptoms of renal failure
	Rectal symptoms including bleeding
	Haemospermia

Symptoms of Bladder Outflow Obstruction

Because the condition is so prevalent most men with prostate cancer have concomitant histological, benign prostatic hyperplasia (BPH). Although in some cases outflow-obstruction symptoms may be attributable to the cancer (especially if it is locally advanced), in many cases the BPH, which arises within the transition zone close to the prostatic urethra, is much more likely to cause lower urinary tract symptoms. Since prostate cancer most often arises in the peripheral zone, it is less likely to cause obstructive symptoms until it is of considerable volume, and by which time will also be extra-capsular. It is interesting to note that in spite of exhaustive pre-operative investigation, approximately 10% of men undergoing transurethral resection (TURP) for supposed BPH are found to have foci of prostate cancer within the resected chips. It is unlikely that such small volume 'sub-clinical' prostate cancers contribute significantly to outflow obstruction.

Bladder outflow obstruction symptoms have been extensively investigated in BPH, and symptom scores devised by the American Urologic Association[1] endorsed by the World Health Organization; these are shown in **Table 5.2**. Although primarily designed to evaluate patients with BPH and their response to various treatments, the International Prostate Symptom Score (IPSS) (**Table 5.2**) can also be used to measure the severity of obstructive and irritative lower urinary tract symptoms in prostate cancer, and also to gauge response to local and systemic treatments.

The symptoms of bladder outflow obstruction are usefully divided into two groups: obstructive and irritative. Obstructive symptoms, namely reduced uroflow, hesitancy and incomplete emptying, result from occlusion of the prostatic urethra by tumour. Urinary retention – the ultimate obstructive symptom – is a common occurrence in locally advanced prostate cancer; it necessitates urgent decompression by either urethral or suprapubic catheterization. Irritative symptoms such as urinary frequency and urgency result from secondary detrusor instability as a response to obstruction and are usually due to BPH; they may, however, also occur with prostate cancer. In addition, irritative symptoms may occur in prostate cancer because of invasion of the trigone of the bladder and pelvic nerves.

Bladder outflow obstruction may lead to secondary problems such as recurrent urinary tract infec-

Table 5.2   International Prostate Symptom Score (IPSS)

Patient Name:	Date:	Not at all	Less than 1 time in 5	Less than half the time	About half the time	More than half the time	Almost always
1. Incomplete emptying Over the past month, how often have you had a sensation of not not emptying your bladder completely after you finish urinating?		0	1	2	3	4	5
2. Frequency Over the past month, how often have you had to urinate again less than two hours after you finished urinating?		0	1	2	3	4	5
3. Intermittency Over the past month, how often have you found you stopped and started again several times when you urinated?		0	1	2	3	4	5
4. Urgency Over the past month, how often have you found it difficult to postpone urination?		0	1	2	3	4	5
5. Weak stream Over the past month, how often have you had a weak urinary stream?		0	1	2	3	4	5
6. Straining Over the past month, how often have you had to push or strain to begin urination?		0	1	2	3	4	5

	None	1 time	2 times	3 times	4 times	5 times or more
7. Nocturia Over the past month, how many times did you most typically get up to urinate from the time you went to bed at night until the time you got up in the morning?	0	1	2	3	4	5

	Delighted	Pleased	Mostly satisfied	Mixed – about equally satisfied and dissatisfied	Mostly dissatisfied	Unhappy	Terrible
Quality of life due to urinary symptoms If you were to spend the rest of your life with your urinary condition just the way it is now, how would you feel about that?	0	1	2	3	4	5	6

The International Prostate Symptom Score (IPSS) is based on the answers to seven questions concerning urinary symptoms. Each question is assigned points from 0 to 5 indicating increasing severity of the particular symptom. The total score can range from 0 to 35 (asymptomatic to very symptomatic). Although there are presently no standard recommendations for grading patients with mild, moderate or severe symptoms, patients can be tentatively classified as follows: **0–7 = mildly symptomatic; 8–19 = moderately symptomatic; 20–35 = severely symptomatic**. The International Consensus Committee (ICC) recommends the use of only a single question to assess a patient's quality of life. The answers to this question range from 'delighted' to 'terrible', or 0–6. Although this single question may or may not capture the global impact of BPH symptoms on quality of life, it can serve as a valuable starting point for a doctor–patient conversation.

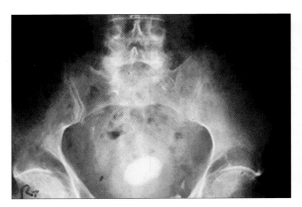

5.2 A large bladder stone seen on plain x-ray.

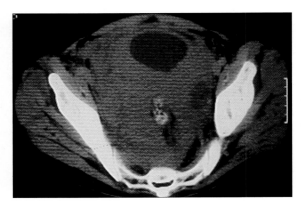

5.3 CT scan showing an enormous prostate cancer encircling the rectum; this patient presented with subacute large bowel obstruction.

tions, which in turn result in frequency, dysuria and sometimes also haematuria. Urinary stasis within the bladder can result in the formation of bladder calculi, which can themselves predispose the patient to recurrent urinary sepsis (**5.2**). Irritation of the trigone by stones may cause suprapubic pain, strangury and haematuria, especially towards the end of micturition. Haemospermia is a symptom that is only occasionally associated with prostate cancer, but the description of this by a patient should prompt both a digital rectal examination with PSA determination and transrectal ultrasonography, together with prostatic biopsy if indicated on other clinical grounds.

Symptoms of Local Invasion

Carcinomatous infiltration of the prostate and local invasion of adjacent structures can lead to an assortment of symptoms. Direct invasion of the prostatic urethra may lead to haematuria, which may on occasions be profuse with clots. The haematuria may be associated with dysuria due to malignant infiltration of the urothelium within the prostatic urethra.

Urinary incontinence may rarely be a consequence of local invasion of the distal urethral sphincter mechanism, which may be so debilitating that it necessitates permanent catheterization. It is, however, important to be sure in such circumstances that incontinence is not due to chronic retention with overflow, which could potentially be remedied by TURP or by other local therapeutic procedures such as intraprostatic stent insertion.

Extraprostatic posterolateral extension of prostate cancer may lead to invasion and destruction of the neurovascular bundles, and erectile impotence (see **2.5**). It is important to bear this unusual presentation of prostate cancer in mind when investigating men of middle-age or beyond for symptoms of erectile dysfunction. Extracapsular extension of cancer may also invade other nerves, leading to pain which is characteristically located in the perineum and suprapubic areas. This differential diagnosis should be borne in mind when investigating prostatitis. Invasion of the seminal vesicles may result in haemospermia.

Extension of prostate cancer posteriorly can lead to lower bowel symptoms and, rarely, prostate cancer may present in such a way. The fascia of Denonvillier is generally protective against direct invasion of the rectal wall by prostate cancer, but it is not unknown for locally advanced prostate cancer to encircle the distal rectum completely, leading eventually to large bowel obstruction (**5.3**). Prostate cancer patients presenting in this way may sometimes be referred to the colorectal clinic with symptoms such as constipation and rectal bleeding. At sigmoidoscopy, the tumour may mimic a primary rectal tumour and biopsy will show adenocarcinoma. In such circumstances, specific immunohistochemical PSA staining of the biopsies will identify the prostate as the origin of the tumour (**2.27**), and serum PSA will almost always be markedly elevated.

Symptoms of Metastatic Disease

Internationally, in spite of efforts to detect early disease by increasing the public awareness of

Table 5.3 Presenting symptoms of metastatic prostate cancer	
Local metastatic	Bone pain (consider pathological fracture when acute) Paraplegia (secondary to cord compression) Lymph node enlargement Lymphoedema (particularly lower limb) Loin pain (ureteric obstruction)
Systemic metastatic	Lethargy (due to anaemia, uraemia and non-specific effects) Weight loss and cachexia Haemorrhage (cutaneous and bowel)

symptoms attributable to prostate diseases and the screening of asymptomatic men (see Chapter 7), more than half of men with prostate cancer still present with spread of disease beyond the confines of the prostate.

Currently, in Europe, at least a quarter of men with prostate cancer will also have bone metastases detectable on an isotope bone scan at presentation[2]. These individuals may have a number of symptoms (**Table 5.3**). Local pain is the commonest complaint caused by bone metastases, and since these are most frequently found within the pelvic bones and lumbar spine, sudden onset of progressive, low-back pain is a cardinal symptom of metastatic prostate cancer. Bony metastases from prostate cancer may be seen in almost every bone in the skeleton, and can lead to pathological fractures, especially as a result of local trauma. The neck of the femur is not an uncommon site for metastatic prostate cancer, and is particularly prone to pathological fracture, often necessitating orthopaedic surgical correction by prosthetic arthroplasty. Acute, severe, hip pain, and inability to bear weight on the affected limb in an elderly male with bladder outflow symptoms, suggests this diagnosis. Metastatic disease within the vertebral bodies is common in prostate cancer, and compression of the spinal cord causing neurological symptoms (especially within the lower limbs) may occur in 1–12% of patients[3] (**5.4**); in one series, in 17% of cases of acute spinal-cord compression due to metastatic prostate cancer, this was the initial presentation of the disease[4]. Although opinions are divided between the comparative benefits of radiotherapy and surgical decompression, it is important to emphasize the importance of prompt local treatment accompanied by urgent androgen deprivation

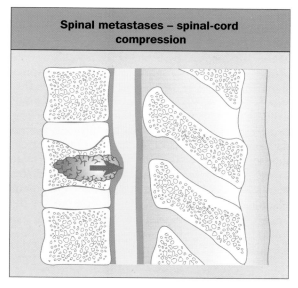

Spinal metastases – spinal-cord compression

5.4 Spinal-cord compression resulting from metastases of prostate cancer in the lumbar spine.

therapy in all cases of cord compression that is secondary to bony metastases, to improve the overall outcome[5]. Extensive metastatic disease within the bone marrow may lead to normochromic, normocytic anaemia, due to both the replacement of marrow as well as to cachexia.

While metastatic prostate cancer within the skeleton may present with dramatic symptoms, the presentation of lymph-node metastases is usually less overt. Enlarging nodal masses may become apparent to the patient, particularly within the inguinal lymph nodes, but also within the cervical and axillary nodes. Intra-abdominal, lymphatic, metastatic spread initially involves the obturator and internal iliac lymph nodes, and may result in ureteric obstruction. Later, tumour may spread to common iliac, external iliac, inguinal and para-aortic nodes; eventually, lymphatic involvement may spread as far as thoracic, cervical and axillary lymph node chains. Lymphatic involvement from prostate cancer may cause a variety of symptoms, including palpable swellings noticed by the patient, loin pain due to upper urinary tract obstruction, and lymphoedematous lower limb swelling.

PHYSICAL EXAMINATION

Routine, external physical examination may reveal no abnormality suggesting an underlying diagnosis of prostatic carcinoma. However, since prostate cancer is such a commonly encountered disease in men (and especially in the older male), not only urologists but also primary health-care physicians should be aware of the salient physical signs that should alert their attention towards this important diagnosis. More precise physical examination is usually guided by the presenting medical history, and hence, symptoms of bladder outflow obstruction should raise a suspicion of underlying prostate cancer. On physical examination, the search for prostate cancer should include an inspection for bladder distension (assisted by percussion of the lower abdomen), as well as examination of the lower limbs for lymphoedema and lymph nodes for enlargement and induration.

Digital Rectal Examination

Examination of the prostate digitally per rectum (DRE) is the most useful clinical method for the diagnosis of prostate cancer, provided the tumour is of sufficient volume to be palpable (**5.5**).

The precise technique for examining the prostate varies from one country to another. In the UK, patients are usually examined in the left lateral position with the knees brought up to the chest. In the USA, DRE is more often performed from behind the patient, with the patient standing and leaning forwards. There is now some evidence to suggest that the positioning of the patient does make a difference in the diagnostic yield of DRE, with the knee–elbow position proving superior[6].

It is fortuitous that the majority (approximately 70%) of prostate cancers arise from within the peripheral zone and hence are more likely to be

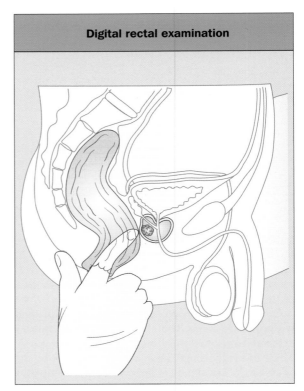

Digital rectal examination

5.5 Digital rectal examination (DRE) of a posteriorly located prostatic nodule.

palpable by DRE. In a recent series of 6630 men, DRE detected 55% of prostate cancers while transrectal ultrasound (TRUS) detected 82%[7]; this difference reflects the impalpability of small prostate cancers. However, other prostatic pathologies may result in a false positive diagnosis of prostate cancer when a firm palpable nodule or induration is felt. Histological examination of such areas reveals prostate cancer in about only one third of cases[8] (**5.6**). The differential diagnoses of such abnormal palpable lesions are summarized in **Table 5.4**.

STAGING OF PROSTATE CANCER BY DRE

Early stages of prostate cancer (T2a or Stage B1), if palpable, often appear as a peripheral, firm nodule, that is not apparently distorting the capsule. More extensive cancers (T2b or Stage B2) feel hard and less discrete, with unilateral enlargement when confined to one side of the gland. Stage T3 (Stage C) prostate cancer is again palpably hard; irregular distortion of the prostate outline is often apparent,

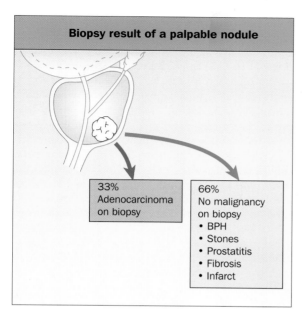

Biopsy result of a palpable nodule

33% Adenocarcinoma on biopsy

66% No malignancy on biopsy
• BPH
• Stones
• Prostatitis
• Fibrosis
• Infarct

5.6 Probability of a palpable nodule proving positive for adenocarcinoma on pathological examination after transrectal biopsy.

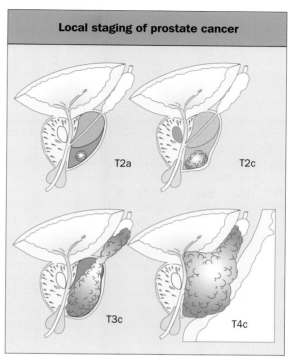

Local staging of prostate cancer

T2a

T2c

T3c

T4c

5.7 Local staging of prostate cancer.

Table 5.4 Causes of false positive diagnosis of prostate cancer on digital rectal examination

BPH nodule
Prostatic calculi
Prostatitis
Ejaculatory duct anomaly
Seminal vesicle anomaly
Rectal wall phlebolith
Rectal wall polyp/tumour

but the prostate as a whole remains mobile; the seminal vesicles are often involved, and may be palpable as firm cords. In locally advanced T4 prostate cancer, the prostate is grossly enlarged, hard, irregular throughout, and immobile due to fixation to adjacent structures (5.7).

Loss of palpability of the median sulcus of the prostate is a non-specific finding that may be found in T2–T4 disease. BPH can usually be differentiated from prostate cancer on DRE by virtue of the softer, springier, and more symmetrical nature of the benign gland. However, peripheral-zone calcification, which is a common feature of BPH, parti-

cularly when associated with chronic prostatitis, may masquerade as prostate cancer since hard and often discrete nodules may be palpable. Acute prostatitis (which may lead to a rise in the PSA and hypoechoic TRUS findings), in which the prostate is soft and exquisitely tender, is easier to differentiate from prostate cancer; chronic prostatitis, particularly granulomatous prostatitis, however, is often clinically indistinguishable[9].

Digital Rectal Examination as a Guide to Biopsy
Digital rectal examination (DRE) can be used to guide biopsies of the prostate that utilize fine-needle aspiration techniques or trucut/biopty biopsies. It is difficult to guide biopsies of small, palpable lesions digitally, and this technique has largely been superseded by TRUS-guided biopsy with an automatic device. All palpably abnormal lesions should be considered for biopsy, taking into account the patient's age and life expectancy. The decision regarding the necessity for biopsy of the prostate when no suspicious lesions are palpable is guided by the level of serum PSA and the presence or absence of any abnormal findings on TRUS. This topic is discussed

in more detail in the chapters dealing with imaging, PSA and screening. Although misleading in some cases, and not diagnostic for prostate cancer in isolation, DRE remains the crucial first step towards making the diagnosis of prostate cancer. Palpation of the prostate should not be considered as exclusively within the realm of the urologist. Primary health-care physicians should also be encouraged to develop expertise in DRE, and to use their acquired skill to contribute towards earlier detection of prostate cancer, especially in men under the age of 70 years who are most likely to benefit from this.

Incidental Prostate Cancer

A not infrequent presentation of localized prostate cancer remains the 'incidental' diagnosis of the disease at TURP[10]. However, the recent decline in the number of transurethral resections performed for what is presumed to be benign disease, and the increase in the pre-operative PSA testing and ultrasound-guided transrectal prostatic biopsy, seems likely to reduce the frequency with which the larger volume, more clinically significant incidental prostate cancers are diagnosed in this way.

Currently, of those incidental cancers that are detected, roughly two thirds are well-differentiated tumours involving 5% or less of the resected chippings; this has been termed T1a (A1) stage disease.

In the remaining one third of cases, there is evidence of less well-differentiated (Gleason grade > 4) tissue and/or involvement of more than 5% of the resected tissue (T1b (A2) stage disease).

Although the T1a/T1b classification is easy to apply clinically, and correlates reasonably well with the subsequent risk of disease progression, it does possess some obvious drawbacks in terms of prognosis for the individual patient. The tissue sampled at TURP is predominantly that of the transition zone, from whence less than 30% of prostate cancers stem. More importantly, the 5% of curettings involved by the 'cancer cut-off point' employed do carry a substantial risk of underestimation, or sometimes overestimation, of the residual disease present after TURP (especially when the disease is multifocal)[11]. The nature of the problem is illustrated in **5.8**.

There may not always be a good correlation between the volume and grade of cancer excised with that of the extent and nature of tumour remaining. However, the means to circumvent this problem are now available: a reasonable estimate of that volume and grade of residual disease can be obtained by post-operative PSA determination and transrectal ultrasound-guided biopsy. Those patients with biopsy-proven residual cancer of a volume > 0.5 cm³, and who have a life expectancy of more than 10 years,

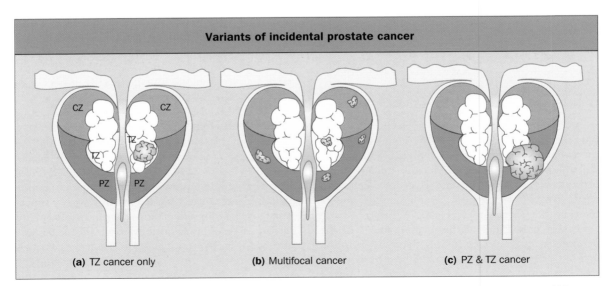

Variants of incidental prostate cancer

(a) TZ cancer only   **(b)** Multifocal cancer   **(c)** PZ & TZ cancer

5.8 Variations in anatomical locations of prostatic tumours diagnosed incidentally at TURP. Case (**a**) the cancer would be completely excised; case (**b**) is multifocal and small residual areas of cancer would remain; case (**c**) TURP simply samples the 'tip of the iceberg' of a larger, predominantly peripheral-zone, cancer.

might be considered for definitive therapy – either radical surgery or radical radiotherapy. By contrast, those with no evidence of either significant-volume or moderate to high-grade residual disease can be managed by so-called 'watchful waiting'[12]. A rise in serum PSA of more than 0.75 ng/ml per annum in men younger than 75 years of age, however, should set alarm bells ringing and should prompt repeat ultrasound-guided transrectal biopsies which, if positive, might suggest the need for further therapy[13].

CONCLUSIONS

Careful history and examination, including, crucially, DRE, remain the cornerstone of the clinical evaluation of patients suspected of harbouring prostate cancer. The diagnosis of prostate cancer, however, may have a profound effect on the affected individual and his family. Caution should therefore be exercised in setting the wheels in motion of confirming the presence of prostate cancer in very elderly men, since active treatment may not always be indicated. In men younger than 75 years whose life expectancy exceeds 5–10 years, however, accurate diagnosis, staging and appropriate therapy may prevent the development of extensive metastatic disease with its severely negative impact on quality of life. A high index of suspicion and diagnostic acumen is necessary to identify correctly those individuals harbouring disease that truly constitutes a genuine threat to their lives at a stage when it is still potentially curable.

REFERENCES

1 Barry MJ, Fowler FJ, O'Leary MP, *et al*. The American Urologic Association index for benign prostatic hyperplasia. *J Urol* 1992;**140**:1549–1557.

2 Johansson JE, Adami MD, Andersson SO, *et al*. Natural history of localised prostate cancer: a population-based study in 223 untreated patients. *Lancet* 1989;**1**:799–801.

3 Liskow A, Chang CH, De Sanctis P. Epidural cord compression in association with genito-urinary neoplasms. *Cancer* 1986;**58**:949–954.

4 Rosenthal MA, Rosen D, Raghavan D, *et al*. Spinal cord compression in prostate cancer. A 10-year experience. *Br J Urol* 1992;**69**:530–533.

5 Iacovou JW, Marks JC, Abrams P, *et al*. Cord compression and carcinoma of the prostate; is laminectomy justified? *Br J Urol* 1985;**57**:733–736.

6 Frank J, Andrews S, Oliver S, Emerton M. Digital rectal examination in the left-lateral or in the knee-elbow position: a randomised trial. *Br J Urol* 1999;**63**:365.

7 Catalona WJ, Richie JP, Ahmann FR, *et al*. Comparison of digital rectal examination and serum prostate-specific antigen in the early detection of prostate cancer: results of a multicentre clinical trial of 6630 men. *J Urol* 1994;**151**:1283–1290.

8 Catalona WJ. Yield from routine prostatic needle biopsy in patients more than 50 years old referred for urologic evaluation. *J Urol* 1980;**124**:844–846.

9 Lui S, Miller PD, Kirby RS. Eosinophilic prostatitis and prostate-specific antigen. *Br J Urol* 1992;**69**:61–63.

10 Matzkin H, Patel JP, Altwein JE, *et al*. Stage T_{1a} carcinoma of the prostate. *Urol* 1994;**43**:11–21.

11 Voges GE, McNeal JE, Redwine EA, *et al*. The predictive significance of substaging stage A prostate cancer (A_1 versus A_2) for volume and grade of total cancer in the prostate. *J Urol* 1992;**147**:858–863.

12 Cantrell BB, De Klerk DP, Eggleston JC, *et al*. Pathological factors that influence prognosis in stage A prostatic cancer: the influence of extent versus grade. *J Urol* 1981;**125**:516–520.

13 Feneley MR, Webb JAW, McLean A, Kirby RS. Post-operative serial prostate-specific antigen and transrectal ultrasound for staging incidental carcinoma of the prostate. *Br J Urol* 1995;**75**:14–20.

Chapter 6

Tumour markers in prostate cancer

Serum tumour markers are often a most helpful tool in the evaluation and management of patients with any type of neoplasm. They complement the measurement of serum testosterone levels and other hormonal factors such as dihydrotestosterone (DHT) and follicle-stimulating hormone (FSH) that provide diagnostic and monitoring information. New tumour markers will be developed but one caveat must be remembered as we look realistically towards the future: in a qualitative sense, no analyte has been associated with a human neoplasm that has not been shown to be present in a normal cell. It thus seems unlikely that absolute specificity for cancer will ever be realized.

ACID PHOSPHATASE

There is a long history of interest in the application of tumour markers to the prostate. Indeed, the first clinical use of *any* serum marker was the report of Gutman and Gutman[1], who measured acid phosphatase in men with prostatic carcinoma. Many studies have appeared since that time, using first enzymatic and later immunometric assays for initially non-specific, and subsequently prostate-specific, acid phosphatase. At one point it was even claimed that this test would serve as an equivalent to the cervical smear or the 'male Pap test'; with further research, it has been shown that owing to a lack of sensitivity to early-stage disease, this test has little or no role in diagnosis.

While formerly used widely, prostatic acid phosphatase (**Table 6.1**) has largely been replaced by prostate-specific antigen (PSA) for clinical staging. Although a correlation occurs between the pathological stage and the serum acid phosphatase levels, a substantial overlap precludes any useful stratification. In addition, acid phosphatase is abnormal in

Table 6.1 Serum acid phosphatase vs clinical stage					
		Per cent abnormal by stage			
	Assay type	OC	C	C&D	D
Foti et al.[102]	E	14	29		60
Cooper et al.[103]	E	9		46	
Bruce, Mahan and Belville[104]	E	9	17		73
Murphy, Chu and Carr[105]	E	11	17		51
Van Cangh, Opsomer and de Nayer[106]	E	21	31		78
Foti et al.[102]	I	60	71		92
Cooper et al.[103]	I	43		94	
Bruce et al.[107]	I	22	24		78
Murphy, Chu and Carr[105]	I	36	49		69
Van Cangh, Opsomer and de Nayer[106]	I	21	54		89

E, Enzymatic assay; I, Immunologic assay; OC, Organ confined; D, Disseminated; C, Capsular penetration

only about two thirds of patients with organ-confined carcinoma. The one group where acid phosphatase remains useful, at least in the eyes of many investigators, is patients with clinically localized disease with an abnormal enzymatic acid phosphatase level[2]; this category, referred to as M_o (or D_o) by some, has been shown to have an ominous prognosis, with clinical evidence of progression in the majority of patients in a relatively short time.

Recently, the group from Johns Hopkins University[3] has shown that it is unusual for acid phosphatase to provide unique information with respect to PSA in staging of prostatic carcinoma (less than 1% of patients). In general, there is now little justification for the primary-care provider or urologist to use this marker.

PROSTATE-SPECIFIC ANTIGEN

Prostate-specific antigen represents the best serum marker for prostatic carcinoma, and indeed could be argued to be the best tumour marker available today. It has established utilities both as an immuno-histochemical marker, and as a method of monitoring patients with established malignancy. The utility of PSA for staging and diagnosis, especially in the early-detection arena, is currently undergoing detailed investigation.

PSA is a 34 kilodalton glycoprotein, which is specific to prostatic epithelium (**6.1**). It is a neutral serine protease whose function is to lyse seminal-vesicle protein. Although most PSA remains within the prostatic ducts, a proportion is absorbed into the blood stream where to a large extent it is bound mainly to two proteins: alpha-1-antichymotrypsin (ACT) and alpha macroglobulin (**6.2**). Initial reports of a serum assay for PSA using simple electrophoresis[4] were insensitive, demonstrating elevated levels in only 17 out of 219 patients with prostatic carcinoma (8%). More sensitive assays were developed later.

Assay Variability

One of the problems with PSA assays is the lack of an international standard. Different manufacturers may report dramatically different results on the same serum specimen[5-12]. Recently the World Health Organization has begun the process of adopting the standard reference material based on 90% complex and 10% free PSA[13]. The availability of numerous different assays for the determination of PSA has thus created substantial problems in interpretation, particularly in Europe where over 80 PSA assays are available – this is a considerable problem for the clinician and patient alike[12]. There are a number of reasons for potential differences between different manufacturers assay including assay calibration; incubation time (particularly for the automating format assays); as well as non-equilibrium or different affinities of the various isoforms of PSA (free PSA, complex PSA, etc.)[14-19].

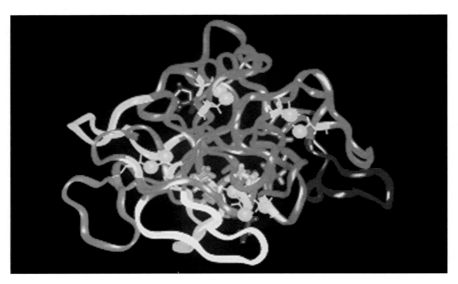

6.1 Three-dimensional molecular model of PSA. (Figure kindly supplied by Dominique P Bridon of Abbott Laboratories.)

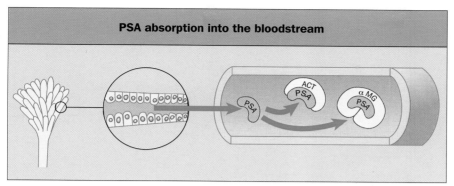

PSA absorption into the bloodstream

6.2 PSA is exclusively secreted from the epithelial cells of the prostatic ducts. A small proportion is absorbed into the blood stream where it is largely bound to either anti-chymotrypsin (ACT) or alpha macroglobulin (αMG), leaving only a small proportion of free, uncomplexed PSA.

This latter finding has been recently dramatically demonstrated by Semjonow et al.[15]. Because of the widespread use of the Hybritech assay in which 4.0 ng/ml was established as the upper limit of normal[20,21], other manufacturers have recommended this as their cutoff without clearly demonstrating equivalence between their assay and the Hybritech method[15-17]. Indeed some manufacturers have not specified a reference range or have established their reference range with young men or even females as normal. An additional problem is that even if different manufacturers report substantially equivalent results on identical patient's sera, the ability for that particular assay to identify carcinoma may differ. Certainly the need for reliably determined reference ranges is obvious. Laboratory workers must not only document in the report which assay was used, but the manufacturers should provide correlation data to other widely used assays, not only obtaining a similar analyte concentration, but also in demonstrating substantial equivalent risk assessment for carcinoma.

The magnitude of this problem is staggering. Semjonow and associates demonstrated as much as a twofold factor in different concentrations of PSA when different assays were used[5,19]. Further,

Semjonow demonstrated that the greatest accuracy in diagnosis of carcinoma varied between a level of 4.4 and 8.9 ng/ml depending upon which assay was used[19].

Early reports demonstrating that PSA was elevated in a proportion of patients with benign prostatic hyperplasia[22-25] (**Table 6.2**) in fact hindered interest in the use of PSA for the diagnosis of carcinoma. Because of the virtual certainty that men being evaluated for prostate cancer would have at least histological benign prostatic hyperplasia (BPH), it was reasoned that the specificity of an elevated PSA would be simply too low.

Prostate-specific antigen levels in prostatic fluid are approximately one million-fold higher than serum PSA values. An epithelial layer, a basal-cell layer, and a basement membrane separate the intra-ductal PSA from the capillary and lymphatic drainage of the prostate. Disruption of these barriers may allow increased PSA leakage into the interstitial tissue spaces and the systemic circulation resulting in elevated serum PSA levels (**6.3**).

The specificity for prostatic tissue of antibodies to PSA makes it a uniquely suitable marker for immunohistochemically identifying prostate as the site of origin for poorly differentiated neoplasms of

Table 6.2 Serum PSA in patients with histologically confirmed benign prostatic hyperplasia (%)

Author	Assay	PSA >4.0 ng/ml	PSA >10.0 ng/ml
Ercole et al[108]	Tandem-R	75 (21)	10 (3)
Ferro et al[109]	Tandem-R		13 (33)
Hudson, Bahnson and Catalona[110]	Tandem-R	35 (21)	3 (2)
Stamey et al[82]	Pros-check	70 (88)	

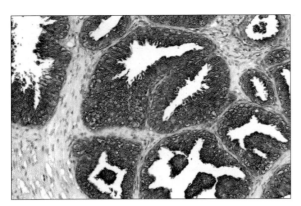

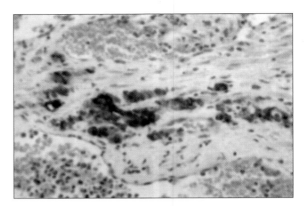

6.3 Anti-PSA stain showing strong positive (brown) staining of columnar epithelial cells of normal prostatic acini. (Reproduced with permission from Weiss MA, Mills SE. *Atlas of Genitourinary Tract Disorders*. London: Gower; 1988.)

6.4 Immunohistochemical staining of PSA demonstrated in a poorly differentiated metastatic lesion from the prostate.

unknown aetiology. Primary and metastatic lesions almost invariably continue to express PSA, albeit in variable degrees, and the presence of PSA staining infers that the prostate is the site of origin. This may be exceedingly useful in cases of metastatic carcinoma of unknown origin (**6.4, Table 6.3**).

In attempts to further establish the relationship of serum PSA to the underlying prostate pathology, simple prostatectomy specimens were studied from 81 men with bladder outlet obstruction symptoms which were considered to be secondary to BPH[26]. In this study, pre-operative serum PSA was correlated with the pathology observed on histological section of all tissue removed. It was found that 36 of the 81 men (44%) had a PSA > 4.0 ng/ml. However, 35 had significant pathology which could allow leakage

of PSA into the systemic circulation (**6.5**). This observation suggests that significant pathological lesions associated with disruption of the basal-cell layer, rather than the presence of BPH itself, explains the majority of elevations of serum PSA.

Several clinical parameters need to be considered when evaluating serum PSA levels. Brawer *et al.* reported that digital rectal examination was not associated with erroneous elevation of PSA[27], and Crawford and associates[28] as well as Yuan *et al.*[29] confirm this.

More significant prostatic perturbations, such as prostate needle biopsy, urethral instrumentation and transurethral resection *will* cause significant elevation of serum PSA. Yuan and associates[29] noted that prostate needle biopsy resulted in a significant elevation of PSA that lasted for more than two weeks in 27 of 89 men. Brawer *et al.* studied 127

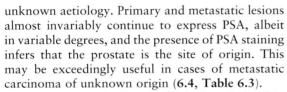

Table 6.3 PSA immunohistochemistry				
Author	**Primary prostate cancer**	**Metastatic prostate cancer**	**Irradiated prostate cancer**	**Other tumours**
Nadji *et al.*[111]	73/73	49/49		0/78
Stein *et al.*112	13/15			
Vernon and Williams[113]	30/30		5/5	
Ford *et al.*[114]	63/65	16/17		0/13
Brawer *et al.*[115]			33/33	
Sohlberg *et al.*[116]	23/23			
Total	202/206	65/66	38/38	0/91

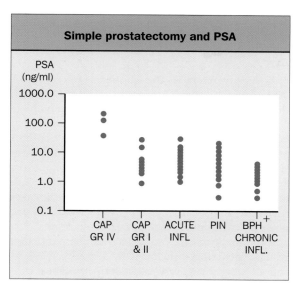

6.5 Pre-operative PSA values grouped for various pathologies identified at prostatectomy. (Reproduced with permission from Brawer MK, *et al*. Serum prostate-specific antigen and prostate pathology in men having simple prostatectomy. *Am J Clin Path* 1989;**92**(6):760–764.

men following six-sector ultrasound-guided trans-rectal prostate needle biopsies, and noted a 20% or greater elevation in PSA levels 28 days after the procedure, when compared to prebiopsy level[30].

Table 6.4 Serum PSA versus age in screened population

Age (yrs)	PSA (ng/ml)			
	No. (%)	Mean	Median	SD
50–59	222 (17.8)	1.62	1.0	6.5
60–69	600 (48.0)	2.7	3.8	1.4
70–79	365 (29.2)	3.1	5.0	1.7
> 79	62 (5.0)	8.8	11.9	2.2
Total	1249	2.9	2.2	10.4

(Reproduced with permission from Brawer *et al*.[33])

Patient age also has an effect on the PSA level; in a screening study of 1249 healthy men, PSA correlated significantly with patient age (**Table 6.4**). Oesterling has made similar observations (**6.6**).

PSA was initially approved in the USA for the monitoring of men with established malignancy and although it has application in staging and prognostic information, the most important indication is for use in the early detection and screening for prostatic carcinoma. This is discussed in more detail in Chapter 7.

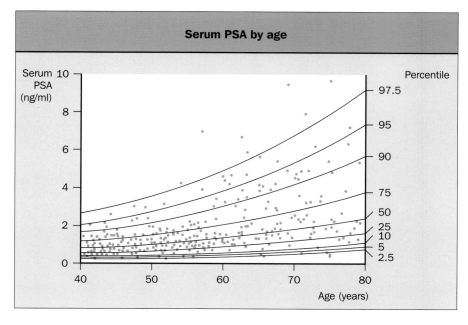

6.6 Serum PSA versus patient age in a cohort of patients without evidence of prostate cancer. (Modified with permission from Oesterling JE, *et al*. Serum prostate-specific antigen in a community-based population of healthy men. *JAMA* 1993;**270**:840–864.)

Methods to Enhance PSA Performance

Despite the impressive results of a series in which early detection for prostatic carcinoma was made using PSA alone or in conjunction with the digital rectal examination[20,31–36], PSA is not the perfect test. Although the sensitivity is quite impressive, the widely accepted cutoff of 4.0 ng/ml is the upper limit of normal; however, approximately 18–25% of those who are found to have carcinoma in contemporary biopsy series have serum PSA levels below this threshold. A greater problem has been the lack of specificity. Approximately two-thirds to three-quarters of men who have a serum PSA greater than 4.0 ng/ml will have benign histology on initial prostate biopsy. Because of the problems of lack of specificity, namely that they mandate further testing, and this is expensive (both economically owing to the need for antibiotics, ultrasound biopsy, pathology charges, etc., and psychologically owing to the anxiety a man experiences when told that he has an elevated PSA), efforts have primarily been directed to enhancement of specificity. A number of approaches have been used including PSA density, PSA velocity, age-specific PSA levels and more recently measurement of the different isoforms of PSA present in the systemic circulation.

PSA Density

PSA density refers to the quotient of serum PSA divided by the volume of the prostate gland[37]. Given the fact the biggest component of prostate volume is benign prostatic hyperplasia, it makes sense that normalizing to the gland volume may make PSA more specific. Several investigators have carried out studies in this regard[37–41] (**Table 6.5**). The authors demonstrated enhancement in specificity with minimal reduction in sensitivity when PSA density was used[42,43]. The Seattle group, along with others, however, was unable to replicate these results[44–46].

A number of factors could explain these different results, including differences in accuracy in ultrasound measurement, the prostate volume, variability of the histological makeup in the cohort of men being tested as well as biopsy sampling error and PSA assay variability[17,47]. We have noted that in all of the papers in which PSA density indicated a benefit that the glands with carcinoma were significantly smaller that those without a benefit. In studies in which the cancer glands were larger or if

Table 6.5 PSA results					
Author	**Biopsy**	**No. of patients**	**PSA (ng/ml)***	**Prostate volume (cc)***	**PSA density***
Benson et al.[38]	Positive	98	7.0 (1.7)[†]	28.9 (14.6)[†]	0.30 (0.15)[†]
	Negative	191	6.8 (1.8)	40.1 (20.2)	0.21 (0.11)
Seaman et al.[39]	Positive	115	6.87 (1.70)	29.2 (14.2)[†]	0.285 (0.147)[†]
	Negative	311	6.77 (1.71)	42.2 (21.8)	0.199 (0.108)
Brawer et al.[44]	Positive	68	10.7 (11.4)[†]	40.5 (16.6)	0.29 (0.41)
	Negative	159	5.2 (5.0)	42.6 (25.6)	0.14 (0.14)
Bazinet et al.[40]	Positive	217	21.4 (29.6)[†]	37.6 (21.4)[†]	0.63 (0.86)[†]
	Negative	317	9.1 (8.1)	51.6 (27.3)	0.21 (0.25)
Rommel et al.[41]	Positive	612	15.5 (21.6)[†]	42.7 (27.2)[†]	0.47 (0.11)[†]
	Negative	1394	4.9 (4.7)	47.0 (31.6)	0.105 (0.09)
Mettlin et al.[45]	Positive	171	12.0 (16.0)[†]	38.9 (16.4)	0.35 (0.5)[†]
	Negative	650	2.1 (2.3)	33.5 (14.2)	0.08 (0.09)
Ohori et al.[46]	Positive	110	9.3 (0.3–1320)[‡]	28.1 (15.1–228.7)[‡]	0.21 (0.009–39.3)[‡]
	Negative	134	4.8 (0.2–64.1)[‡]	47.3 (13.3–332.6)[‡]	0.09 (0.007–1.82)[‡]

*Data reported as mean (standard deviation).
[†]p <0.05
[‡]data reported as median (range), p <0.05

there was no diffference, PSA density did not seem to work. Sampling bias would favour detection of cancer in smaller glands, which have higher PSA density. Recently, we demonstrated a decrease in cancer detection in men with larger prostates[48].

Transition Zone Density

In a further attempt at enhancement of PSA, a number of authorities have examined so-called transition zone density with a normalization of the serum PSA by the volume of the transition zone of the prostate. Initial reports by Djavan *et al.*[49] and Maeda *et al.*[50] indicated increased efficacy when this derivative was used. We have been unable to to reproduce these results[51]. We have theorized that this may be because of an artefact of sampling mistakes in larger glands. In addition, measurement of transition zone density is obviously operator dependent and this could play an even more marked role in this derivative. Generally the cost and inconvenience of performing transrectal ultrasound probably renders density calculation in all men unwarranted.

PSA Velocity

Another approach to the assay specificity enhancement has been so-called PSA velocity. This is the change in PSA over time and certainly this makes intrinsic sense. A person who develops prostatic carcinoma may eventually have a PSA level in the hundreds or indeed thousands. Certainly the rate of change in his PSA would be expected to be far greater than that in a man who never develops a significant malignancy. This concept was first reported on by Carter and associates in their evaluation of a cohort of men in which serum had been banked as part of an aging study[52]. These investigators demonstrated that if the PSA increased more than 0.75 ng/ml for a year it helped predict those men who had carcinoma.

The Seattle group has been unable to reproduce the results of Carter[35,53]. The biggest differences certainly were the fact that in the Baltimore longitudinally aging study a minimum of 7 years was required between PSA determinations. In our study, we could not see stratification of men with and without carcinoma with PSA measurements between 1 and 2 years apart. Similarly, Catalona and associates using relatively short intervals were unable to support the observation of Carter and associates[54]. In subsequent analysis, Carter and associates demon-

strated that PSA velocity was only useful when a minimum of three consecutive measurements were taken over at least a 2-year time interval[55].

A major limitation of PSA velocity is the significant degree of biological variation observed in PSA levels in normal men. We have demonstrated that there has to be approximately a 30% change in the serum PSA before one can attribute this change to disease of the prostate[56].

Age-specific PSA

Another so-called PSA derivative is the age-specific reference range. Establishment of the upper limit of normal for PSA was initially based on the 97.5% confidence interval of so-called normal men[21]. Although there was no scientific basis in establishment of this threshold, it has stood the test of time owing to the fact that a relatively high percentage of men with a greater level will be shown to have carcinoma. In a biopsy population, this level approximates the cutoff, optimizing sensitivity and specificity[34]. It is widely recognized that PSA increases with age (**6.6**; **Table 6.4**). Oesterling and associates initially suggested that we should increase the PSA level of normal for older men. Theoretically this approach would enhance sensitivity in the younger man and specificity in older patients[57]. Reissigl and associates echoed this concept[36].

Other investigators have reported dissimilar results including Etzioni *et al.*[58] and Borer *et al.*[59]. They and others have pointed out that dimunition in sensitivity in the older cohort is problematic given that the prevalence of disease increases so dramatically. Indeed, Etzioni and associates demonstrated not only significant decrease in cancer detection if age-specific cutoffs were used, but even normalizing for age and life expectancy in a screening cohort would be significantly reduced.

Molecular Forms of PSA

The most significant advance in PSA testing has been the recognition that PSA circulates in a variety of molecular forms. The majority does not occur in the free form found in the ejaculate, but rather is complexed to protease inhibitors. These protease inhibitors including alpha-2-macroglobulin, alpha-1-antichymotrypsin (ACT), alpha-1-antitrypsin or protein C inhibitor render the circulating PSA inactive[60–63]. The majority of PSA in the systemic circulation is complexed to ACT. It is perplexing that there is any free or noncomplex PSA identified in the circulation given that ACT occurs in significant molar excess to the amount of PSA generally found in the bloodstream. When PSA is complexed with alpha-2-macroglobulin it is not identified by commercial assays owing to the steric hindrance of the epitopic sites[64,65].

We know very little about the site of complexation of PSA. A great deal is owed to the Scandinavian investigators who were the first to report that the ACT-complexed PSA occurs in a greater proportion of men with carcinoma. Stenman and associates in 1991 demonstrated a correlation between the complex PSA and cancer[61]. Christensson and Lilja upheld these findings[66]. Subsequent reports from Luderer *et al.*[67], Higashihara *et al.*[68], and Chen *et al.*[69] have offered confirmatory evidence.

Difficulty in development of assays that could specifically measure ACT-complex PSA resulted in the use of the free-to-total PSA ratio to approximate this marker. The definitive trial of this was reported by Catalona and associates[70]. This was a seven institution trial in which men undergoing ultrasound-guided prostate needle biopsy who had a total PSA between 4.0 and 10.0 ng/ml and benign feeling prostates were evaluated. When the free-to-total PSA ratio was less than 25%, the sensitivity for cancer detection was 95% and the specificity enhanced by 20% over what was realized with total PSA alone. In other words, one out of five negative prostate needle biopsies could be avoided if the clinician was willing to miss 5% of cancers (**6.7**; **Table 6.6**) Hugosson and associates[71] reported that 44% of men with benign biopsies could be eliminated if a free PSA less than 18 was used as the indication for biopsy. However, this enhanced specificity relative to that reported by Catalona and associates was associated with reduced sensitivity (11% of men with carcinomas would be missed).

Use of the percent free-to-total PSA has also been shown to be effective in men who have serum PSA less than 4.0 ng/ml[65] as well as in men undergoing repeat biopsy[72–75]. These and other studies clearly indicate enhanced specificity when the free-to-total PSA ratio is used.

Several concerns with this exist, however. Preanalytic handling of the specimens is important because the free form of PSA has been shown to be unstable during improper storage[76]. For details, the reader is referred to the summary of Woodrum and associates[77].

Different manufacturers' assays have been shown

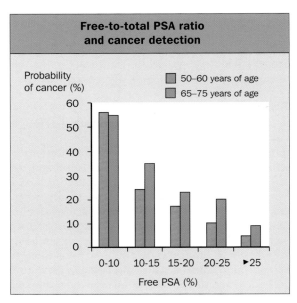

6.7 Free-to-total PSA and probability of cancer. (Data with permission from Catalona *et al.*[70])

Table 6.6 Sensitivity and specificity of free-to-total PSA		
Sensitivity (%)	**Cutoff (%)**	**Specificity (%)**
90	22	29
95	25	20
98	32	6

(Data with permission from Catalona *et al.*[70])

to give staggeringly different results for the free-to-total PSA ratio. The quotient nature of this makes such a bias particularly problematic[78,79]. **Tables 6.7 and 6.8** demonstrate the significant findings from these studies indicating manufacturer variability of the free PSA assays. Of major concern is the fact that measurement of the free and total PSA mandates two tests and effectively doubles the cost of PSA testing.

Complex PSA

Given these concerns with the free-to-total PSA there is increasing interest in assays that measure

Table 6.7 Free-to-total PSA using different assays

Assay	Cutoff for 95% sensitivity	Specificity (%)
Hyb. F/Hyb T	22	38
Dia. F/Hyb. T	35	19
Chi. F/Hyb. T	35	33

(Data with permission from Nixon et al.[79])
Hyb, Hybritech; Dia, Dianon; Chi, Chiron; F, free PSA; T, total PSA

the complex form of PSA. Recently the Bayer Corporation has demonstrated a specific assay for ACT–PSA complex[64].

The Seattle group performed a study on archival serum in men who had undergone previous ultrasound-guided prostate needle biopsy using the Bayer complex PSA assay[80]. We compared this with the Hybritech Tandem R free and total assays. The significant findings are shown on **Table 6.9**. At the 95% sensitivity level, the specificity of the total

PSA was 22%. The free-to-total PSA ratio required a 28% cutoff to afford the sensitivity and provided only a 15.6% specificity. In contrast, the complex PSA ratio of 2.52 offered a 26.7% specificity.

Similar results have recently been reported in a multicenter trial with the Bayer assay[81] (**Table 6.10**). Assuming that other institutions report similar results it is likely that complex PSA will replace not only the free-to-total PSA ratio in testing, but given the fact that it is a more specific analyte for cancer will be widely adopted for staging and monitoring men who have established malignancy.

PSA AND STAGING

PSA correlates with the clinical and, more reliably, the pathological stage of prostatic carcinoma (**Table 6.11**). Furthermore, the Stanford group correlated the volume of prostatic carcinoma with serum PSA level[82]; these authors demonstrated that each gram of prostatic carcinoma contributed around 3.5 ng/ml to the serum PSA level, and these data have been confirmed by others[83]. While there is a good correlation between the serum PSA level and the pathological stage in groups of patients, PSA is a relatively poor predictor of pathological stage for an

Table 6.8 Sensitivity and specificity of total PSA and the free-to-total PSA includes data from all patients in the benign prostatic hyperplasia and prostate cancer groups

Assay	Sensitivity (%)	Specificity (%) Total PSA	Specificity (%) F/T PSA	Cutoff total PSA (ng/ml)	Cutoff F/T PSA (%)
ACS:180 PSA2 and free PSA	100	0	0	0.02	90
	95	10	17	1.7	25
	90	25	54	3.3	15
Enzymun PSA and free PSA	100	0	0	0.02	100
	95	5	7	1.1	43
	90	24	32	3.0	23
Tandem-R PSA and free PSA	100	1	1	0.4	52
	95	7	22	2.1	25
	90	17	31	3.4	21

(Data with permission from Roth et al.[78])
F, free PSA; T, total PSA

Table 6.9 Specificity of the cutoff values of different PSA assays at selected sensitivities over the entire PSA range

Sensitivity (%)	Total PSA		Complex PSA		Free-to-total PSA	
	Cutoff (ng/ml)	Specificity (%)	Cutoff (ng/ml)	Specificity (%)	Cutoff (%)	Specificity (%)
80	4.11	35.6	3.98	51.6	19	46.2
85	3.86	31.1	3.34	38.7	22	32.4
90	3.4	25.3	2.94	33.8	24	26.2
95	3.06	21.8	2.52	26.7	28	15.6
97.5	2.28	12.9	1.67	14.7	32	8.9
100	1.0	3.1	0.89	6.2	67	0

(Data from Brawer et al.[80] © 1998, with permission from Elsevier Science.)

Table 6.10 Specificity of total and complexed PSA, and the free-to-total PSA ratio for all samples within the sensitivity range of 80% to 95%, as determined by ROC analysis

Sensitivity (%)	Total PSA		Complexed PSA		Free-to-total PSA Ratio	
	Cutoff (ng/ml)	Specificity (%)	Cutoff (ng/ml)	Specificity (%)	Cutoff (ng/ml)	Specificity (%)
80	4.64	41	4.09	46	17.1	52*[†]
85	4.33	33	3.79	41*	18.9	42*
90	3.99	28	3.40	32	20.9	31
95	3.06	18	2.75	24*	23.9	23*

*Significantly different from total PSA.
[†]Significantly different from complexed PSA.
(Data with permission from Brawer et al.[81])

individual patient[84] because of substantial overlap of PSA levels within any stage. PSA values vary widely among disease stage, and overlapping of stages further confounds the predictive value of PSA to pathological stage.

As mentioned earlier, PSA values can be greatly affected by any invasive prostatic manipulation. For this reason, prebiopsy PSA values are much better correlated to pathological stage than are postbiopsy PSA values. In our study, where PSA determinations were carried out prior to significant prostatic perturbation and then radical prostatectomy was performed, none of the fourteen tumours found in men with prebiopsy values greater than 10.0 ng/ml was organ-confined on pathological examination. A recent study by the Washington University group confirms these observations[85]. In this study, 14 out of 16 patients with biopsy-proven prostate carcinoma and a serum PSA of greater than 10.0 ng/ml were found to have extracapsular disease. These observations suggest that a correlation exists between serum PSA values of greater than 10.0 ng/ml by the Hybritech method and the presence of extracapsular tumour extension.

Serum PSA values have also proven useful in the determination of bone metastases in untreated prostate cancer patients. The Mayo Clinic group[86] found that only 1 of 306 patients with serum PSA

Table 6.11 PSA and pathological stage

Author	Assay	PSA > 4.0 ng/ml				PSA > 10.0 ng/ml			
		OC	CP	SV	LN	OC	CP	SV	LN
Ercole et al.[108]	TANDEM-R	12 (40)	14 (74)	8 (100)	17 (100)	2 (7)	6 (32)	8 (100)	12 (71)
Hudson et al.[110]	TANDEM-R					3 (11)	5 (56)	0	2 (100)
Oesterling et al.[87]	TANDEM-R	47 (46)	26 (65)	13 (72)	17 (100)	10 (10)	8 (20)	11 (61)	12 (71)
Stamey et al.[117]	PROSCHECK	NS	23 (82)	20 (95)	13 (100)				

OC, organ confined; CP, capsular penetration; SV, seminal vesicle involved; LN, node positive

values of less than 20 ng/ml (Tandem-R) had a positive bone scan. The probability of a positive bone scan with a serum PSA of 10.0 ng/ml or less was estimated at 1.4%. PSA was found to be a more reliable and accurate indicator of bony metastases than clinical stage, tumour grade, acid phosphatase or PAP. It should be noted, however, that only 7 of the 852 men studied actually had a positive bone scan. Of course, any patient with skeletal pain or other indications of extraprostatic spread should be fully staged by radionucleotide bone scan, but the need for cost savings may lead to a more selective approach to ordering bone scans in asymptomatic men and during follow-up.

PSA AFTER RADICAL PROSTATECTOMY

Within a few weeks following a radical prostatectomy with negative surgical margins, the serum PSA should theoretically be zero; this level should be attained within 3–4 weeks post-operatively[87] as the half-life of PSA is between 2.2 and 3.2 days. Unfortunately, none of the currently available assays for PSA can measure levels down to zero. The biological sensitivity of the assay (that level of serum PSA which can be distinguished from zero with 95% certainty) varies between commercial assays, and must be determined in an individual laboratory by repetitive testing.

After radical prostatectomy or radiotherapy, serum PSA is generally the first indicator of 'recurrent' disease. Carter et al.[88] noted that no patient with undetectable PSA level after radical prostatectomy had clinical evidence of active prostate cancer. Carter further noted that all patients with clinically detectable distant recurrences had elevated PSA post-operatively. Stamey et al.[82] added to these findings by noting that no patients who failed to normalize serum PSA within 3 weeks of radical prostatectomy had a subsequent decrease in PSA levels to undetectable range without adjuvant therapy.

Several studies imply that the majority of patients with undetectable PSA values following radical prostatectomy will remain without evidence of recurrence, whereas those whose PSA levels remain detectable will almost always experience some type of recurrence. Lange et al.[89] measured PSA levels three to six months after radical prostatectomy and correlated the results with clinical outcome: in men with PSA levels ≤ 0.2 ng/ml, only 11% recurred; for those who had PSA > 0.4 ng/ml, 100% recurred. In following 86 patients who had undetectable PSA levels after radical prostatectomy, seven (8.1%) had a subsequent rise in PSA levels to a mean of 70.6 ng/ml. Stein et al.[90] reported that in all cases of a group of 230 patients with pathological stage T1–T2, non-metastatic disease followed for a mean of 48 months after radical retropubic prostatectomy; elevations of serum PSA preceded the clinical recurrence of disease. However, in 41 out of 175 patients with detectable PSA values and no clinical evidence of recurrent prostate cancer, elevated serum PSA levels suggested a recurrence. The 5-year and 10-year clinical disease-free survivals were 82% and 72% respectively. If an elevated serum PSA value was taken to indicate recurrent disease, then the 5-year and 10-year disease-free survival decreases to 62% and 41% respectively. Thus, even 10 years after radical prostatectomy, a significant percentage of patients with apparent, recurrent, prostate cancer by biochemical parameters remain without other clinical evidence of the disease.

Detecting the location of low-volume, persistent disease can be difficult. Digital rectal examinations are often inconclusive, and bone scan and computerized tomography scan are generally negative in these patients. Lightner and associates[91], in evaluating needle biopsy of the anastomosis (NBA) in a group of men with serum PSA value >0.4 ng/ml after radical prostatectomy, found that 42% of the patients had a positive needle biopsy but negative bone scans and computed tomography (CT) scans. No patient with an undetectable PSA value had a positive needle biopsy of the anastomosis. Foster et al.[92] and Abi-Aad and associates[93] observed similar findings, reporting positive biopsies among 45% and 40%, respectively of those patients with elevated PSA values following radical prostatectomy.

The development of more sensitive assays for PSA should allow earlier detection of persistent disease[94]. Takayama et al.[95] found a 9–12 month lead time in detecting persistent disease using 0.1 ng/ml rather than 0.4 ng/ml of serum PSA to indicate persistent disease. All patients in this group whose serum PSA reached a level of 0.1 ng/ml continued to show a rise in PSA levels. No patient who had a serum PSA value <0.1 ng/ml at 36 months after radical prostatectomy developed recurrent disease; the Stanford group[96] has reported similar findings.

Whether the early treatment of patients with biochemical evidence of recurrent disease will result in prolonged survival remains to be determined.

There is some evidence indicating that patients who fail to normalize their PSA initially are more likely to have distant metastases, while those who develop delayed PSA elevations after radical prostatectomy more often have a local recurrence. The PSA doubling time has been correlated with the risk of distant versus local recurrence[97]. Lange et al.[89] treated 29 patients who had elevated PSA values and negative CT scans and bone scans with pelvic irradiation. PSA values decreased by more than 50% in 82% of the patients. Forty-three percent of the patients had an accompanying decrease in serum PSA within six months, to an undetectable range. Link et al.[22] reported similar findings in an evaluation of 2 groups of patients with adjuvant radiation therapy. They found that only 1 out of 12 patients (8%) receiving radiation treatment for elevated PSA immediately after prostatectomy, versus 7 of 15 (54%) patients receiving radiation treatment for a delayed elevation in PSA after radical prostatectomy, had continued suppression of PSA levels at undetectable levels during an average 33 month follow-up.

PSA AFTER RADIATION THERAPY

PSA also offers new information on the behaviour of prostate cancer following radiation therapy. Serum PSA has been found to decrease following radiation therapy, with a half life estimated at between 1.4 and 2.6 months[24,25]. The Stanford group[26] followed 183 patients after completion of radiation therapy (most of whom had localized disease) for a mean of 61 months. Serum PSA was reduced to undetectable levels in 11% of the patients; 25% of patients had a decrease in serum PSA values to the normal range (less than 2.5 ng/ml, Pros-check). Elevated PSA levels persisted in 65% of patients. Radiation therapy during the first year caused a reduction in PSA values in 82% of patients. Continued reduction after the first year of therapy occurred in only 8% of patients. PSA values rose in 51% of the patients.

Russell et al.[98] reported that pretreatment PSA values are associated with the chance of complete response (normalization of PSA with no tumour detectable by radiographic studies or digital rectal examination). In an evaluation of 143 men who were treated with external-beam irradiation (either photon or fast neutron) for clinically localized prostate cancer with a median follow-up of 27 months, patients with a pretreatment PSA value that was less than 4 times the normal had an 82% chance of complete response. Those with a PSA value greater than 4 times the normal value were associated with only a 30% chance of complete response. Furthermore, the time to normalization of PSA also appears to be important. In Russell and colleagues' study, 94% of those with normalization of PSA within 6 months remained complete responders during the study, compared with 8% of men with persistently elevated PSA values after 6 months.

Meek and associates[23] conducted a similar study of serum PSA and radiotherapy for prostate cancer. They found a post-treatment PSA nadir in the normal range to be the most important prognostic variable. Pretreatment PSA was not predictive of outcome if serum prostatic acid phosphatase (PAPs) were considered. They also noted that the initial rate of PSA decrease was unrelated to outcome.

Kabalin[26] conducted transrectal ultrasound-guided sextant biopsies on 27 men 18 months after external-beam radiation therapy. Persistent prostate carcinoma was detected in 25 of the 27 patients, including 20 of 22 men in whom it was also detectable with normal digital rectal examination. All four patients with normal PSA levels (<2.5 ng/ml, Proscheck), including one patient with an undetectable PSA, had positive biopsies. This suggests that rising PSA levels after radiation therapy do in fact indicate persistent disease. Such rises should prompt further evaluation with prostate needle biopsy if the patient is a candidate for salvage radical prostatectomy or hormonal ablation.

PSA AND HORMONAL THERAPY

The PSA nadir also appears to be an important indicator of response to hormonal therapy. Stamey et al.[99] followed a cohort of patients with metastatic prostate cancer after initiation of hormonal therapy. Twenty-two percent of the patients had a decrease in serum PSA levels to the normal range, while 9% had a decrease to undetectable levels. Of 11 patients who were followed with frequent PSA determinations following the induction of hormonal therapy, the PSA nadir was reached within 5 months in 9 of the 11. Seventy-two percent of the patients were noted to have increasing PSA values after 6 months. The effect of hormonal ablation on serum PSA is extremely variable.

Miller et al.[100] studied serum PSA levels of 48 patients with metastatic prostate cancer who achieved an objective response to hormonal therapy. They found that patients who reached a PSA nadir of less than 4.0 ng/ml had a significantly longer duration of remission than those who failed to normalize their PSA levels. No patient gave evidence of progressive disease while the PSA level was decreasing or at the nadir level. They also noted that a rise in serum PSA predated other evidence of disease progression by a mean of 7.3 months. Gillatt et al.[101] also reported that PSA levels are significantly related to survival after initiation of hormonal therapy in his study of 136 men with metastatic prostate cancer whose PSA levels were determined at 3 and 6 months following therapy initiation.

SUMMARY

It is widely accepted now that PSA is the most valuable of all tumour markers in oncology. This analyte is useful in diagnosis, staging and monitoring men who have established carcinoma. Considerable efforts have been made to enhance the specificity of PSA testing. In this regard, the ratio of the free-to-total PSA and the complex PSA show the most promise. It is highly likely that complex PSA, owing to the fact that it is the more specific form of PSA for carcinoma, will replace PSA testing in most applications. Finally, additional markers will be developed that will be useful in the management of men who have prostatic carcinoma. However, it is unlikely that these will replace PSA. Rather, they will primarily be used, in our opinion, to provide improved staging and prognostic information.

REFERENCES

1 Gutman AB, Gutman EB. 'Acid' phosphatase activity of the serum of normal human subjects. *Proc Soc Exp Biol Med* 1938;**38**:470.

2 Whitesel J, Donohue R, Mani J et al. Acid phosphatase: Its influence on the management of carcinoma of the prostate. *J Urol* 1984;**131**:70–72.

3 Burnett AL, Chan DW, Brendler CB, et al. Is it necessary to measure serum enzymatic acid phosphatase prior to radical prostatectomy? *J Urol* 1992;**147**[Abstract]:361.

4 Papsidero L et al. A prostate antigen in sera of prostatic cancer patients. *Cancer Res* 1980;**40**:2428–2432.

5 Chan DW, Bruzek DJ, Oesterling JE, Rock RC, Walsh PC. Prostate-specific antigen as a marker for prostatic cancer: a monoclonal and polyclonal immunoassay compared. *Clin Chem* 1987;**33**:1916.

6 Graves HCB, Wehner N, Stamey TA. Comparison of a polyclonal and monoclonal immunoassay for PSA: need for an international antigen standard. *J Urol* 1990;**144**:1516.

7 Jolley NL, Bacarese Hamilton. SR1 assays of alpha-fetoprotein, carcinoembryonic antigen, and prostate-specific antigen compared with corresponding established commercial assays. *Clin Chem* 1994;**40**:895–899.

8 Dnistrian AM, Schwartz MK, Smith CA, Nisselbaum JS, Fair WR. Abbott L1Mx evaluated for assay of prostate-specific antigen in serum. *Clin Chem* 1992;**38**:2140–2142.

9 Thorne T, Duncan M. Evaluation of Ciba Corning ACS 180: prostate-specific antigen assay. *Clin Chem* 1994;**40**:1008.

10 Gibbons AB, Jonza JJ, Hart T, Hohnadel DC, D'Souza JP, Mayer TK. Three-way comparison of prostatic specific antigen (PSA) using Hybritech Photon ERA-QA, Abbott 1Mx, and Ciba-Corning ACS-180. *Clin Chem* 1994;**40**:1012–1013.

11 Schambeck CM, Schmeller N, Steiber P, *et al.* Methodological and clinical comparison of the ACS PSA assay and the Tandem-E PSA assay in prostate cancer. *Urology* 1995;**46(2)**:195–199.

12 Semjonow A, Brandt B, Oberpenning F, Roth S, Hertie L. Discordance of assay methods creates pitfalls for the interpretation of prostatic-specific antigen values. *Prostate* 1996;**7(Suppl)**:3–16.

13 Stamey TA. Some comments on progress in the standardization of immunoassays for prostate-specific antigen. *Br J Urol* 1997;**79**:49–52.

14 Zhou AM, Tewari PC, Bluestein BI, Caldwell GW, Larsen FL. Multiple forms of PSA in serum. Differences in immunorecognition by monoclonal and polyclonal assays. *Clin Chem* 1993;**39**:2483–91.

15 Graves HC. Standardization of immunoassays for PSA: a problem of PSA complexion or a problem of assay design? *Cancer* 1993;**72**:3141–3144.

16 Wener MH, Daum PR, Close B, Brawer MK. Method-to-method and lot-to-lot variation in assays for prostate-specific antigen. *Am J Clin Pathol* 1994;**101**:387–388.

17 Brawer MK, Daum P, Petteway JC, Wener MH. Assay variability in serum PSA determination. *Prostate* 1995;**27(1)**:1–6.

18 Graves HCB. Issues on standardization of immunoassays for prostate-specific antigen: a review. *Clin Invest Med* 1993;**16**:415–424.

19 Semjonow A, Weining C, Oberpenning F, *et al.* Application of assay-specific cut-off values: results of the assay comparison study for PSA. *Eur Urol* 1999;**19(Suppl 2)**:18–21.

20 Catalona WJ, Richie JP, Ahmann FR, *et al.* Comparison of digital rectal examination and serum prostate-specific antigen in the early detection of prostate cancer: results of a multicenter clinical trial of 6,630 men. *J Urol* 1994;**151**:1283–1290.

21 Myrtel JF, Klimley PG, Ivor LP, Bruni JF. Clinical utility of prostate-specific antigen (PSA) in the management of prostate cancer. *Adv Cancer Diagn* 1986:1–4.

22 Link P, Freiha F, Stamey T. Adjuvant radiation therapy in patients with detectable prostate-specific antigen following radical prostatectomy. *J Urol* 1991;**145**:532–534.

23 Meek AG, Park TL, Oberman E, *et al.* A prospective study of PSA levels in patients receiving radiotherapy for localized carcinoma of the prostate. *Int J Radiat Oncol Biol Phys* 1990;**75**:1982.

24 Ritter MA, Messing EM, Shanahan TG, *et al.* Prostate-specific antigen as a predictor of radiotherapy response and patterns of failure in localized prostate cancer. *J Clin Oncol* 1992;**10**:1208–1217.

25 Stamey TA, Kabalin JN, Ferrari M. Prostate-specific antigen in the diagnosis and treatment of adenocarcinoma of the prostate. III. Radiation treated patients. *J Urol* 1989;**141**:1083–1087.

26 Kabalin J, Hodge K, McNeal J, *et al.* Identification of residual cancer in the prostate following radiation therapy: role of transrectal ultrasound guided biopsy and prostate-specific antigen. *J Urol* 1989;**142**:326.

27 Brawer M, Schifman R, Ahmann F, *et al.* The effect of digital rectal examination on serum levels of prostatic-specific antigen. *Arch Pathol Lab Med* 1988;**112**:1110.

28 Crawford E, Schutz M, Drago J, *et al.* The effect of digital rectal examination on PSA. *J Urol* 1991;**145**:398A.

29 Yuan JJ, Catalona WJ. Effect of digital rectal examination, prostate massage, transrectal ultrasonography and needle biopsy of the prostate on serum prostate-specific antigen levels. *J Urol* 1991;**145**:213A.

30 Ellis WJ, Brawer MK. The role of tumor markers in the diagnosis and treatment of prostate cancer. In: *Prostate Diseases.* Lepor H (ed.) W.B. Saunders: Philadelphia, 1993.

31 Brawer MK, Lange PH. PSA in the screening, staging and follow up of early-stage prostate cancer: a review of recent developments. *World J Urol* 1989;**7**:1–11.

32 Catalona WJ, Smith DS, Ratliff TL, *et al.* Measurement of PSA in serum as a screening test for prostate cancer. *N Engl J Med* 1991;**324**:1156–1161.

33 Brawer MK, Chetner MP, Beatie J, *et al.* Screening for prostatic carcinoma with PSA. *J Urol* 1992;**147**:841–845.

34 Brawer M. How to use PSA in the early detection or screening for prostatic carcinoma. *CA Canc J Clin* 1995;**45(3)**:148–164.

35 Brawer M, Beatie J, Wener M, Vessella R, Preston S, Lange P. Screening for prostatic carcinoma with PSA: results of the second year. *J Urol* 1993;**150(1)**:106–109.

36 Reissigl A, Pointer J, Horninger W, *et al.* Comparison of different prostate-specific antigen cutpoints for early detection of prostate cancer: results of a large screening population. *Urology* 1995;**46**:662–665.

37 Benson MC, Whang IS, Pantuck A, *et al.* Prostate-specific density: a means of distinguishing benign prostatic hypertrophy and prostate cancer. *J Urol* 1992;**147**:815–821.

38 Benson MC, Whang IS, Olsson CA, McMahon DJ, Cooner WH. The use of PSA density to enhance the predictive value of intermediate levels of serum PSA. *J Urol* 1992;**147**:817–821.

39 Seaman E, Whang M, Olsson CA, Katz A, Cooner WH, Benson MC. PSA density (PSAD): role in patient evaluation and management. *Urol Clin North Am* 1993;**20**:653.

40 Bazinet M, Meshref AW, Trudel C, *et al.* Prospective evaluation of prostate-specific antigen density and

systematic biopsies for early detection of prostatic carcinoma. *Urology* 1994;**43**:44–51.

41 Rommel FM, Augusta VE, Breslin J, *et al.* The use of PSA and PSAD in the diagnosis of prostate cancer in a community based urology practice. *J Urol* 1994;**151**:88–93.

42 Littrup PJ, Kane RA, Mettlin CJ, *et al.* Cost-effective prostate cancer detection: reduction of low-yield biopsies. *Cancer* 1994;**74(12)**:3146–3158.

43 Bangma CH, Kranse R, Blijenberg BG, Schroder FH. The value of screening tests in the detection of prostate cancer. Part I: results of a retrospective evaluation of 1726 men. *Urology* 1995;**46(6)**:773–778.

44 Brawer MK, Aramburu EAG, Chen GL, Preston SD, Ellis WJ. The inability of PSA index to enhance the predictive value of PSA in the diagnosis of prostatic carcinoma. *J Urol* 1993;**150**:369–373.

45 Mettlin C, Littrup PL, Kane RA, *et al.* Relative sensitivity and specificity of serum PSA level compared with age-referenced PSA, PSA density and PSA change. *Cancer* 1994;**74**:1615–1620.

46 Ohori M, Dunn JK, Scardino PT. Is prostate-specific antigen density more useful than prostate-specific antigen levels in the diagnosis of prostate cancer. *Urology* 1995;**46**:666–671.

47 Wener MH, Daum PR, Brawer MK. Variation in measurement of PSA. The importance of method and lot variability. *Clin Chem* 1995;**41(12)**:1730–1737.

48 Letran J, Meyer G, Loberiaz F, Brawer M. The effect of prostate volume on the yield of needle biopsy. *J Urol* 1998;**160(5)**:1718–1721.

49 Djavan B, Zlotta AR, Byttebier G, *et al.* Prostate-specific antigen density of the transition zone for early detection of prostate cancer. *J Urol* 1998;**160**:411–418.

50 Maeda H, Ishitoya S, Maekawa S, *et al.* Prostate-specific antigen density of the transition zone in the detection of prostate cancer. *J Urol.* 1997;**2193**:58A.

51 Lin DW, Gold MH, Ransom S, Ellis WJ, Brawer MK. Transition zone PSA density. Lack of utility in prediction of prostatic carcinoma. *J Urol* 1998;**160**:77–82.

52 Carter H, Morell CH, Pearson JD, *et al.* Estimation of prostatic growth using serial PSA measurements in men with and without prostate disease. *Cancer Res* 1992;**52**:3323–3328.

53 Porter JR, Hayward R, Brawer MK. The significance of short-term PSA change in men undergoing ultrasound guided prostate biopsy. *J Urol* 1994;**264**:293A.

54 Catalona WJ, Smith DS, Ratliff TL. Value or measurement of the rate of change of serum PSA levels in prostate cancer screening. *J Urol* 1993;**150**:300A.

55 Carter HB, Pearson JD, Chan DW, Guess HA, Walsh PC. Prostate-specific antigen variability in men without prostate cancer: effect of sampling interval on prostate-specific antigen velocity. *Urology* 1995;**45**:591.

56 Mantzoros CS, Tzonou A, Signorello LB, Stampfer M, Trichopoulos D, Adami HO. Insulin-like growth factor 1 in relation to prostate cancer and benign prostatic hyperplasia. *Br J Cancer* 1997;**76**:1115–1118.

57 Oesterling JE, Cooner WH, Jacobsen SJ, Guess JA, Lieber MM. Influence of patient age on the serum PSA concentration: an important clinical observation. *Urol Clin North Am* 1993;**20(4)**:671–680.

58 Etzioni R, Shen Y, Petteway JC, Brawer MK. Age-specific PSA: a reassessment. *Prostate* 1996;**7**:70–77.

59 Borer JG, Serman J, Solomon MC, *et al.* Age-specific reference ranges for prostate-specific antigen and digital rectal examination may not safely eliminate further diagnostic procedures. *J Urol* 1996;**155**:48A.

60 Christensson A, Laurell CB, Lilja H. Enzymatic activity of prostate-specific antigen and its reaction with extracellular serine proteinase inhibitors. *Eur J Biochem* 1990;**194**:755.

61 Stenman U, Leinonen J, Alfthan H, Rannikko S, Tuhkanen K, Althan O. A complex between PSA and a 1-antichymotrypsin is the major form of PSA in serum of patients with prostatic cancer: Assay of the complex improves clinical sensitivity for cancer. *Cancer Res* 1991;**51**:222.

62 Espana F, Sanchez CJ, Vera CD, Estelles A, Gilabert J. A quantitative ELISA for the measurement of complexes of prostate-specific antigen with protein C inhibitor when using a purified standard. *J Lab Clin Med* 1993;**122**:711–719.

63 Christensson A, Lilja J. Complex formation between protein C inhibitor and prostate-specific antigen *in vitro* and in human semen. *Eur J Biochem* 1994;**220**:45–53.

64 Zhang WM, Finne P, Leinonen J, *et al.* Characterization and immunological determination of the complex between prostate-specific antigen and alpha-2-macroglobulin. *Clin Chem* 1998;**44(12)**:2471–2479.

65 Lilja H, Haese A, Bjork T, *et al.* Significance and metabolism of complexed and non-complexed prostate-specific antigen (PSA) forms and human glandular kallikrein 2 (hK2) in localized prostate cancer before and after radical prostatectomy. *J Urol* 1999 (in press).

66 Christensson A, Bjork T, Nilsson O, *et al.* Serum prostate-specific antigen complexed to alpha 1-antichymotrypsin as an indicator of prostate cancer. *J Urol* 1993;**150(1)**:100–105.

67 Luderer AA, Chen Y, Thiel R, *et al.* Measurement of the proportion of free to total PSA improves diagnostic performance of PSA in the diagnostic gray zone of total PSA. *Urology* 1995;**46(2)**:187–194.

68 Higashihara E, Nutahara K, Kohima M, *et al.* Significance of serum free prostate-specific antigen in the screening of prostate cancer. *J Urol* 1996;**156**:1964–1968.

69 Chen Y, Luderer AA, Thiel RP, Carlson G, Cuny CL, Soriano TF. Using proportions of free to total prostate-specific antigen, age, and total prostate-specific antigen to predict the probability of prostate cancer. *Urology* 1996;**47(4)**:518–524.

70 Catalona WJ, Partin AW, Slawin KM, *et al.* Use of the percentage of free prostate-specific antigen to enhance differentiation of prostate cancer from benign prostatic

disease: a prospective multicenter clinical trial. *JAMA* 1998;**279**(19):1542–1547.

71 Hugosson J, Aus G, Bergdahl S, *et al.* Population based screening for prostate cancer by measurements of free and total concentrations of prostate-specific antigen (PSA). *Urology* 1999 (submitted).

72 Letran JL, Blase AB, Loberiaz FR, Meyer GE, Ransom SD, Brawer MK. Repeat ultrasound-guided prostate needle biopsy: The utility of free to total PSA ratio in predicting those men with or without prostatic carcinoma. *J Urol* 1998;**160**(2):426–429.

73 Djavan B, Remzi M, Seitz C, Marberger M, Zlotta A, Hammerer P. Serum-PSA, F/T PSA, PSAD, PSA-TZ and PSA, velocity: Early detection of prostate cancer in men with serum PSA levels of 2.5 to 4.0 ng/ml. *J Urol* 1999;**161**(Suppl):95.

74 Sokoll LJ, Bruzek DJ, Dunn W, Jones KA, Partin AW, Chan DW. Cancer detection rate for patients with total PSA concentrations, 4 ng/ml: Comparison of total, free, and complexed PSA. *J Urol* 1999;**161**(Suppl):318.

75 Yu E, McNight S, Ferreri LF, Brawer MK. Prostate specific biopsy in men with total prostate-specific antigen (PSA) less than 4.0 ng/ml: The role of complex PSA (cPSA). *J Urol* 1999;**161**(Suppl):321.

76 Piironen T, Pettersson K, Suonpaa M, *et al.* In vitro stability of free prostate-specific antigen (PSA) and prostate-specific antigen (PSA) complexed to alpha-1-antichymotrypsin in blood samples. *Urology* 1996;**48**(6A):81–87.

77 Woodrum DL, Brawer MK, Partin AW, Catalona WJ, Southwick PC. Interpretation of free prostate-specific antigen clinical research studies for the detection of prostate cancer. *J Urol* 1998;**159**:5–12.

78 Roth HJ, Christensen-Stewart S, Brawer MK. A comparison of three free and total PSA assays. *PCPD* 1998;**1**(6):326–331.

79 Nixon RG, Gold MH, Blase AB, Meyer GE, Brawer MK. Comparison of three investigative assays for the free form of prostate-specific antigen. *J Urol* 1998;**160**:420–425.

80 Brawer MK, Meyer GE, Letran JL, *et al.* Measurement of complexed PSA improves specificity for early detection of prostate cancer. *Urology* 1998;**52**(3):372–378.

81 Brawer MK, Cheh CD, Neaman IE, *et al.* Complexed prostate-specific antigen provides significant enhancement of specifity compared with total prostate-specific antigen for deteching prostate cancer. *J Urol* 2000 (in press).

82 Stamey TA, Yang N, Hay AR, *et al.* Prostate-specific antigen as a serum marker for adenocarcinoma of the prostate. *N Engl J Med* 1987;**317**:909–916.

83 Partin A, Carter H, Chan D, *et al.* Prostate-specific antigen in the staging of localized prostate cancer: Influence of tumor differentiation, tumor volume and benign hyperplasia. *J Urol* 1990;**143**:747–752.

84 Brawer MK, Lange PH. Prostate-specific antigen in management of prostatic carcinoma. Suppl to *Urol* 1989;**33**:11.

85 Catalona W, Smith D, Ratcliff T, *et al.*. Measurement of prostate-specific antigen in serum as a screening test for prostate cancer. *N Engl J Med* 1991;**324**:1156–1161.

86 Oesterling JE, Martin SK, Bergstraih EJ, *et al.* The use of prostate-specific antigen in staging patients with newly diagnosed prostate cancer. *JAMA* 1993;**269**(1):57–60.

87 Oesterling J, Chan D, Epstein J, *et al.* Prostate-specific antigen in the preoperative and postoperative evaluation of localized prostatic cancer treated with radical prostatectomy. *J Urol* 1988;**139**:766–772.

88 Carter HB, Partin AW, Oesterling JE, *et al.* The use of PSA in the management of patients with prostate cancer: The Johns Hopkins experience. *Clinical Aspects of Prostate Cancer* 1989;247–254.

89 Lange PH, Lightner DJ, Medini E, *et al.* The effect of radiation therapy after radical prostatectomy in patients with elevated PSA levels. *J Urol* 1990;**144**:927.

90 Stein A, deKernion JB, Smith RB, Dorey F and Patel H. PSA levels after radical prostatectomy in patients with organ confined and locally extensive prostate cancer. *J Urol* 1992;**147**:942.

91 Lightner D, Lange P, Reddy P, *et al.* Prostate-specific antigen and local recurrence after radical prostatectomy. *J Urol* 1990;**144**:921.

92 Foster LS, Shinahara K, Carol P, *et al.* The value of PSA and transrectal ultrasound-guided biopsy in accurately detecting prostatic fossa recurrences following radical prostatectomy. *J Urol* 1993;**149**:1024.

93 Abi-Aad AS, Macfarlane MT, Stein A *et al.* Detection of local recurrence after radical prostatectomy by PSA and TRUS. *J Urol* 1992;**147**:952.

94 Vessella RL, Noteboom J, Lange PH. Evaluation of the Abbott IMX (R) automated immunoassay of PSA. *Clin Chem* 1992;**38**:2044.

95 Takayama TK, Vessella RL, Brawer MK, *et al.* The enhanced detection of persistent disease after radical prostatectomy with a new PSA immunoassay. *J Urol* 1993;**150**:374.

96 Stamey TA, Graves H, Wehner N, *et al.* Early detection of residual prostate cancer after radical prostatectomy by an ultrasensitive assay for prostate-specific antigen. *J Urol* 1993;**149**:787–792.

97 Patel A, Doney F, Fanklin J, Dekernion JB. Recurrence patterns after radical retropubic prostatectomy: clinical usefulness of prostate-specific antigen doubling times and log slope prostate-specific antigen. *J Urol* 1997;**158**:1441–1445.

98 Russell KJ, Dunatov C, Hafermann JT, *et al.* Prostate-specific antigen in the management of patients with localized adenocarcinoma of the prostate treated with primary radiation therapy. *J Urol* 1991;**146**:1041–1052.

99 Stamey TA, Kabalin JN, Ferrari M, *et al.* Prostate-specific antigen in the diagnosis and treatment of adenocarcinoma of the prostate: IV. Anti-androgen treated patients. *J Urol* 1989;**141**:1088–1090.

100 Miller JI, Ahman FR, Drach GW, *et al.* The clinical

usefulness of serum PSA after hormonal therapy of metastatic prostate cancer. *J Urol* 1992;**147**:956.

101 Gillatt D, Gingell C and Smith PJB. Serum PSA for the assessment of response to hormonal therapy. *J Urol* 1990;**143**:207A.

102 Foti AG, Cooper JF, Herschman H, *et al*. Detection of prostatic cancer by solid-phase radioimmunoassay of serum prostatic acid phosphatase. *N Engl J Med* 1977;**297**:1357–1361.

103 Cooper JF, Foti AG, Herschman HH, *et al*. A solid phase radioimmunoassay for prostatic acid phosphatase. *J Urol* 1978;**119**:388.

104 Bruce AW, Mahan DE, Belville WD. The role of the radioimmunoassay for prostatic acid phosphatase in prostatic carcinoma. *Urol Clin N Amer* 1980;**7**:645.

105 Murphy GP, Chu TM, Karr JP. Prostatic acid phosphatase – the developing experience. *Clin Biochem* 1979;**12**:226.

106 Van Cangh PJ, Opsomer R, de Nayer P. Serum prostatic acid phosphatase determination in prostatic diseases: a critical comparison of an enzymatic and a radioimmunologic assay. *J Urol* 1982;**128**:1212.

107 Bruce A, Mahan D, Sullivan L, *et al*. The significance of prostatic acid phosphatase and adenocarcinoma of the prostate. *J Urol* 1981;**125**:357.

108 Ercole C, Lange P, Mathisen M, *et al*. Prostate-specific antigen and prostatic acid phosphatase in the monitoring and staging of patients with prostatic cancer. *J Urol* 1987;**138**:1181–1184.

109 Ferro M, Barnes I, Roberts J, *et al*. Tumor markers in prostatic carcinoma. A comparison of prostate-specific antigen with acid phosphatase. *Br J Urol* 1987;**60**:69.

110 Hudson M, Bahnson R, Catalona W. Clinical use of prostate-specific antigen in patients with prostate cancer. *J Urol* 1989;**142**:1011.

111 Nadji M, Tabei S, Castro A, *et al*. Prostatic-specific antigen: An immunohistologic marker for prostatic neoplasms. *Cancer* 1981;**48**:1229–1232.

112 Stein BS, Petersen RO, Vangore S, *et al*. Immunoperoxidase localization of PSA. *Am J Surg Path* 1982;**6**:553.

113 Vernon S, Williams W. Pre-treatment and post-treatment evaluation of prostatic adenocarcinoma for prostatic specific acid phosphatase and prostatic specific antigen by immunohistochemistry. *J Urol* 1983;**130**:95–98.

114 Ford T, Butcher D, Masters J, *et al*. Immunocytochemical localization of prostate-specific antigen: specificity and application to clinical practice. *Br J Urol* 1985;**57**:50.

115 Brawer M, Nagle R, Pitts W, *et al*. Keratin immunoreactivity as an aid to the diagnosis of persistent adenocarcinoma in irradiated human prostates. *Cancer* 1989;**63**:454.

116 Sohlberg OE, Bigler SA, Brawer MK. PSA immunohistochemistry in PIN. *J Urol* 1990;**143**:202A.

117 Stamey TA, Kabalin JN. Prostate-specific antigen in the diagnosis and treatment of adenocarcinoma of the prostate: I. Untreated patients. *J Urol* 1989;**141**:1070–1075.

Chapter 7

Screening for prostate cancer

INTRODUCTION

In the USA especially, both the general interest in prostatic carcinoma and the early detection/screening for this common neoplasm have already achieved staggering levels. The recommendations by the American Cancer Society[1], as well as the American Urologic Association, of an annual digital rectal examination (DRE) and prostate-specific antigen (PSA) test for all men over 50 for early detection of prostate cancer has further fostered interest in this area. The rest of the world has watched with some bemusement the machinations of urologists, oncologists, and primary-care practitioners, along with health planners, economists and the lay press in the US wrestling with the complex issues of early detection and screening. The need to resolve these conflicts for the sake of the patients has prompted both European and US randomized studies in screening for this most prevalent of neoplasms in men beyond middle age.

Despite a very real increase in the depth of our knowledge of prostatic carcinoma, which ranges from epidemiological insight into the perplexing increase in both incidence and mortality from this cancer, to our increasing understanding of the molecular basis of the disease, therapeutic advances, and improvement in diagnostic technology – the *sine qua non* of any screening protocol, proof that cancer-related mortality can be decreased – has not yet been achieved.

This has led many to assume a negative, if not nihilistic attitude towards early detection. However, one may be sobered by the reality that prostatic cancer is the number one malignancy in incidence in US men, and the second most common cause of cancer-related death[2,3].

It is clearly not feasible to wait 10–15 years, when the efficacy of early detection and treatment may be provided by the several international studies currently underway. Urologists worldwide must at least understand the lessons to be gleaned from the *existing* data, and apply this information wisely in order to help their patients make informed and rational decisions when faced with the threat of this insidious, and often lethal, disease.

It may sometimes be difficult to distinguish between screening and early detection. In the broad sense, *screening* represents the physician-initiated search for disease by invitation in an asymptomatic subject, and is distinct from *early detection,* which attempts to identify a condition in patients seeking medical care – albeit for an unrelated malady. From an epidemiological and ethical perspective these are certainly separable. However, by the time a patient presents to a clinician, the differences pale and the physician is in fact involved in early detection.

Historically, we have observed that the clinical diagnosis of prostate cancer is insensitive for identifying men with curable malignancies. Approximately 30% of patients detected clinically had disseminated disease with a median duration of survival of less than three years[4–7], and 30% of patients had clinical evidence of tumour extension beyond the confines of the prostate at the time of presentation[8,9]. Among such men, irrespective of the therapeutic approach employed, evidence of disease progression occurs generally well within 10 years[8,10,11].

Thus, if clinical parameters are relied upon, only approximately 40% of patients have potentially curable malignancy at the time of presentation. Of these, 10% have minimal cancer which is found upon transurethral prostatectomy, and which most clinicians believe does not require aggressive management. Therefore, without screening, less than one-third of all men presenting with carcinoma are suitable candidates for curative therapy. Among this third, pathological upstaging at radical prostatectomy occurs in approximately half[4,8,9,12].

Without early detection or screening, therefore,

only about 15% of those presenting clinically with prostate cancer have potentially curable neoplasm. Even among these most favourable patients, significant cancer-related mortality occurs, even with aggressive radiation therapy[13,14] or radical prostatectomy[15–17]. It is therefore clear that routine clinical approaches to the identification of men with prostate cancer are woefully inadequate. Most patients present with advanced local or metastatic disease, and even among those with favourable clinical parameters, cancer progression with its long, drawn-out morbidity and negative effects on the quality of life occurs all too often.

Prostate cancer clearly represents a significant problem. How, then, can we decrease cancer-related mortality? In general, for all neoplasms, we have three options: we can prevent the incidence of the disease; we can improve curative therapy; or we may enhance early detection – that is, identify more patients with cancers amenable to cure (**Table 7.1**). We do not know what causes prostate cancer, and until we do it is unlikely that we can significantly reduce the incidence. A large-scale chemoprevention trial utilizing the 5 alpha-reductase finasteride is currently underway in the USA, and other chemopreventative approaches are being considered. These investigations may result in a decrease in the incidence of prostate cancer, but the data will not be forthcoming for many years.

The second option in the battle to reduce prostate cancer-related mortality is to improve the efficacy of therapy. This is discussed in subsequent chapters on treatment. Suffice it to say here that while significant strides have been made in decreasing the morbidity of radiation therapy, radical prostatectomy as well as hormonal manipulation, whether any of these approaches has truly decreased cancer-related mortality remains to be proven. Thus we are left with early detection or screening in an attempt to reduce the death rate from this malignancy. If treatment for localized carcinoma is indeed effective, then identification of a greater percentage

of men with early disease makes intuitive sense. The widespread application of the early detection of prostate cancer stems from this logic.

For early detection, or indeed screening, to make sense, the disease in question must fulfill a number of criteria (**Table 7.2**). First, it should have a high prevalence; in a disease with a low prevalence, too many subjects must be tested for each carcinoma found, resulting in significant logistic as well as economic problems. Certainly prostatic carcinoma fulfills the requirement of high prevalence. Confounding this, however, is a unique feature of prostate cancer: the fact that the autopsy prevalence far exceeds that of clinically manifest disease. As previously cited, approximately 30% of men undergoing post-mortem examination without a clinical history of prostate cancer can be demonstrated to have histological evidence of prostatic cancer on serial sections of their prostate[15–18]. Cystoprostatectomy specimens from men with transitional-cell carcinoma of the urinary bladder have confirmed these findings[19–22]. For example, in 1985, 86 000 diagnoses of prostatic carcinoma were made in the United States. This represented only 1.05% of the estimated 8 193 000 men with 'autopsy' or latent carcinoma. Thus, in 1985, 0.31% of those who we can assume had microscopic foci of prostate cancer actually died of the disease[23]. However, these data do not take into consideration the importance of the prolonged period of risk in a man's life for either cancer development or progression. Scardino[23] 'factored in' the important variable of time and concluded that the lifetime risk of developing 'autopsy cancer' was 42%; the lifetime risk of developing 'clinical cancer' based on data from Seidman[3] was 9.5%, and the lifetime risk of dying of prostatic carcinoma was 2.9%.

The second requirement for an early detection or screening regimen is that the natural history of the disease be known. For prostate cancer, this is inextricably related to the dilemma associated with

Table 7.1 Approaches to reduce cancer-related mortality
• Decrease incidence
• Improve therapy
• Provide early detection

Table 7.2 Screening essentials
• Significant disease
• Known natural history
• Effective therapy
• Availability of diagnostic tests
• Subject acceptance
• Cost effectiveness

the discrepancy between histological evidence of disease and cancer-related morbidity and mortality. Of all human malignancies, prostate cancer exhibits the greatest variability in natural history, and it is in this arena that our ignorance makes recommendations about screening most troublesome.

A number of institutions have reported on the natural history of untreated prostatic carcinomas[24–29] (see **Table 7.3**). While one may derive information from these studies with respect to the outcome of untreated prostate cancer, the reader must be cautioned that all are hampered by methodological constraints; no report derives from a randomized controlled trial. Clearly, given the prevalence, we do not want to identify in early detection or screening programmes all of the men with cancers in their prostates. One might ask how many should be diagnosed? That is, how many cancers in men must we identify in order to offer treatment to the majority of patients whose malignancies would go on to affect the quantity or quality of their lives? While no definitive answer can be provided, Scardino and associates in a review of the features separating cancers with and without likely clinical sequelae have concluded that optimal efficiency would result if we could identify approximately 20% of the men with prostate cancer[30]. Thus, 6% (20% of the 30% autopsy prevalence) of men subjected to early detection/screening should have a cancer diagnosis. In the USA currently, it is estimated that around 3% of men will die eventually of prostate cancer. Implicit in this is the assurance that we can identify those cancers which possess a lethal potential during the course of the individual patient's lifetime, and successfully intervene. Moreover, we must not detect those much more prevalent malignancies that have low malignant potential. This is the most important issue in the early detection of prostatic carcinoma, and has already been discussed in the chapters on pathology and basic science issues.

The yield of any diagnostic test for detecting carcinoma obviously depends upon the prevalence of the disease in the population being evaluated. Because of variable study populations (i.e. whether patients present in a screening or early detection trial, are referred from other clinicians, or are gleaned from a urological practice) the prevalence of carcinoma may vary significantly; thus, meaningful comparison of studies of prostate cancer diagnosis is almost impossible. This must be remembered as we begin to examine the efficacy of screening tests.

Another essential for screening is the availability of diagnostic tests for the disease in question. In a sense, the elucidation of symptoms may be considered a test. Constitutional symptoms such as bone pain, weakness, weight loss, anaemia and uraemia may prompt the clinician to consider prostate carcinoma in the older man. Certainly such patients do not comprise an early detection or screening population. Symptomatic patients do, however, constitute a potential bias in the evaluation of the efficacy of early detection, because such patients generally have advanced disease. Comparison of the outcomes of those who present with symptoms, with those of healthy subjects participating in screening trials, almost universally results in the latter performing better. In general, neoplasms detected by screening are of smaller volume, lower stage, and better differentiated than carcinomas that give rise to symptoms. This phenomenon constitutes the so-called 'length–time' bias (**Table 7.4**).

Historically the most widely used test for the detection of prostate cancer was the digital rectal examination (DRE). The subjectivity of the DRE,

Table 7.3 Results of expectant management of prostatic carcinoma					
Author	**Number of patients**	**Mean F.U. (years)**	**Overall mortality (%)**	**CaP mortality (%)**	**CaP progression (includes CaP death)**
Johansson et al.[24]	223	10.2	56	8	34
Whitmore, Warner and Thompson[25]	75	9.5	39	15	69
Hanash et al.[26]	179	15	55	45	NA
George[27]	120	15	44	4	83
Madsen et al.[28]	50	10	52	6	18

Table 7.4 Length-time bias	
'Screened' patients	**'Clinical' patients**
Asymptomatic	Symptomatic
Earlier cancer	More advanced cancer
Slower growing	Rapidly growing
Lower stage	Higher stage
Lower grade	Higher grade

differing skills among examiners and our increasing suspicion of subtle abnormalities, have resulted in great variability in the yield of cancer detected in men with an abnormality on digital rectal examination. Detection rates of 0.8–25.2% have been reported, along with positive predictive values of 6.3–50% (see **Table 7.5**).

In the experience in Seattle, carcinoma has been detected in 40 of 229 men (17.5%) with normal-feeling prostates undergoing biopsy because of elevated prostate-specific antigen level, or being evaluated for alternative therapies to bladder-outlet obstruction owing to presumed benign prostatic hyperplasia (BPH) (**Table 7.6**). Twenty-four of 185 men (13.0%) with asymmetry as their only abnormality and 112 of 456 (24.6%) with prostatic induration revealed carcinoma. In contrast, 79 of 150 men (52.7%) with clearly palpable nodules or areas of marked induration strongly suggestive of carcinoma actually demonstrated malignancy.

Transrectal ultrasound (TRUS) is the most common approach for imaging the prostate; it offers several advantages to other imaging modalities. TRUS is a readily accepted, fairly simple procedure affording excellent visualization of the gland. It has the advantage of being able to identify suspicious lesions in the prostate which are non-palpable. A number of authorities, including Cooner et al.[31], Lee et al.[32] and Drago et al.[33], reported a 1.3–2 fold increase in the detection rate of carcinoma when digital rectal examination was compared to TRUS (**Table 7.7**). In early detection and screening studies, detection rates of 1.7–37.5%, and positive predictive values of 6.8–58.3%, have been reported. However, the procedure is hampered by its high cost, and this, in conjunction with overall inadequate performance (sensitivity and specificity), makes this test unsuitable for the early detection of carcinoma (**7.1 and 7.2**). Despite these limitations, transrectal ultrasound-guided prostate needle biopsy employing a spring-loaded biopsy device is undoubtedly the best way of providing histological samples of the prostate. The procedure is simple and rapid with low, acceptable morbidity (around 2–3% infective complications) presuming that appropriate antimicrobial prophylaxis is administered for a sufficient period.

Prostate-specific antigen (PSA) has already been reviewed in Chapter 6. Here we shall confine our

Table 7.5 Results of prostate cancer screening by digital rectal examination		
Source	**No. of cancer/no. of patients screened (%)**	**Positive predictive value**
Catalona, Smith and Ratliff[59]	146/6630 (2.2)	146/683 (21.4)
Cooner et al.[31]	203/807 (25.2)	203/470 (43.2)
Chodak and Schoenberg[60]	36/2131 (1.7)	36/144 (25.0)
Faul[61]	1951/1,500,000 (0.1)	1951/11,308 (17.3)
Gilbertsen[62]	75/5856 (1.3)	–
Jenson, Shahon and Wangensteen[63]	36/4367 (0.8)	–
Lee et al.[64]	10/784 (1.3)	10/29 (34.5)
McWhorter et al.[65]	4/34 (1.8)	4/8 (50.0)
Mettlin et al.[66]	33/2425 (13.6)	33/118 (28.0)
Mueller et al.[67]	312/11,523 (2.7)	122/312 (39.1)
Thompson et al.[68]	17/2005 (0.8)	17/65 (26.2)
Vihko et al.[69]	6/771 (0.8)	6/27 (22.2)
Waaler et al.[70]	1/480 (0.2)	1/16 (6.3)

| Table 7.6 Yield for DRE in which all men underwent TRUS biopsy irrespective of the DRE result |||
DRE	Biopsy	Carcinoma (%)
Normal	224	40 (17.9)
Asymmetry	181	24 (13.3)
Induration	448	111 (24.8)
Malignant	148	78 (56.7)

| Table 7.7 Results of prostate cancer screening by TRUS |||
Author	No. of cancer/ No. of subjects screened (%)	Positive predictive value (%)
Cooner et al.[31]	263/1807 (14.6)	263/835 (31.5)
Devonec, Chapeleon and Cathignol[71]	42/213 (19.7)	42/132 (31.8)
Fritzsche et al.[72]	41/228 (18.0)	41/121 (33.9)
Hunter et al.[73]	29/508 (5.7)	29/119 (24.4)
Lee et al.[32]	20/748 (2.7)	20/64 (31.3)
McWhorter et al.[65]	7/34 (20.6)	7/12 (58.3)
Mettlin et al.[66]	44/2425 (1.8)	44/290 (15.2)
Perrin et al.[74]	11/666 (1.7)	11/162 (6.8)
Ragde et al.[75]	50/765 (6.5)	50/138 (36.2)
Rifkin, Friedland and Shortliffe[76]	3/112 (2.7)	3/8 (37.5)

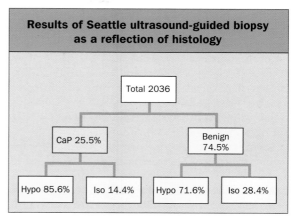

7.1 Results of Seattle ultrasound-guided biopsy as a reflection of histology. Yield of transrectal ultrasonography-guided pelvic node biopsy by patient. CaP, prostatic carcinoma; Hypo, hypoechoic peripheral zone lesion; Iso, no hypoechoic peripheral zone lesion. (Reproduced with permission from Walsh PC, Retik AB (eds) *Campbell's Urology* 7th edn, Vol. 3, Philadelphia: W.B. Saunders; 1998.)

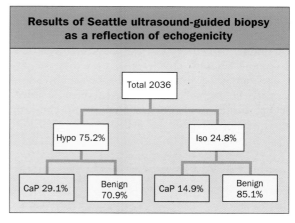

7.2 Results of Seattle ultrasound-guided biopsy as a reflection of echogenicity. Yield of transrectal ultrasonography-guided pelvic node biopsy by patient. CaP, prostatic carcinoma; Hypo, hypoechoic peripheral zone lesion; Iso, no hypoechoic peripheral zone lesion. (Reproduced with permission from Walsh PC, Retik AB (eds) *Campbell's Urology* 7th edn, Vol. 3, Philadelphia: W.B. Saunders; 1998.)

comments to its utility in early detection and screening. After the development of sensitive assays for serum PSA detection, considerable enthusiasm was generated for the utility of this test for the detection of prostate cancer. Several investigators have utilized PSA as the initial test in an early-detection programme. Catalona and associates[34], employing the Hybritech Tandem-R assay and utilizing a 4.0 ng/ml cut off, examined 1653 men over the age of 50. The overall detection rate was 2.2% and positive predictive value 33%.

At Seattle, Brawer et al. have conducted a similar study examining 1249 men over age 50 with the Hybritech Tandem-R assay as the initial test in an early-detection programme[35]. The overall detection rate was 2.6% and the positive predictive value 30.5%. Two smaller screening studies in the UK also reported a detection rate of around 2%[36,37].

In an effort to understand how we should follow-up men with an initially normal PSA, Brawer et al.

elected to perform digital rectal examination and transrectal ultrasound, as well as ultrasound-guided biopsy, in men in the original screening cohort who, on evaluation one year later, had a 20% increase in their PSA level[38]. Schmid and associates[39] demonstrated that the PSA doubling time in untreated localized prostate cancer is around 4–5 years, offering some biological rationale to our selection of a 20% cut off to select subjects for biopsy.

Seven hundred and one patients returned for the second year of our screening study. Two hundred and sixty (37.1%) demonstrated a greater than 20% increase in PSA value (**Table 7.8**). Biopsies were performed on 82 of these men and carcinoma detected in 14 (17.1%). Twelve of the men with carcinoma (86%) had a second year PSA <4.0 ng/ml. Radical prostatectomy was performed on 8 patients. Seven of these had organ-confined disease or tumour penetrating the capsule with negative surgical margins[38].

In the third year of studying the original cohort. Seven hundred and thirty-eight men returned; 260 (35.2%) had a 20% annualized PSA elevation, 70 (50.8%) underwent biopsy, and carcinoma was detected in 13 (18.6%). The observed prostatic carcinoma detection rates for years 1–3 were 2.6, 2.0 and 1.8% respectively.

Despite the reasonable performance of PSA in an early-detection realm, one caveat must be noted. A significant number of men in whom prostatic carcinoma is detected have PSA < 4.0 ng/ml. For instance, in a recent compilation of our ultrasound-guided prostate needle biopsy series, carcinoma was noted in 542 of 2197 men (24.7%) who had undergone six systematic random biopsies. Sixty-nine of these 542 patients (12.7%) had a pre-operative PSA level <4.0 ng/ml.

Comparison of these three diagnostic tests may be best achieved using the receiver-operating characteristic curve. When we applied this to our series, PSA had the best performance characteristics (7.3).

A number of investigators have examined PSA in conjunction with other diagnostic techniques, primarily DRE and TRUS. Most studies have confirmed that approximately one out of three men with a PSA greater than 4.0 ng/ml has carcinoma (**Table 7.8**). A review of these and other series demonstrates the minimal importance of transrectal ultrasonography if there is an abnormality on DRE or elevated PSA. This has led to the widespread practice of performing TRUS only in men with either a palpable prostatic abnormality or an elevation in serum PSA or both.

One of the definitive trials on screening in the USA was that reported by Catalona and associates in 1994[40]. This multi-institutional trial evaluated 6630 men aged 50 years or older who underwent testing with DRE and serum PSA determination. Biopsy was performed in a quadrant fashion for those men who had a PSA greater than 4.0 ng/ml or abnormality of the DRE: 15% of men had a PSA greater than 4.0 ng/ml and 15% had a

Table 7.8 Yield of DRE, TRUS and PSA

DRE	TRUS	PSA	Catalona et al.[34] BX/CaP (% CaP)	Cooner et al.[31] BX/CaP (% CaP)	Lee et al.[32] BX/CaP (% CaP)	Mettlin et al.[66] BX/CaP (% CaP)	Brawer et al.[77] BX/CaP (% CaP)	Catalona et al.[40] BX/CaP (% CaP)	Total BX/CaP (% CaP)
–	–	–	11/0 (0)				23/0 (0)		37/0 (0)
–	–	+	37/6 (16)				53/10 (19)	686/216 (32)	776/242 (31)
+	–	–	17/0 (0)			30/5 (17)	78/5 (6)	683/146 (21)	808/156 (19)
–	+	–	35/2 (6)	204/19 (9)	44/2 (5)	164/9 (6)	55/4 (7)		502/36 (7)
–	+	+	63/14 (22)	161/41 (25)	92/31 (34)	37/9 (24)	96/26 (27)	191/57 (30)	640/178 (28)
+	–	+	49/16 (33)			8/3 (38)	50/8 (16)	63/26 (41)	170/53 (31)
+	+	–	53/11 (21)	195/33 (17)	23/6 (26)	48/7 (15)	305/44 (14)	232/32 (14)	856/133 (16)
+	+	+	81/49 (60)	275/170 (62)	89/63 (71)	25/17 (68)	352/157 (45)	117/64 (55)	939/520 (55)

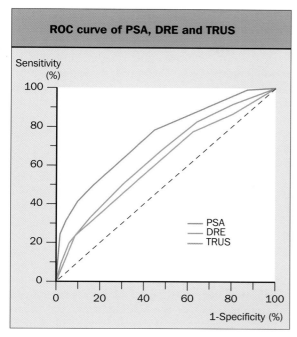

ROC curve of PSA, DRE and TRUS

Sensitivity (%)

- PSA
- DRE
- TRUS

1-Specificity (%)

7.3 Receiver operating characteristic (ROC) curve comparing PSA, DRE and TRUS in a biopsy population. Note that overall PSA is the best predictor of carcinoma. (Reproduced with permission from Ellis WJ, Chetner M, Preston S, *et al.* Diagnosis of prostatic carcinoma: the yield of serum PSA, DRE and TRUS. *J Urol* 1994;**152(5)**:1520–1525.)

suspicious digital rectal examination, and 26% had an abnormality of one or both tests.

Overall 1167 men underwent biopsy and carcinoma was detected in 264 (positive biopsy rate 22.6%). Serum PSA was identified in 82% of the men who had malignancy, whereas DRE was abnormal in only 55%. Cancer detection rates for DRE, serum PSA level and both were 3.2, 4.6, and 5.8%, respectively. The positive biopsy rate was 32% for PSA and 21% for DRE. Of the 160 men who underwent radical prostatectomy, the cancer was organ confined in 71%. The authors concluded that serum PSA in combination with DRE significantly enhanced early prostate cancer detection.

One interesting group presenting symptomatically comprises those men complaining of bladder outlet obstruction. Incidental carcinoma of the prostate is found in 10–20% of men undergoing transurethral prostatectomy (TURP) for presumed benign disease[41]. In the American College of Surgeons review, nearly one half of all prostate cancer

was found incidentally[42]. With the increasing utility of non-surgical or lesser-surgical approaches to the treatment of BPH, such as alpha-adrenergic blockade, 5 alpha-reductase inhibitors, laser prostatectomy, thermotherapy, and so on, there is a genuine need for methods to discriminate between those patients with potentially clinically significant carcinoma and those with BPH alone.

We have evaluated 91 men seeking treatment in Seattle for bladder outlet obstruction with transrectal ultrasound (TRUS) and biopsy[43] (**Table 7.9**). The overall cancer-detection rate in this group was greater than that found in screening studies of asymptomatic men (13.2%). All cancers were found in men with either an abnormality on the DRE (including asymmetry), or a PSA greater than 4.0 ng/ml. Lepor has recently reported similar data[44].

SUMMARY OF SCREENING TESTS

Improvements in our diagnostic armamentarium have increased the sensitivity for subtle abnormalities on rectal examination, TRUS ultrasound-

Table 7.9 Histology of men with bladder-outlet obstruction undergoing TRUS biopsy

DRE	PSA (ng/ml)	Biopsy	CaP	% CaP
Normal	<4.0	47	0	0
	4.0–10.0	8	1	12.5
	>10.0	1	1	100.0
Asymmetry	<4.0	3	0	0
	4.0–10.0	0	0	0
	>10.0	0	0	0
Induration	<4.0	10	2	20.0
	4.1–10.0	8	2	25.0
	>10.0	6	3	50.0
'Malignant'	<4.0	5	1	20.0
	4.1–10.0	3	2	66.7
	>10.0	0	0	0
Total		91	12	

guided biopsy and most importantly PSA, have truly revolutionized the detection of prostatic carcinoma. Several observations emerge from the numerous reports on the application of these to screening and early detection. As a single diagnostic test, PSA offers the best performance characteristics. Utilizing PSA, significantly higher positive predictive values are realized than that reported for mammography[45,46]. Even greater efficacy (positive predictive value) is realized if PSA is combined with DRE. PSA index, while intuitively making sense, seems in at least some settings to offer little more stratification of men who do or do not harbour malignancy than PSA alone. Transrectal ultrasound, while invaluable for performing biopsy, seems to add little to DRE and PSA in selecting men for biopsy.

Moreover, patients whose carcinomas are detected utilizing these modalities tend to have more favourable stage. For example, in Catalona et al.[34] as well as Brawer's PSA-based series[35], virtually all men had clinically localized malignancies (**Table 7.10**). While significant pathological upstaging was noted in the first year, with serial monitoring of the cohort, the vast majority of patients have organ-confined disease (**Table 7.11**).

EARLY DIAGNOSIS AND SCREENING FOR PROSTATE CANCER

Early detection and screening is now commonplace throughout the USA. The impact, however, is difficult to assess. As is shown in Chapter 1, early detection resulted in a peaking in the incidence of prostate cancer in 1991 in Western Washington and by 1992 in the rest of the USA[47]. Although the ultimate impact of such efforts cannot be assessed, it is heartening to realize as recently reported by Mettlin and associates that for the first time the mortality rate of prostate cancer in the USA is beginning to decrease[48]. Although a number of factors may result in this encouraging statistic, this may be an early indication of the efficacy of screening.

The early clinical and pathologic stage at diagnosis observed in the early PSA screening studies shown in **Tables 7.10 and 7.11** have been echoed in a compilation of the findings from the Mayo Clinic[49]. These authors report on 5568 radical prostatectomies performed between 1987 and 1995. Stage T1c increased from 2 to 37% during this interval while T3 disease decreased from 25 to 7%.

Table 7.10 Clinical stage in PSA screening patients				
Clinical stage	**Catalona et al.[34] (Year 1)**	**Brawer et al.[35] (Year 2)**	**Brawer et al.[36] (Year 3)**	**Brawer et al.[38]**
		PSA > 4.0 ng/ml (%)		
T1c	–	4 (33.3)	1 (14.3)	
T2	–	8 (67.8)	6 (85.7)	
T3	–	–	–	
N+, M+	–	–	–	
		PSA 4.0–10.0 ng/ml (%)		
T1c	19 (100)	6 (26.1)	1 (50.0)	2 (40.0)
T2	–	16 (69.6)	1 (50.0)	3 (60.0)
T3	–	1 (4.3)	–	–
N+, M+	–	–	–	–
		PSA < 10.0 ng/ml (%)		
T1c	10 (58.8)	2 (22.2)	1 (50.0)	1 (100.0)
T2	–	6 (67.3)	1 (50.0)	–
T3	7 (41.2)	1 (11.1)	–	–
N+, M+	–	–	–	–

Table 7.11 Pathological stage in PSA screening patients				
Pathological stage	Catalona *et al.*[34]	Brawer *et al.*[35] (Year 1)	Brawer *et al.*[36] (Year 2)	Brawer *et al.*[36] (Year 3)
			PSA less than 4.0 ng/ml	
PT1–T2	–		6/8 (75/0)	2 (66.7)
PT1–T2	–	–	–	
			PSA 4.0 to 10.0 ng/ml	
PT1–T2	10/17 (58.8)	9/12 (75.0)	1/8 (12.5)	1 (33.3)
PT3–T4, N+	7/17 (41.2)	3/12 (25.0)		1/8 (12.5)
			PSA more than 10.0 ng/ml	
PT1–T2	2/16 (12.5)	–	–	
PT3–T4, N+	14/16 (87.5)	4/4 (100.0)	–	

The Stanford group has reported similar findings comparing radical prostatectomies performed between 1988 and 1996[50]. They noted that although there was a shift toward T1c carcinoma, cancer volume percent Gleason grade 4 or 5, serum PSA, the incidence of very small cancers did not change during this interval. Other reports have similarly indicated an important stage shift associated with early detection programmes[51–53].

PROBLEMS WITH SCREENING

Despite these encouraging observations, screening for prostate cancer may potentially give rise to significant problems (**Table 7.12**). Briefly, these may be divided into scientific, ethical, legal, and economic. In each of these domains, unfortunately, more questions remain about the efficacy of screening for prostate cancer than we have answers.

Problems in the scientific issues of screening include 'lead-' and 'length-time' bias as well as the very real potential of overdetection. Length-time bias has already been discussed. Lead-time bias occurs because, if we do nothing to alter the natural history with therapy, patients whose cancers are diagnosed as part of a screening programme will have a survival advantage (the lead time). However, no actual increased longevity may in fact be realized.

Overdetection is a significant issue in screening for prostatic carcinoma, perhaps more so than for any other malignancy. The discrepancy between

Table 7.12 Prostate carcinoma screening: what we need to know
• Does treatment for localized prostate cancer result in a reduction in morbidity and mortality?
• Do screening tests identify patients who are curable and who need to be cured?
• What are the best screening tests to use, in whom and how often?
• Can we afford it?

prevalence and clinically manifest disease and the implications of this in screening have already been alluded to.

Additional support for the potential lack of utility of early detection comes from the reports indicating the long natural history and the low cancer-related death rate owing to prostatic carcinoma in series of untreated patients previously described. It must be reiterated, however, that these derive from highly selected populations. Patient-selection bias, concurrent disease, tumour characteristics, and so on, make clear conclusions from these series difficult.

It seems obvious that some older men in whom cancer of the prostate is discovered may be better off untreated; however, one must balance this observation with the fact that all of the 3% of men destined to die of prostatic carcinoma at one point surely had curable neoplasms.

Many ethical dilemmas surround screening for prostate cancer. Society must decide the appropriate level of health resources to be applied to this disease. Certainly, the administration in Washington is scrutinizing the current approach in the US. Legal issues primarily surround the concept of informed consent. Should a man undergo explanation of not only the potential benefits to be derived by application of screening tests but also the potential costs in terms of discomfort, morbidity, anxiety, as well as fiscal?

One of the biggest problems associated with prostate cancer screening is the tremendous potential cost incurred. The actual economic implications become increasingly significant when one realizes that the cost of early detection and screening is not merely the cost of the diagnostic test, even when it includes biopsy, pathology, staging and so forth. The true cost includes such factors as patient education, advertising for screening, treatment of complications of the diagnostic tests staging, definitive therapy, secondary therapy, monitoring of patients, and treatment of complications. Although several authors have estimated the cost likely to be incurred by widespread screening programmes based on various modelling approaches, the lack of unanimity of their conclusions mandates actual cost analysis of ongoing trials.

Labrie and associates[54] calculated the cost of cancer detection using combination of PSA greater than 3.0 ng/ml and DRE for the initial evaluation was $2665 at the first visit. This is contrasted with estimates of $10 000 for detection of a case of cervical cancer and $30 000 for carcinoma of the breast.

Several critical issues need to be answered before widespread recommendation of prostate cancer screening can be made (**Table 7.13**). We need prospective studies to definitively answer whether treatment for prostate cancer results in a decrease

in mortality. This demands randomization of men into treatment and no-treatment arms with long follow-up, with both all-cause and cancer-related mortality being ascertained. Several studies are underway or have been planned. The Swedish Oncology Group is randomizing men to radical prostatectomy versus watchful waiting. In Denmark, men are being randomized to external-beam radiation or expectant management. These studies are well-designed in that they offer randomization, but are unfortunately limited in the number of patients to be evaluated. Moreover, their Scandinavian setting may instil biases as we try to extrapolate the result of these investigations to populations in the rest of the world.

The 'Prostatectomy Versus Observation for Clinically Localized Carcinoma of the Prostate' (PIVOT) trial, will randomize 1050 men in the USA to radical prostatectomy versus expectant management. This trial, under the auspices of the Veterans Affairs Cooperative Study Program and the National Cancer Institute, is powered to detect a decrease in cancer-related mortality of 15%, and an overall decrease in mortality of 45%, and should definitively answer the question of whether radical prostatectomy works in men with clinically localized disease[55]. Unfortunately, the results of the trial will not be known for many years; moreover, there are worries about the problems of recruiting into a study with a no-treatment arm.

Whether screening results in decreased cancer-related mortality remains to be proven. Obviously, as noted, this presupposes effective therapy, which should be answered by the above-mentioned studies. The PLCO trial (Prostate, Lung, Colon, Ovarian), funded by the National Cancer Institute and currently underway, randomizes men to screening with PSA and DRE versus no screening[56]. This large, cohort, multi-institutional trial utilizes cancer mortality as an endpoint, and is an attempt to answer the question of whether early detection works. Unfortunately, no standard therapeutic regimens are provided, potentially resulting in significant biases. The biggest problem associated with this trial is whether indeed a non-screen population can still be identified in the USA where PSA testing is already so prevalent.

Recently Labrie and associates[57] reported on a prospective randomized control trial of prostate cancer screening in Quebec, Canada. In this investigation, 46 193 men gathered from the electoral

Table 7.13 Problems with screening
• Overdetection
• Unknown natural history
• Therapy unproven
• Economic
• Ethical
• Legal

rolls of Quebec were randomized in November of 1988 between screening and no screening.

The evaluation included PSA testing and a level greater than 3.0 ng/ml was an indication for further work-up along with digital rectal examination. Transrectal ultrasound was performed if there was an abnormality in either of these two tests and biopsy performed if the PSA was above the predicted value based on gland volume. In evaluations, PSA alone was used for screening.

The authors noted that there were 137 deaths due to prostate cancer among the 38 056 men who did not undergo screening, but only five deaths among the 8137 men who were screened. The calculated death rate per 100 000 man years in the unscreened and screened groups was 48.7 vs 15, respectively. The authors concluded that expectation of men at risk for prostate cancer with DRE and PSA in combination with effective treatment of localized disease resulted in a 'dramatic decrease in deaths from prostate cancer'. The authors are to be commended for reporting on the first true randomized trial in screening. Obviously, their results are impressive. However, several methodologic problems exist in this study. There was a significant crossover in the cohorts – that is, men who were not randomized to screening but were screened, and of equal concern, men who were randomized to screening, but were not screened, and thus were counted in the nonscreen cohort. This comprised 76.9% of the men originally scheduled for screening. In an attempt to screen subanalysis, comprising the 23.1% of men actually screened, only a 6% decrease in prostate cancer death rate was observed between screened and not screened. This may indeed be a pivotal study given the fact that it was initiated before widespread application of PSA was realized in Canada or elsewhere. Another very important trial currently underway is the European Randomized Study of Screening for Prostate Cancer (ERSPC)[58]. Seven countries and 17 centers are participating. and 60% of accrual has been completed. As with the PLCO trial, results will not be available for approximately 5 more years.

In conclusion, screening for prostatic carcinoma is associated with the potential for both considerable problems and substantial benefits. How should the individual clinician proceed today? It seems appropriate that the gatekeeper – the individual who should make the decision whether or not early detection is warranted – should not be the urologist, but, more appropriately, that this decision should fall on the primary-care practitioner. He or she can weigh all of the evidence and factors surrounding the costs and benefits to accrue to the individual man. Factors to consider include the patient's overall health and intercurrent disease, socioeconomic considerations as well as physiological and chronological age and life expectancy. Only after appropriate and detailed counselling of the patient with regard to both the benefits and the potential risk of early detection of prostatic carcinoma can an appropriate decision be made.

If it is determined that it is in the best interests of the patient to be evaluated for prostatic cancer, then a carefully performed digital rectal examination and serum PSA determination should be accomplished. Biopsy should be performed for abnormality in either, ideally under sonographic guidance. The appropriate interval for such testing remains to be defined, but is probably less frequently than annually.

If, after an analysis by the primary-care practitioner, it is not in the best interests of the patient to have an early diagnosis of prostatic carcinoma, because, for example, comorbidity suggests a life expectancy of < 10 years, then we believe no testing should be performed and the patient informed accordingly.

REFERENCES

1 American Cancer Society. Guidelines for the cancer-related health checkup: Recommendations and rationale. *CA* 1980;**30**:194.

2 Landis SH, Murray T, Bolden S, Wingo PA. Cancer statistics. *CAJ* 1999;**49**:8–31.

3 Seidman H, Mushinski MH, Geib SK *et al.* Probabilities of eventually developing or dying of cancer – United States, 1985. *CA* 1985;**35**:36–56.

4 Crawford ED. A controlled trial of leuprolide with and without flutamide in prostatic carcinoma. *N Engl J Med* 1989;**321**:419–424.

5 Scardino PT, Gervasi L, Mata LA. The prognostic significance of the extent of nodal metastasis in prostatic cancer. *J Urol* 1989;**142**:332–336.

6 Austenfield MS, Davis BE. New concepts in the treatment of stage D1 adenocarcinoma of the prostate. *Urol Clin North America* 1990;**17**:867–884.

7 Zincke H, Utz D, Thule Pi, *et al.* Treatment options for patients with stage DI (T0–3, N1–2, M0) adenocarcinoma of the prostate. *Urology* 1987;**30**:307–315.

8 Smith J Jr, Haynes T, Middleton R. Impact of external irradiation on local symptoms and survival free of disease in patients with pelvic lymph node metastasis from adenocarcinoma of the prostate. *J Urol* 1984;**131**:705–707.

9 Mench HR, Garfinkel L, Dodd GD. Preliminary report of the National Cancer Data Base. *CA* 1991;**41**:7–18.

10 Carlton CEJ, Scardino PT. Long-term results after combined radioactive gold seed implantation and external beam radiotherapy for localized prostatic cancer. In: *A Multidisciplinary Analysis of Controversies in the Management of Prostate Cancer.* Coffey D, Resnick M, Dorr R (ed.) Plenum: New York; 1988.

11 Bagshaw MA. Radiation therapy for cancer of the prostate In: *Diagnosis and Management of Genitourinary Cancer.* Skinner D, Lieskovsky S (ed.) W.B. Saunders: Philadelphia; 1988.

12 Lepor H, Kimball AW, Walsh PC. Cause-specific actuarial survival analysis: A useful method for reporting survival data in men with clinically localized prostatic cancer: Long term results. *J Urol* 1989;**141**:82–84.

13 Gibbons R, Correa R Jr, Brannen G, *et al.* Total prostatectomy for clinically localized prostatic cancer: long-term results. *J Urol* 1989;**131**:564–566.

14 Paulson DF, Moul JW, Walter PJ. Radical prostatectomy for stage T1–2 N0 M0 prostatic adenocarcinoma, long term results. *J Urol* 1990;**144**(5):1180–1184.

15 McNeal JE, Bostwick DG, Kindrachuck RA, *et al.* Patterns of progression in prostate cancer. *Lancet* 1986;**1**:60–63.

16 Franks LM. Latency and progression in tumors: The natural history of prostatic cancer. *Lancet* 1956;**2**:1037.

17 Dhom G. Epidemiologic aspects of latent and clinically manifest carcinoma of the prostate. *J Cancer Res Clin Oncol* 1983;**106**:210.

18 Scott R Jr, Mutchnik DL, Laskowski TZ *et al.* Carcinoma of the prostate in elderly men: Incidence, growth characteristics and clinical significance. *J Urol* 1969;**101**:602–607.

19 Kabalin JN, McNeal JE, Price HM, *et al.* Unsuspected adenocarcinoma of the prostate in patients undergoing cystoprostatectomy for other causes: Incidence, histology and morphometric observations. *J Urol* 1989;**141**:1091–1094.

20 Montie JE, Wood DP Jr, Pontes JE, *et al.* Adenocarcinoma of the prostate in cystoprostatectomy specimens removed for bladder cancer. *Cancer* 1989;**63**:381–385.

21 Babaian RJ, Troncoso P, Ayala A. Transurethral resection zone prostate cancer detected at cystoprostatectomy. *Cancer* 1991;**67**:1418–1422.

22 Troncoso P, Babaian RJ, Ro JY, *et al.* Prostatic intraepithelial neoplasia and invasive prostatic adenocarcinoma in cystoprostatectomy specimens. *Urology* 1989;**34**(Suppl):52–56.

23 Scardino PT. Early detection of prostate cancer. *Urol*

Clin North Am 1989;**16**:635–655.

24 Johansson J-E, Adami H, Andersson S-O, *et al.* High 10-year survival rate in patients with early, untreated prostatic cancer. *JAMA* 1992;**267**:2191–2196.

25 Whitmore W Jr, Warner J, Thompson I Jr. Expectant management of localized prostatic cancer. *Cancer* 1991;**67**:1091–1096.

26 Hanash K, Cooke E, Taylor W, *et al.* Carcinoma of the prostate: A 15-year follow-up. *J Urol* 1972;**107**: 450–453.

27 George NJR. Natural history of localized prostate cancer managed by conservative therapy alone. *Lancet* 1988;**110**: 95–100.

28 Madsen PO, Graverson PH, Gasser TC, *et al.* Treatment of localized prostatic cancer: Radical prostectomy vs. placebo: A 15-year followup. *Scand J Urol Nephrol Suppl* 1988;**110**:95–100.

29 Johansson JE, Adami HO, Andersson SO, *et al.* Natural history of localized prostatic cancer. A population-based study in 223 untreated patients. *Lancet* 1989;**1**:799–803.

30 Scardino PT, Weaver R, Hudson MA. Early detection of prostate cancer. *Human Pathology* 1992;**23**(3):211–222.

31 Cooner W, Mosley R, Rutherford CJ, *et al.* Prostate cancer detection in a clinical urological practice by ultrasonography, digital rectal examination and prostate-specific antigen. *J Urol* 1990;**143**:1146–1152.

32 Lee F, Littrup PJ, Torp-Pederson ST, *et al.* Prostate cancer: Comparison of transrectal US and DRE for screening. *Radiology* 1988;**168**: 389–394.

33 Drago JR. The role of new modalities in the early detection and diagnosis of prostate cancer. *CA* 1990;**40**:77.

34 Catalona W, Smith D, Ratcliff T, *et al.* Measurement of prostate-specific antigen in serum as a screening test for prostate cancer. *N Engl J Med* 1991;**324**:1156–1161.

35 Brawer M, Chetner M, Beatie J, *et al.* Screening for prostatic carcinoma with prostate-specific antigen. *J Urol* 1992;**147**: 841–845.

36 Kirby RS, Kirby MG, Feneley MR, *et al.* Screening for prostate cancer: a GP based study. *Br J Urol* 1994;**74**:64–71.

37 Chadwick DJ, Kemple T, Astley JP, *et al.* Pilot study of screening for prostate cancer in general practice. *Lancet* 1991;**338**:613–616.

38 Brawer MK, Beattie J, Wener MH, *et al.* Screening for prostatic carcinoma with prostate-specific antigen: Results of the second year. *J Urol* 1993;**150**:106–109.

39 Schmid HP, McNeal JE, Stamey TA. Observations on the doubling time of prostate cancer: The use of serial prostate-specific antigen in patients with untreated disease as a measure of increasing cancer volume. *CA* 1993;**71**(6):2031.

40 Catalona WJ, Richie JP, Ahmann FR, *et al.* Comparison of digital rectal examination and serum prostate-specific antigen in the early detection of prostate cancer: Results of a multicenter clinical trial of 6,630 men. *J Urol* 1994;**151**:1283–1290.

41 Altwein JE, Faul P, Schneider W. *Incidental Carcinoma*

of the Prostate. 1991, Springer-Verlag, Berlin.

42 Schmidt JD, Mettlin CJ, Natarajan N, *et al.* Trends in patterns of care for prostatic cancer, 1974–1983: Results of surveys by the American College of Surgeons. *J Urol* 1986;**136**:416–421.

43 Ploch NR, Ellis WJ, Brawer MK. Transrectal ultrasound guided prostate needle biopsies in men presenting with obstructive voiding symptoms. 1994 AUA Annual Meeting. 1993.

44 Lepor H, Owens RS, Rogenes V, *et al.* Detection of prostate cancer in men with prostatism. *Prostate* 1994;**25**:132–148.

45 Kinne DW, Kopans DB. Physical examination and mammography in the diagnosis of breast disease. *Breast Disease* 1987;54–86.

46 Moskowitz M. Cost-benefit determinations in screening mammography. *CA Suppl* 1987;**60**:1680–1683.

47 Brawer MK. Prostate cancer: epidemiology and screening. *PCPD* 1999;**2**(Suppl):2–6, 1999.

48 Mettlin CJ, Murphy GP, Rosenthal DS, Menck HR. The National Cancer Data Base report on prostate carcinoma after the peak in incidence rates in the U.S. The American College of Surgeons Commission on Cancer and the American Cancer Society. *Cancer* 1998;**83**(8):1679–1684.

49 Drachenberg DE, Brawer MK. Screening for prostate cancer. In: Vogelsang NJ, Scardino PT, Shipley WU, Coffey DS (eds). *Comprehensive Textbook of Genitourinary Oncology,* 2nd ed. Philadelphia: Lippincott Williams & Wilkins; 2000 (submitted).

50 Stamey TA, Donaldson AN, Yemoto CE, McNeal JE, Sozen S, Gill H. Histological and clinical findings in 896 consecutive prostates treated only with radical retropubic prostatectomy: epidemiologic significance of annual charges. *J Urol* 1998;**160**(6):2412–2417.

51 Mettlin C, Murphy G, Babian R, *et al.* Observations on the early detection of prostate cancer from the American Cancer Society National Prostate Cancer Detection Project. *Cancer* 1997;**80**:1814–1817.

52 Smart CR. The results of prostate carcinoma screening in the US as reflected in the Surveilance, Epidemiology, and End Results Program. *Cancer* 1997;**80**:1835–1844.

53 Standaert B, Denis L. The European randomized study of screening for prostate cancer. *Cancer* 1997;**80**:1830–1834.

54 Labrie F, Dupont A, Suburu R, *et al.* Optimized strategy for detection of early stage, curable prostate cancer: role of prescreening with prostate-specific antigen. *Clin Invest Med* 1993;**16**:425–439.

55 Wilt TJ, Brawer MK. Prostate cancer intervention versus observation trial: randomized trial comparing radical prostatectomy versus expectant management for the treatment of clinically localized cancer. *J Urol* 1994;**152**:1910–1921.

56 Gohagan JK, Prorok PC, Kramer BS, *et al.* Prostate cancer screening in prostate, lung, colorectal and ovarian cancer screening trial of National Cancer Institute. *J Urol 1994;152:1905–1909.*

57 Labrie F, Candas B, Dupont A, *et al.* Screening decreases prostate cancer death: first analysis of the 1988 Quebec prospective randomized controlled trial. *Prostate* 1999;**38**:83–91.

58 Kranse R, Beemsterboer P, Rietbergen J, Habbema D, Hugosson J, Schroder FH. Predictors for biopsy outcome in the European Randomized Study of Screening for Prostate Cancer (Rotterdam region). *Prostate* 1999;316–322.

59 Catalona WJ, Smith DS, Ratliff TL. Value of measurements of the rate of change on serum PSA levels in prostate cancer screening. *J Urol* 1993;**149**(4): 300A.

60 Chodak GW, Schoenberg HW. Progress and problems in screening for carcinoma of the prostate. *World J Surg* 1989;**13**:60–64.

61 Faul P. Experience with the German annual preventive checkup examination. In: *Prostate Cancer* 1982;57.

62 Gilbertsen VA. Cancer of the prostate gland: Results of early diagnosis and therapy undertaken for cure of the disease. *JAMA* 1976;**215**: 81–84.

63 Jenson CB, Shahon DB, Wangensteen OH. Evaluation of annual examinations in the detection of cancer: Special reference to cancer of the gastrointestinal tract, prostate, breast, and female reproductive tract. *JAMA* 1960;**174**: 1783–1788.

64 Lee F, Littrup P, Torp-Pedersen S, *et al.* Prostate cancer: Comparison of transrectal US and digital rectal examination for screening. *Radiology* 1988;**168**:389–394.

65 McWhorter WP, Hernandez AD, Meikle AW, *et al.* A screening study prostate cancer in high risk families. *J Urol* 1992;**148**: 826.

66 Mettlin C, Lee F, Drago J, *et al.* The American Cancer Society National Prostate Cancer Detection Project: Findings on the detection of early prostate cancer in 2425 men. *Cancer* 1991;**67**:2949–2958.

67 Mueller EJ, Crain TW, Thompson IM, *et al.* An evaluation of serial digital rectal examinations in screening for prostate cancer. *J Urol* 1988;**140**:1445.

68 Thompson IM, Rounder JB, Teaque JL, *et al.* Impact of routine screening for adenocarcinoma of the prostate on stage distribution. *J Urol* 1987;**137**:424.

69 Vihko P, Kontturi M, Lukkarinen O, *et al.* Screening for carcinoma of the prostate: Rectal examination, and enzymatic and radioimmunologic measurements of serum acid phosphatase compared. *Cancer* 1985;**56**:173–177.

70 Waaler G, Ludvigsen TC, Runden TO, *et al.* Digital rectal examination to screen for prostatic cancer. *Eur Urol* 1988;**15**:34.

71 Devonec M, Chapeleon JY, Cathignol D. Comparison of the diagnostic value of sonography and rectal examination in cancer of the prostate. *Eur Urol* 1988;**14**:189.

72 Fritzche PJ, Axford PO, Ching VC, *et al.* Correlation of transrectal sonographic findings in patients with suspected and unsuspected prostatic disease. *J Urol* 1983;**30**:272.

73 Hunter PT, Butler SA, Hodge GB, *et al.* Detection of

prostatic cancer using transrectal ultrasound and sonographically guided biopsy in 1410 symptomatic. *J Endourol* 1989;3:167.

74 Perrin P, Mouriquand P, Monsallier M, *et al.* Irradiation of carcinoma of the prostate localized to the pelvis: Analysis of tumor response and prognosis. *Int J Radiat Oncol Biol Phys* 1980;6:555.

75 Ragde H, Bagley CM, Aldpae HC, *et al.* Screening for prostatic cancer with high-resolution ultrasound. *J Endourol* 1989;3:115.

76 Rifkin MD, Friedland GW, Shortliffe L. Prostatic evaluation by transrectal ultrasonography: Detection of carcinoma. *Radiology* 1986;**158**:85.

77 Brawer MK. Unpublished Observation.

Chapter 8

Staging of prostate cancer

INTRODUCTION

An accurate assessment of the clinical stage of prostate cancer is important not only for the correct selection of therapy, but also for the estimation of prognosis and the comparison of results of various forms of therapy. However, in spite of many recent advances, the precision with which an individual patient who has prostate cancer can be staged before therapy still remains suboptimal, largely because early extraprostatic extension is generally microscopic. It is therefore not surprising that imaging techniques such as computed tomography (CT) and magnetic resonance imaging (MRI) have limited accuracy in this context. Progress is being made, however, and future technological advances seem likely to enable us to distinguish more precisely those patients who have truly localized disease, who are most likely to derive benefit from curative local therapy, from those who have more advanced disease in whom systemic therapy may be more effective. This chapter reviews the current state of the art and looks forward to the future of this important component of prostate cancer evaluation.

CURRENT TUMOUR (T), NODE (N), M (METASTASIS) STAGING

Current tumour TNM staging is shown in **Tables 8.1–8.5.**

DIGITAL RECTAL EXAMINATION IN THE DIAGNOSIS AND STAGING OF PROSTATE CANCER

For decades, digital rectal examination (DRE) has been the cornerstone in the diagnosis and assessment of prostatic cancer. Determination of serum prostate-specific antigen (PSA) is, however, more sensitive and specific than DRE for both the diagnosis and staging

Table 8.1 Clinical staging of primary tumour (T)	
TX	Primary tumour cannot be assessed
T0	No evidence of primary tumour
T1	**Clinically inapparent tumour not palpable or visible by imaging**
T1a	Tumour incidental histological finding in 5% or less of tissue resected
T1b	Tumour incidental histological finding in more than 5% of tissue resected
T1c*	Tumour identified by needle biopsy (e.g. because of elevated PSA)
T2	**Tumour confined within the prostate**
T2a	Tumour involves one lobe
T2b	Tumour involves both lobes
T3**	**Tumour extends through the prostate capsule**
T3a	Unilateral extrapsular extension
T3b	Bilateral extracapsular extension
T3c	Tumour invades the seminal vesicle(s)
T4	**Tumour invades any of bladder neck, external sphincter, or rectum**
T4a	Tumour invades any of bladder neck, external sphincter or rectum
T4b	Tumour invades levator muscles and/or the pelvic wall

*Tumour found in one or both lobes by needle biopsy, but not palpable or reliably visible by imaging, is classified as T1c
**Invasion into the prostatic apex or into (but not beyond) the prostatic capsule is not classified as T3 but as T2

of prostate cancer. A combination of an abnormal DRE and elevated PSA defines a group of patients at high risk for extraprostatic extension of disease.

At the time of DRE, the examining clinician

Table 8.2 Pathological staging of primary tumour (pT)

*pT2	**Organ confined**
T2a	Unilateral
T2b	Bilateral
pT3	**Extraprostatic extension**
T3a	Extraprostatic extension
T3b	Seminal vesicle invasion
pT4	**Invasion of bladder, rectum and tissues listed above**

*There is no pathological T1 stage

Table 8.5 TNM stage grouping

Stage	T	N	M	Grade
I	T1a	N0	M0	G1
II	T1a	N0	M0	G2,3
	T1b	N0	M0	Any G
	T1c	N0	M0	Any G
	T1	N0	M0	Any G
	T2	N0	M0	Any G
III	T3	N0	M0	Any G
IV	T4	N0	M0	Any G
	Any T	N1	M0	Any G
	Any T	Any N	M1	Any G

Table 8.3 Staging by regional lymph node involvement (N)

NX Regional lymph nodes cannot be assessed
N0 No regional lymph node metastasis
NI Metastasis in regional node or nodes

Table 8.4 Staging by presence of distant metastasis (M)*

MX	Presence of distant metastasis cannot be assessed
M0	No distant metastasis
M1	**Distant metastasis**
M1a	Non-regional lymph node(s) metastasis
M1b	Bone(s) metastasis
M1c	Other sites(s) metastasis

*When more than one site of metastasis is present, the most advanced category (pM1c) is used

dimensional diagram of the prostate and seminal vesicles should ideally be used to document the DRE findings. The classical DRE sign of a prostate cancer is an irregular, indurated or nodular area with indistinct margins. Cancer should also be considered in the presence of any change in consistency or configuration of the gland. It must be remembered, however, that tuberculosis, infarction granulomatous prostatitis and prostatic calculi, as well as a post-biopsy reaction, can also cause palpable alterations.

Clearly a definite diagnosis of prostate cancer cannot be based solely upon DRE, but always requires histopathological confirmation. Conversely, a negative biopsy does not exclude the presence of carcinoma. Patients who have an abnormal DRE should usually be re-evaluated periodically by DRE and PSA determination, and rebiopsy considered.

In a recent report by Brawer et al.[1], carcinoma was histologically confirmed in only 39% of needle biopsies of patients performed on the basis of abnormal DRE findings. Cancer detection was highest in the presence of a markedly indurated or nodular area highly suspicious for cancer (54%), when compared with the presence of induration (25%), or asymmetry (12%). These percentages of cancer detection denote the continuing importance of DRE in suggesting the possibility of prostate cancer. Digital rectal examination accuracy depends upon the individual examiner's experience, and there is a considerable inter- and intra-examiner variability[2,3].

Digital rectal examination as a method to assess the local extension of disease (8.1) lacks sensitivity and specificity to determine accurately tumour volume and periprostatic extension. Often DRE

should consider size, consistency and shape of the gland, and also evaluate the integrity of the median furrow or sulcus and lateral sulci. The presence, location and configuration of nodules, induration or irregular areas should be recorded, along with the extension of these abnormalities, and whether or not extraprostatic disease is suspected. A two-

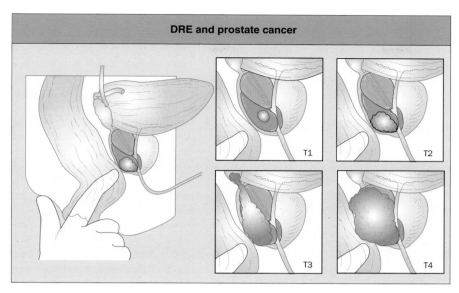

DRE and prostate cancer

T1

T2

T3

T4

8.1 Digital rectal examination (DRE) as a staging manoeuvre.

underestimates extension of intracapsular cancer and focal extraprostatic invasion. Therefore, distinction between T2a and T2b based on DRE is unreliable. The same is true in distinguishing between T2 and T3 tumours. In this regard, suspected extraprostatic extension and seminal vesicle involvement may sometimes be suggested when none is in fact present. Only extensive T3 tumours can be reliably diagnosed and staged by DRE. This finding mandates complementary tests, such as ultrasound-guided tissue sampling to confirm, for example, seminal vesicle invasion[4] or MRI. By contrast, DRE is clearly of no value for patients who have stage T1 and particularly those patients whose impalpable tumours are discovered as a result of an elevated serum PSA (stage T1c) because, by definition, no palpable DRE abnormality is present.

PSA IN THE DIAGNOSIS AND STAGING OF PROSTATE CANCER

As already discussed PSA is glycoprotein of the kallikrein family (kallikrein 3) and is widely used for early detection, staging and follow-up of patients who have prostate cancer (**8.2**). Several detailed biochemical and clinical reviews are available about this marker[5–8]. Serum PSA increases progressively with advanced stage of disease. However, there is considerable overlap between benign prostatic hyperplasia (BPH) and localized prostate cancer, which makes a single level of PSA unreliable in this

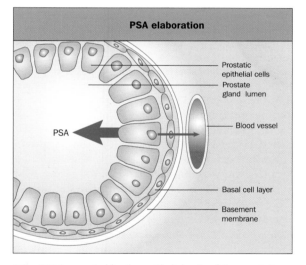

PSA elaboration

Prostatic epithelial cells

Prostate gland lumen

PSA

Blood vessel

Basal cell layer

Basement membrane

8.2 PSA is secreted by the epithelial cells of the prostatic acini. The majority of the PSA enters the lumen of prostatic acini, a minority is absorbed and enters the blood stream.

context. Serum PSA levels in isolation have limited value, although it has been proposed that patients who have localized prostate cancer and PSA less than 10 ng/ml do not need additional metastatic work up with a bone scan because of the low positive yield[9]. The most recent comprehensive study published by D'Amico *et al.* correlated PSA levels and Gleason scores and number of positive biopsies with outcomes for curative treatment of localized prostate cancer. The authors defined a low-risk, an intermediate-risk and a high-risk pretreatment group, which show excellent correlation with PSA value[10,11].

Two new markers are now under investigation: human kallikrein-2 (hK-2) and prostate-specific membrane antigen (PSMA)[12,13]. Kallikrein-2 has 80% homology with PSA, is specific for prostate and associated more often with high-grade malignancies. Initial studies using Western blot for the selection of PSMA in the serum reveals the potential use of this marker as a prognostic marker, especially for hormonally unresponsive cases[13]. New immunological assays for detection of PSMA in the serum are presently undergoing clinical trials.

COMBINING CLINICAL PARAMETERS: PARTIN'S TABLES AND NEURAL NETWORKS

Although a number of clinical staging studies are available for patients who have prostate cancer, they all have appreciable limitations when they are used as stand-alone tests.

Digital rectal examination is of value in identifying some patients who have localized disease, although it is well recognized that there is significant under- and overstaging. For obvious reasons the study is highly examiner dependent and may be further biased by the clinical orientation of the physician. For instance, surgeons may identify disease as being localized more commonly than radiotherapists who may be inclined to diagnose extraprostatic disease more frequently. Experience indicates that the staging accuracy of DRE alone is approximately 50% in men who have palpable disease[14–16].

Although PSA has been of value in identifying patients who have prostate cancer, this test has been of limited value when used in isolation for staging. Prostate-specific antigen is prostate specific, but not prostate cancer specific, and, because most men who have prostate cancer also have BPH, staging errors are inevitable. Although it is recognized that patients who have initially high levels of PSA have a greater risk of recurrence after therapy, the relatively poor sensitivity and predictive value, and the fact that almost one-quarter of the patients who have positive surgical margins have a PSA level less than 10 ng/ml, confirm that PSA by itself cannot be used to define clinical stage or predict poor outcome after surgery[17]. Use of free/total PSA ratio does not appear to add additional value to PSA alone when combined with clinical stage and Gleason score for staging purposes[18].

Gleason grade (score) is also useful in predicting the risk of extraprostatic disease and lymph node metastases[19,20], but the scoring system is not without limitations. Preoperative Gleason score does not always correlate with final pathological score after surgery (a phenomenon resulting from limited tumour sampling on biopsy). Moreover most men who have prostate cancer have intermediate Gleason scores (5–7). This limits this scoring system as a stand-alone test to determine accurately the preoperative tumour stage[21,22].

In an attempt to improve the accuracy of preoperative staging several authors have analysed various 'independent' parameters in combination by a variety of statistical analysis. Ackerman and associates found that pre-treatment PSA level and the number of positive core biopsies correlated well with the risk of positive surgical margins[23]. Hammer *et al.* calculated the sensitivity and specificity of the number of positive sextant cores and the total linear percent involvement for predicting lymph node metastasis, and Bostwick *et al.* accurately predicted extracapsular extension using percent cancer on biopsy, PSA and Gleason score[24,25]. Daniels *et al.* improved the predictive value of prostate needle biopsies by correlating bilaterality of neoplastic disease to final pathological stage and Stamey's group both demonstrated that small tumours less than 4 cc were associated with a good prognosis whereas tumours greater than 12 cc were invariably surgically incurable[26–28].

Several authors have attempted to combine some or all of these parameters (serum PSA, Gleason score as determined on biopsy and DRE findings in addition to other parameters) to improve staging accuracy and all apparently accomplished their goal[29–36]. Partin and associates have popularized this approach and recently have refined their method of analysis[37,38] (**8.3, 8.4**). The most recent report evaluated preoperative PSA, Gleason score and digital rectal findings in 4133 men treated for clinically localized prostate cancer at three institutions. Radical prostatectomy specimens and removed lymph nodes were all examined and the findings correlated with the preoperative clinical data. Multinomial log-linear regression techniques were used in the development of the nomograms, and bootstrap statistical procedures provided improved estimates

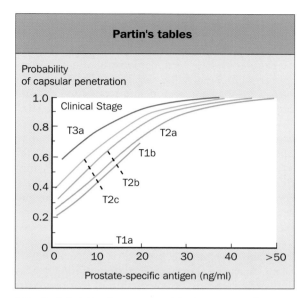

8.3 Partin's tables for assessing risk of extraprostatic extension of cancer: clinical stage and PSA.

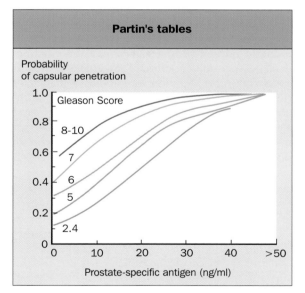

8.4 Partin's tablets for assessing the risk of extraprostatic extension: Gleason score and PSA.

of the medians and 95% confidence intervals of the predicted reported probabilities.

The combination of PSA, clinical stage (TNM) and Gleason score greatly assisted in predicting pathological stage (p <0.001). The probability of accurately predicting pathological stage was 72.4%.

Although even more accurate and predictive data would be ideal, these nomograms are particularly valuable when counselling patients about the probability of their tumour being a specific pathological stage. This enables patients and their clinician to make more informed treatment decisions based on the probability of extraprostatic extension, as well as their risk tolerance and the values they place on various potential outcomes.

Artificial intelligence (AI) based on neural networks has also recently been used for medical applications, and several groups have applied this methodology to predict pathological stage before therapy. An early report by Snow and associates used serum PSA to predict biopsy results and found the neural network accuracy to be 85%[39]. Of particular note, tumour recurrence prediction had an overall accuracy of 90%.

Douglas and Moul recently reviewed artificial neural networks and summarized their application in urological oncology[40], and Naguib and associates also emphasized the potential of this modality for staging assessment when using prognostic markers[41]. Tewari and Narayan[42] compiled data (PSA, systematic biopsy and Gleason score) on 200 men who had clinically localized prostate cancer and found that the sensitivity of the network for predicting pathological margins, seminal vesicle involvement and lymph node metastases was 81–100%. The specificity was 72–75%. Negative predictive values were high and ranged from 92–100%. They concluded the networks avoid unnecessary additional staging tests for 63% of patients who have clinically localized disease.

Bostwick and associates noted that for neural networks to be of value, data must be obtained that include patient factors, serum factors and tissue-specific factors obtained from biopsy[43]. Predictive factors in prostate cancer were classified into four categories:

(1) those in widespread clinical use (e.g., Gleason grade, clinical stage and serum PSA);
(2) factors of unproven significance (e.g., DNA ploidy, volume of cancerous tissue in the needle biopsy);
(3) predictive factors not used routinely (e.g., cell proliferation markers, mitotic figures, proliferating cell nuclear antigen Ki-67 and MIB-1, apoptotic markers, microvessel density and perineural invasion); and

(4) those factors under investigation (e.g., morphometric features such as nuclear roundness, chromatin texture, silver-staining nuclear organizer regions and nuclear size).

Predictive factors in radical prostatectomy specimens included tumour volume and extent and quantification of number and size of metastatic lymph nodes. These multiple parameters when applied to neural networks offer greater potential for predicting pathological stage than traditional statistical models and will likely have more widespread application in the future.

ANGIOGENESIS

The development of a malignant tumour is usually associated with three different stages: growth, infiltration into adjacent tissue and metastasis. In each stage angiogenesis plays an important role (8.5). Whether vascularity of tissue contains information that can be used for differential diagnosis has been investigated with histopathological analysis of resected prostate tissue. It is well known that in order to grow larger than 1 mm^2 in area, cancers must recruit new blood vessels from the host to supply sufficient nutrients to, and remove waste products from tumours[44]. Also, tumour vascularity appears to be associated with tumour aggressiveness[45]. In addition, angiogenesis is necessary for tumour cells to metastasize, and this clearly applies to prostate cancer as well[46].

The hypothesis that tumour growth is dependent

upon the formation of new blood vessels[47] has been evaluated by assessing microvessel density in malignant tissue of the prostate; an increased density of capillaries has been demonstrated in prostate cancer compared with benign prostate tissue[48]. Neovascularity has been demonstrated to be a prerequisite for tumour progression[49] and metastasis.

Currently, most research involves counting microvessels with immunohistochemical assays using an antibody to human von Willebrand factor for assessing intratumour microvessel density. Quantification of tumour angiogenesis carries the potential for stratification of patients to type of treatment and selection of expectant management for men who have low tumour microvessel density; microvessel density is an independent predictor of pathological stage and may provide prognostic information[45,50]. Using microvessel density in combination with PSA and Gleason score, the prediction of extraprostatic extension significantly improved[51]. Topographic analysis of neovascularity in human prostate cancer indicated a high vascularity of the tumour centre, suggesting a high activity of angiogenic promotors in the centre of the neoplasm[52]. The orientation of microvessels was regular along the basement membrane in normal prostates, whereas abnormalities in shape, size and structure of the vessels as well as an increased proliferation were found in malignant tissue[45]. Recent reports confirm the finding of increased microvessel density in tumours that have a higher Gleason score[53]. Borre et al. showed that microvessel density was a significant predictor of disease-specific survival in prostate cancer patients[54].

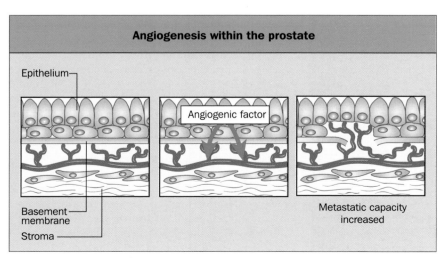

8.5 Angiogenesis: new blood vessels are induced to grow through the basement membrane and are associated with enhanced metastatic capacity.

Angiogenesis within the prostate

Epithelium

Angiogenic factor

Basement membrane

Stroma

Metastatic capacity increased

On the other hand, Gettman *et al.* could not predict prostate cancer recurrence in patients who had $T_2N_0M_0$ prostate cancer treated with radical prostatectomy using microvessel density[55]. More recently, Rubin *et al.* reported that microvessel density did not correlate with Gleason sum, tumour stage, surgical margin status or seminal vesicle invasion, based on data of 87 patients who underwent radical prostatectomy. Also, microvessel density was not significantly correlated with PSA failure[56]. More studies are clearly required in this evolving area.

MOLECULAR STAGING OF PROSTATE CANCER

Following an initial report suggesting that molecular techniques could be adapted for use in the diagnosis of prostate cancer metastases, it was proposed that there might be a role for this technology in staging patients who have clinically localized disease. The molecular technology involved was the reverse transcriptase-polymerase chain reaction (RT-PCR). This technique can be used to identify cells expressing certain genes. Not surprisingly, the gene of interest is PSA or PSMA. The RT-PCR technique involves preparing an RNA sample and reverse transcribing it into DNA. Following this, specific cDNAs can be amplified by the use of primers that are specific for the gene of interest. Amplification can be carried out to the point where the cDNA can be identified by a variety of different probing techniques.

In a study reported by Katz[57], RT-PCR was employed to evaluate the presence of mRNA for PSA. Free mRNA degrades rapidly in the bloodstream, so it is reasonable to assume that if PSA encoding for mRNA is detected, functioning prostate cells must be present in the sample being tested. The PSA primers were designed to isolate a cDNA fragment of the PSA gene containing 710 base pairs. The reason for using such a large fragment was to avoid the identification of partially homologous genes, such as those of the kallikrein family.

The sensitivity of the assay developed has been tested by examining serial dilutions of an LNCaP cell line (a cell line derived originally from a lymph node metastasis of prostate cancer) diluted with cultured B lymphocytes. The initial assay sensitivity allowed the detection of one prostate cell diluted in 10^6 white cells. The assay appears capable of detecting as few as one cell in 10^7. To evaluate the false-positive rates of the assay, peripheral blood samples from more than 100 individuals of both sexes, including men who had histologically proven BPH, have been studied by Cama and co-workers[58].

Application of RT-PCR to prostate cancer staging

The RT-PCR assay developed for PSA-producing cells has been evaluated for its ability to assist in the staging of clinically localized prostate cancer. It was hypothesized that the phenotype of the cell having the ability to escape the prostate capsule might be identical to the phenotype capable of traversing the capillary basement membrane and entering the peripheral circulation. If the blood assay were positive, therefore, there might be extracapsular disease found when the specimen was examined pathologically.

One hundred and thirty-eight patients who had clinically localized prostate cancer and were scheduled to undergo radical prostatectomy were studied. A blood sample was drawn from each patient preoperatively, a minimum of 30 days subsequent to any prostatic manipulation. The sample was processed immediately, and an RNA preparation was made for further sampling.

A comparison was made between the results of the RT-PCR PSA assay and the histology review. Of the 138 cases, 54 (39%) exhibited extraprostatic extension of prostate cancer. Forty patients (29%) were judged to be potential surgical failures, as defined by a positive surgical margin and/or seminal vesicle involvement. A total of 98 patients (71%) had specimen-confined disease, including 84 (61%) who had organ-confined cancer. The RT-PCR assay before radical prostatectomy was negative in 94 patients (68%) and positive in 44 (32%). In patients who had capsular perforation, the assay was positive in 74%, and in seminal vesicle invasion, the assay was positive in 67%. Overall, of the 40 patients who had pathological findings suggestive of potential surgical failure, 70% had a positive pre-operative RT-PCR assay. It was concluded that the blood assay using RT-PCR for PSA was a potentially valuable staging modality in this group of patients[58].

Subsequently the same group reported that preoperative PCR testing could accurately predict PSA progression in patients undergoing radical prostatectomy[59]. Other groups however have not been able to confirm these initially promising findings. There have since been at least nine other publications[60–68], which all report little or no correlation between the pathological stage and the preoperative RT-PCR result. Moreover, a recent publication by Oetelein *et al.*[69] reports that although a significant proportion of men remain positive on RT-PCR testing, follow-up demonstrates reconversion to negative status as the predominant trend. At relatively short follow-up (median 22 months) no significant correlation could be found between the RT-PCR result and the PSA progression-free survival. More work is being actively undertaken in this area.

TRANSRECTAL ULTRASOUND OF THE PROSTATE

Although more uncomfortable to the patient than transabdominal scanning, transrectal ultrasound (TRUS) scanning has the distinct advantage of greater acuity resulting from the very close approximation of the probe to the prostate. Technological advances in ultrasound equipment, grey scale imaging, high-frequency transducers (7–7.5 MHz) and colour Doppler have resulted in significant improvements in the visualization of the prostate. Transrectal ultrasound scanning is performed with a handheld endorectal probe (8.6). Most probes have high-frequency transducers, which provide a spatial resolution down to 0.2 mm. Biplanar scanning in the sagittal and transverse axial planes enables more complete scanning of the prostate. Other technical refinements include colour and power Doppler enhancement and more recently three-dimensional scanning together with the use of contrast agents such as microbubbles, which enable the operator to assess the blood flow within regions of the prostate. This may help with diagnosis, by revealing areas of hypervascularity associated with malignancy, although inflammation, usually due to prostatitis, may also result in increased local blood flow patterns[70].

TRUS findings in prostate cancer

Some, but by no means all, prostate cancers are hypoechoic on TRUS (8.7), but they may also be isoechoic and sometimes hyperechoic[71]. Prostate cancers most commonly develop within the peripheral zone, but can also develop in the transition zone, which is itself hypoechoic, making detection within this zone especially difficult. In the peripheral zone there are several other causes for hypoechoicity and the specificity of this finding for prostate cancer is only 20–25%[72]. Other TRUS characteristics of prostate cancer include asymmetry of prostate size, shape and echogenicity, indefinite differentiation between the central and peripheral zones and bulging or disruption of the capsule. There may also be evidence of abnormal blood flow patterns on colour Doppler ultrasound study although this is more characteristic of prostatitis (8.8).

In patients who are being considered for radical prostatectomy, it is particularly relevant to determine if there is any evidence of extraprostatic extension. Bulging or irregularity of the boundary echo adjacent to a peripheral zone hypoechoic lesion may be a feature of capsular extension[73]. Invasion of the seminal vesicles may also be suggested by TRUS; however, in general TRUS alone has not been a very reliable staging study.

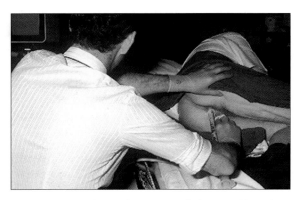

8.6 Patient positioning for transrectal ultrasound (TRUS) scanning.

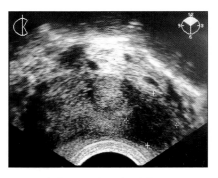

8.7 Transrectal ultrasound study of the prostate; a sizeable hypoechoic lesion is apparent.

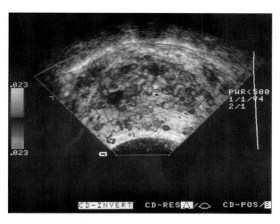

8.8 Hypervascularity within the prostate seen on colour Doppler transrectal ultrasound.

TRUS-guided biopsy

Histological diagnosis is an essential prerequisite before initiating treatment for prostate cancer. A number of different biopsy techniques have been described. Digital guidance can be used to direct biopsy of palpable lesions via the transrectal or transperineal routes. However, TRUS guidance has been shown to be superior in directing biopsy of both palpable and impalpable prostate cancers. Routes for biopsy can vary. The transperineal route carries the advantage that it is less likely to introduce infection, but the disadvantages of requiring local anaesthesia and less easy guidance with the TRUS probe. In contrast, the transrectal route can be used with or without injection of local anaesthesia and can be guided accurately through the biopsy port incorporated in the TRUS probe (**8.9**). By this means systematic sextant biopsies can be accomplished using an automatic biopsy device (**8.10**). It is now standard practice to administer a broad spectrum oral antibiotic before biopsy and to give a 2- or 3-day course of oral antibiotics, usually of the quinolone variety, sometimes in combination with metronidazole, immediately before and continuing after the biopsy. More and more clinicians are now opting to use local anaesthetic prior to biopsy.

There has been some debate about the technique for the biopsy itself. Fine-needle aspiration has been advocated by some; however, the cellular aspirate is sometimes difficult to interpret cytologically, resulting in a false negative diagnosis. One study comparing aspiration cytology with core biopsy in

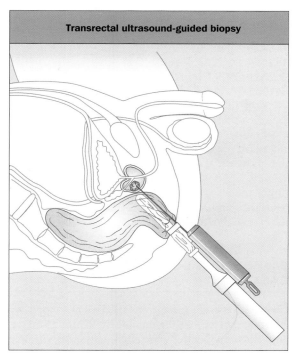

Transrectal ultrasound-guided biopsy

8.9 Transrectal ultrasound-guided prostatic biopsy.

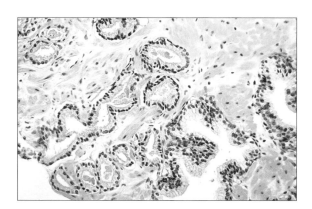

8.10 Core prostate biopsy revealing Gleason 3+3 adenocarcinoma.

30 patients who had prostate cancer showed that whereas core biopsy made the correct diagnosis in all cases, there was a false positive rate of 30% for aspiration cytology[74]. Most sextant prostatic biopsies are now taken using automatic biopsy devices, and additional lateral capsular and seminal

vesicle biopsies can be taken in those judged at high risk of extraprostatic extension. Valuable pre-operative staging information may be gleaned from biopsies taken by this route. In general, the greater the number of biopsies involved, and the greater the percentage involvement of each core, the higher the probability of extracapsular extension. Pathological assessment also permits scrutiny for other markers of biological aggressiveness, such as neo-vascularity[75]. It should be borne in mind, however, that prostate cancer exhibits considerable hetero-geneity[76]. Biopsies therefore may not always accu-rately reflect the entire picture within each given prostate gland, and in general tend to underestimate the eventual pathological stage after radical surgery.

PATHOLOGICAL STAGING OF PROSTATE CANCER

Given the current limitations of clinical staging for prostate cancer, which include both understaging and (less frequently) overstaging, the importance of detailed, accurate and reproducible pathological data for staging is paramount in predicting treatment outcome following radical prostatectomy. The correlation of pathological staging to treatment outcome is crucial in stratifying the risk of bio-chemical failure to a particular therapy for an individual patient. Such knowledge may also iden-tify patients who might potentially benefit from neoadjuvant therapy.

Pathological data can be obtained either before treatment or post-operatively. Information obtained before treatment is used to stage a patient clinically and is useful in recommending the optimal treat-ment for a given individual. Pathological data obtained after surgery can provide the most accurate information about an individual patient's cancer and can be useful in predicting treatment outcome.

The essential information that a pathologist should provide from a biopsy specimen is given in **Table 8.6**. Information about the presence of perineural invasion is not essential because it has not been shown to have prognostic value, although this infor-mation may sometimes be helpful in making a diag-nosis of prostate cancer. If staging biopsies are performed pre-operatively, the pathologist should provide specific information to confirm whether cancer appears to be present in extraprostatic tissue because this finding has clear therapeutic implica-

Table 8.6 What prostatic biopsy report should include
Presence or absence of cancer: if cancer is present, type (i.e., acinar or variant)
Presence of atypical glands that are suspicious for cancer
Presence of high-grade prostatic intraepithelial neoplasia (PIN)
Location of core with any pathologic finding other than benign glands (e.g., atrophy)
Gleason score (i.e., primary and secondary grade)
If only one core is positive, length in millimetres of cancer present
Presence of any cancer in fibroadipose tissue, rectal wall or intraprostatic portion of seminal vesicle

tions. For a histological diagnosis of extraprostatic extension or of seminal vesicle invasion, carcinoma must be present in fibroadipose tissue or in the muscle wall of the seminal vesicle, respectively.

An accurate assessment of pathological informa-tion depends upon the manner in which the pro-statectomy specimen is processed. A comparison of the results of partial sampling versus complete sampling has demonstrated a significant difference between the two sampling methods in detecting positive surgical margins (12 vs 59%, respectively)[77]. The reported incidence of extraprostatic extension has been shown to vary from 40 to 60% based solely on whether standard technique or whole-mount evaluation was used[78]. A practice survey by the American Society of Clinical Pathologists reported in 1994 that 88% of pathologists perform partial sampling of the prostatectomy specimen[79]. It should be noted that even when a prostatectomy specimen is completely embedded a sampling error can occur based on the number of slides reviewed[80]. Of particular interest is the fact that complete sampling can be performed using routine cassettes without the special handling required for whole-mount preparation. Whatever technique is used to review a prostatectomy specimen histologically, it should fulfil all the requirements set out by the College of American Pathologists[80] and the Association of Directors of Anatomic and Surgical Pathology[81]. The recommended information to be reported based on histologic analysis of the prostatectomy specimen

Table 8.7 Information to be reported following histologic evaluation of a radical prostatectomy specimen
Tumour type
Calculation of size of prostate in grams or cubic centimetres
Estimation of the percentage of the gland involved by cancer
Gleason score with grade of primary and secondary pattern of dominant focus
Presence of any other tumour focus with a primary Gleason grade >4
Presence or absence of cancer in either extraprostatic tissue or seminal vesicle
Statement regarding margin status and, if positive, whether or not there is extraprostatic extension at the margin site
Length in millimetres of positive margin
Presence of vascular invasion
Status of removed lymph nodes

is given in **Table 8.7**. The minimum recommended requirements for sampling the prostate have been previously reported[82]. They include complete sectioning of apical and bladder neck margins, all gross tumour with adjacent extraprostatic tissue including the surgical margin, the first slice above the apex in its entirety and the entire posterior third of the prostate at the base with at least one complete level of the proximal portion of each seminal vesicle.

The rationale for reporting information from either a biopsy or radical prostatectomy specimen is that such information can help the urologist make treatment recommendations and provide useful prognostic information to the patient. Information that does not meet these objectives, even if the information has research value, is probably not essential for routine reporting. For example, calculation of tumour volume based on the biopsy specimen has been shown to correlate poorly (r=0.39) with the actual tumour volume in the prostatectomy specimen, and hence such a calculation does not provide clinically useful information[83]. The finding of perineural invasion in either the biopsy specimen or the prostatectomy specimen has been shown to have no independent predictive value[84,85] although not all authors agree[86].

There is good evidence that the presence of extra-prostatic extension and margin status are significant independent predictors of treatment outcome[87–90]. However, the accuracy of the pathological data is predicated on a thorough appreciation of the anatomy of the fibromuscular rim that incompletely surrounds the prostate, the so-called prostatic 'capsule'[91]. A clear distinction between a positive margin with evidence of extraprostatic extension and a positive margin without such evidence is important because it may well have prognostic and therapeutic implications[92]. The presence of Gleason grade 4 or 5 cancer has been shown to be an adverse prognostic factor, and, more recently, the amount of grade 4 has been shown to have a direct relationship to treatment outcome[92–94]. The quantity of extraprostatic extension (i.e., focal versus extensive) has also been shown to have prognostic significance, but more recently an exact quantification of extraprostatic extension by an absolute measurement has shown independent significance in predicting biochemical failure, as has complete excision of the prostate in patients who have pathologically organ-confined disease[85,92]. The presence of vascular invasion has also been shown to have prognostic value. Seminal vesicle invasion has been shown to be a very strong factor influencing treatment outcome[95]. There is no evidence currently to suggest that pathological information after prostatectomy relating to unilateral or bilateral involvement or multicentricity of the cancer in specimens from patients who have organ confined disease, or the presence of bilaterality of extra-prostatic extension (EPE) and the amount of tumour actually present in the seminal vesicle carries valuable prognostic significance.

MAGNETIC RESONANCE IMAGING

Magnetic resonance imaging (MRI) is a rapidly advancing technology that uses a magnetic field rather than ionizing radiation to produce images of impressive clarity. A scanner creates an intense uniform magnetic field that aligns the rotational axes of atomic nuclei, particularly protons. A short powerful pulse of radio-frequency energy is then applied leading to a change in the energy levels of the atomic nuclei. When the radio-frequency pulse stops the nuclei return to their original energy level and in so doing emit energy that can be received and transformed into an image pattern. This return to the previous equilibrium state after the energy pulse is called magnetic relaxation. Two relaxation time measurements can be used to produce varying images. The T1 relaxation time represents the regrowth of the longitudinal component and the T2 relaxation time is the exponential time decay constant. Both T1 and T2 measurements can be used to produce different, but complementary images. Magnetic resonance imaging scanners are capable of producing images in the tranverse axial, coronal and sagittal planes, and endorectal probes have enhanced the definition of intraprostatic and periprostatic anatomy.

Using T1-weighted images, it is not possible to demonstrate the internal architecture of the prostate, although a clear demarcation is apparent between the prostate and seminal vesicles and the surrounding fat. By contrast T2-weighted MRI images are capable of demonstrating the internal architecture of the prostate. Typically the peripheral zone of the prostate returns high-intensity signals, whereas prostate cancer produces relatively low-intensity signals (**8.11**). Most other abnormalities within the prostate such as 'adenomas', calculi and prostatitis also return low-intensity signals so MRI is not accurate at identifying localized prostate cancer (**8.12**). Rather disappointingly MRI, so far has not proven any more accurate than TRUS in local staging of prostate cancer. However, supplementation of transverse axial scans with coronal and sagittal scanning has been shown to enhance local staging accuracy from 61 to 83%. Extracapsular extension may be present if there is apparent asymmetry, irregularity or breaching of the peri-

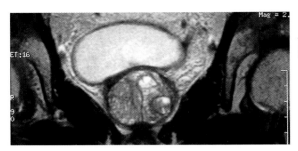

8.12 MRI showing BPH.

prostatic fat, which unlike the prostate itself, sends low-intensity signals. Seminal vesicle invasion is suggested if there are areas of asymmetric low intensity within the normally high-intensity vesicles, but biopsy confirmation is required. It must be borne in mind, however, that previous TRUS-guided biopsies produce perturbation of MRI images for many weeks after the investigation due to local haematoma formation[96] (**8.13**).

An original multicentre trial comparing MRI with TRUS in the staging of localized prostate cancer concluded that there was no statistically significant difference between the two[97]. Endorectal MRI provides better images (**8.14**). However, recent studies have confirmed a rather poor correlation between capsular bulge seen on endorectal MRI and pathological confirmation of extraprostatic extension[98]. Newer technologies, however, including gadolinium enhancement of MRI images, hold promise of improving the sensitivity and specificity of this investigation in the future (**8.15**).

VALUE OF CT SCANNING IN STAGING PROSTATE CANCER

The clinical use of computed tomography (CT) in the staging of prostate cancer has generally been disappointing[99]. Computed tomography has proven to be of little or no value in the assessment of the local disease. It does not display the internal architecture of the gland, is not capable of distinguishing between prostate cancer from benign conditions in the prostate, and is unable to reliably identify extraprostatic penetration or seminal vesicle invasion. It often does not appear to provide significant additional information over and above that obtained by DRE for staging local disease.

There has been more interest in the use of CT to identify the presence of lymphadenopathy in

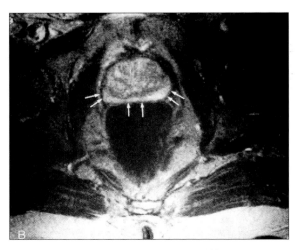

8.11 MRI scan of prostate (T2) showing different signals from peripheral and transition zones.

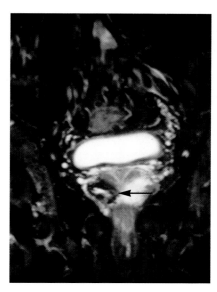

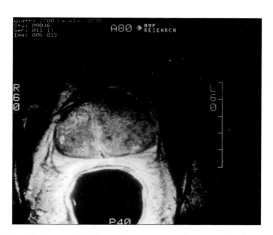

8.14 Endorectal MRI provides images of greater clarity than TRUS.

8.13 MRI showing haemorrhage in the right lobe of the prostate after biopsy.

the pelvis, but because of the current low incidence of positive lymph nodes, the utility of CT is limited. Most nodal metastases are microscopic and do not enlarge or distort the lymph node. There are probably subsets of patients who have a higher risk of having grossly positive nodes. A PSA in excess of 20–30 ng/ml or a poorly differentiated tumour (Gleason >7 on biopsy) may identify a risk for gross involvement and justify a CT scan. It is important to note that if an enlarged lymph node is identified on CT, a tissue diagnosis is necessary to confirm the presence of malignancy (**8.16**).

There is little doubt that the presence of metastases in regional lymph nodes has a profound influence on ultimate prognosis. Historically, around 20% of patients had positive lymph nodes at the time of radical prostatectomy. In the USA, and lately in Europe, the advent of successful earlier detection practices has produced a downward stage shift so that lymph node metastases are identified less and less frequently. Several series identify lymph node metastases in < 2–3% of patients undergoing radical prostatectomy. Data also reaffirm the observation that even micrometastases usually result in PSA-based relapse in almost all patients within 10 years. The low frequency of positive pelvic lymph nodes before radical prostatectomy prompts many surgeons to avoid lymphadenectomy in selected cases. Several studies provide nomograms that allow

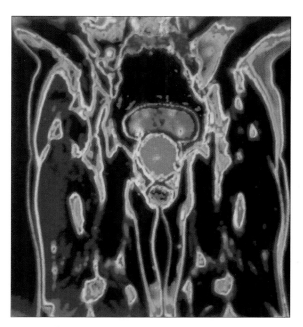

8.15 Colour MRI. The prostate is shown in red.

prediction of risk of metastatic disease[100]. If the risk for metastases is less than 2–3%, lymphadenectomy can often be safely omitted. These nomograms include the variables of clinical stage, histological grade on biopsy and serum PSA level.

Molecular staging of pelvic lymph node tissue may identify extremely small volume metastatic disease[101]. These findings suggest that some patients who have a persisting PSA elevation after radical

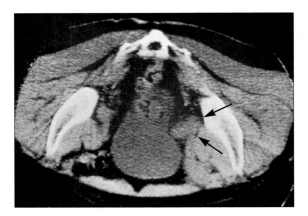

8.16 CT scan showing lymph node involvement (arrowed).

prostatectomy may have micrometastases in pelvic lymph nodes identifiable only by molecular staging.

PELVIC LYMPHADENECTOMY

Perhaps because lymph nodes involved with prostate cancer are often indurated, but not markedly enlarged, non-invasive imaging has often been disappointing as a means of accurate evaluation of the obturator and hypogastric lymph nodes. In the past, lymph node staging has been performed by an open operation, either as a staging procedure before radiotherapy or radical perineal prostatectomy. There now exists, however, the possibility of undertaking this procedure using minimally invasive techniques of laparoscopic technology. Laparoscopic pelvic lymphadenectomy (**8.17–8.19**) and the mini-laparotomy approach are now feasible options, which allow accurate evaluation of the nodal status of patients with minimal attendant morbidity. The post-operative hospital stay is only 24–48 hours and most patients can return to work within 1 week.

Pelvic lymph node dissection (LND) is not appropriate for all patients, but should be confined to individuals who have higher Gleason score (>6) prostate cancer on biopsy and/or a PSA greater than 10 ng/ml, who have no other evidence of metastatic disease and who are candidates, by virtue of both their tumour stage and their life expectancy, for curative therapy.

A further argument in favour of LND is that it permits histological lymph node staging in individuals undergoing non extirpative therapies such as external beam radiotherapy or brachytherapy.

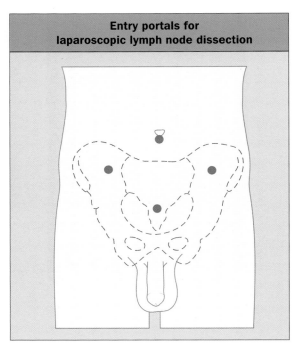

8.17 Laparoscopic pelvic lymph node dissection entry portals.

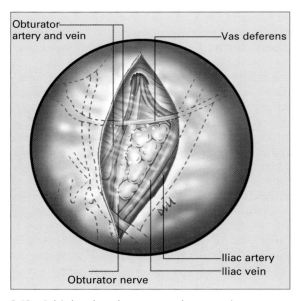

8.18 Pelvic lymph nodes as seen at laparoscopic lymphadenectomy.

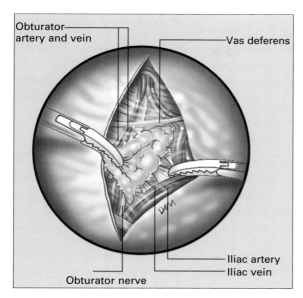

8.19 The lymph node parcel is gently dissected away from the iliac vein and the obturator nerve.

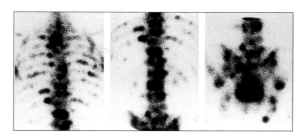

8.20 Positive bone scan. (Left) thorax; (centre) lumbar spine; (right) pelvis.

Lack of accurate staging data in the past have often skewed the results of radiation therapy trials, and now these techniques can facilitate more complete staging, allowing more valid comparisons between surgical and radiotherapeutic treatment[102].

The advantages of LND lie in its accuracy in terms of definitive confirmation of the presence or absence of lymph node involvement. Because a decreasing proportion of patients undergoing radical prostatectomy are now found to have positive lymph nodes, and this is nearly always in the patients who have larger volume, higher stage tumours and significantly raised PSA values[103], it seems logical to restrict LND to this rather rapidly dwindling category of patients.

ROLE OF RADIONUCLIDE BONE SCANS AND CORRELATIVE IMAGING STUDIES IN THE DIAGNOSIS AND TREATMENT OF PROSTATE CANCER

The axial skeleton is the favoured location for metastases from prostate cancer. This 'bone homing' mechanism is a direct consequence of complex, but incompletely understood prostate epithelial–bone stromal interactions. The most sensitive and widely used method to detect bony metastasis is technetium 99m radionuclide bone scanning (**8.20**). Although

false-negative scans are reported in less than 1% of patients (generally due to the presence of widespread symmetrical metastases), false-positive scans are relatively common because the study detects not only metastases but degenerative disease, previous trauma, healing fractures, metabolic disease (e.g., Paget's disease) and inflammatory/infectious lesions. A positive bone scan may be followed by confirmatory plain films, although 50% of bone mineral content must be altered before a lesion can be detected by plain radiographs. Magnetic resonance imaging has been helpful in the differential diagnosis of suspicious areas on scan that are negative on plain radiographs, especially in the axial skeleton.

As the most sensitive staging tool for bone metastases, radionuclide scanning was used routinely in the evaluation of patients who had newly diagnosed prostate cancer in an era when 30–35% of patients presented with metastatic disease. Currently in the USA only 5% of patients have metastases at initial presentation[104]. This fact, along with recent information about the predictive value of serum PSA levels for bone metastases and the high cost of the study (average of $700 in the USA), have led many authorities to advocate skeletal imaging for staging prostate cancer only in select circumstances. Chybowski *et al.*[9] provided the first evidence that radionuclide imaging is unnecessary in a significant proportion of men who have newly diagnosed disease. In a series of 521 patients the negative predictive value for patients who had a PSA of less than 20 ng/ml was 99.7%. No patient who had a PSA less than 15 ng/ml had a positive scan. Although local clinical stage, tumour grade, acid phosphatase and prostatic acid phosphatase all correlated with positivity on a bone scan, PSA was found to be the best predictor. Oesterling's data[104] confirmed these findings. Of 852 newly diagnosed untreated patients who had serum PSA values of less than 20 ng/ml, the negative predictive value for a PSA less than 10 ng/ml was 99.5%. Only seven patients (0.8%) had a positive scan; five of these had correlative skeletal symptoms. Only one patient had no skeletal symptoms, a PSA of less than 10 ng/ml and a positive scan. Other authors have followed with confirmatory data (**8.21**). Gleave *et al.*[105] reported a negative predictive value of 100% in 290 patients who have a PSA of less than 10 ng/ml and of 95.5% in patients who had a PSA of 10–20 ng/ml. They also reported an increased rate of bone positivity in patients who had T3 disease (19%) versus T2 disease (1%), and T1 disease (4%); and, in patients who had poorly differentiated disease (18%) versus moderately (4%) and well-differentiated disease (1.5%). An negative predictive value (NPV) of 100% was obtained by Levran *et al.*[106] for PSA values of less than 20 ng/ml (861 patients). Summarising these and other data, Lee and Oesterling[104] conclude that it is unnecessary to obtain a bone scan in newly diagnosed, previously untreated prostate cancer patients who have a PSA less than 10 ng/ml, a group, which they cite as representing 50–59% of newly diagnosed patients. The American Urological Association Prostate Cancer Guidelines Panel[107] stated that bone scanning 'may no longer be necessary' for the newly diagnosed patient who has a PSA of less than 10 ng/ml and no skeletal symptoms. The National Comprehensive Cancer network recom-

mends a bone scan in patients who have clinical stage T1 and T2 disease only if their PSA is over 10 ng/ml or their Gleason score is 8 or above, and in all patients who have clinical stage T3 or T4 disease or who have bone symptoms[108]. The Society of Surgical Oncology Prostate Cancer Surgical Practice Guidelines recommends bone scanning in a preoperative evaluation only if the PSA is over 8 ng/ml[109]. O'Dowd *et al.*[110] extracted data from 142 articles from the Medline database and concluded that routine bone scanning is necessary in newly diagnosed asymptomatic patients only when the PSA is higher than 10 ng/ml. Many urologists would also consider an elevated serum alkaline phosphatase in such a patient as an indication for bone scanning[111]. Serum alkaline phosphatase is not generally included, however, in the various recommendations for initial staging studies.

It is interesting that, in spite of these data, 52.4% of 1500 randomly selected urologists in the USA (638 responses) continue to order bone scans for all newly diagnosed prostate cancer patients[112]. The reasons generally cited for this practice are:

(1) to document benign abnormalities (e.g. degenerative arthritis of the spine) before treatment; and
(2) as an aid to interpreting scan results in patients who develop bone pain years after treatment[113].

The psychology of an individual patient and his 'need to know' about the possibility of metastases is also an important factor.

The role of radionuclide bone scan in prostatectomy patients who have known metastatic disease elsewhere following definitive treatment is less clear. Some[114] have implied the need for scanning in patents who have metastatic disease elsewhere at presentation as a means of predicting response to therapy and overall survival, and as a means of assessing therapeutic response during treatment. Patients who have bone disease limited to the lumbar spine and pelvis, and those who have a limited number of metastatic foci, have a better response to hormonal therapy and a longer mean survival than those who have more extensive disease. The results of bone scans are infrequently reported in patients who represent biochemical failures after definitive treatment. In 20 such patients following radiation therapy, the median PSA was 6.6 ng/ml; six had a positive bone scan, two of whom had bone symptoms[115]. In 24 such post-prostatectomy patients the

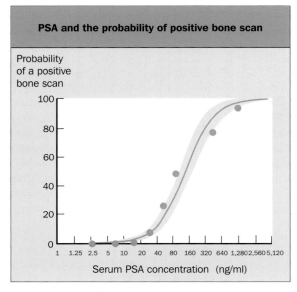

8.21 Probability of positive bone scan versus PSA value.

median PSA was 1.0 ng/ml, one of 20 bone scans was positive, no patient was symptomatic. Lee and Oesterling[104] reported preliminary observations in 84 men who had biochemical failure following radical prostatectomy. Only two patients (2.4%) had metastases on bone scan; no patient who had a PSA less than 2 ng/ml had bone metastases. They recommended against scanning before salvage therapy in the asymptomatic patient who has a PSA less than 2 ng/ml. Miller et al.[116] assessed the value of PSA and bone scanning in 66 patients following various types of curative and palliative treatment. Eleven patients (17%) became bone scan positive and all had a PSA value of higher than 20 ng/ml. Although further data need to be accumulated on this topic, logic would seem to dictate that the answer about whether a bone scan is indicated for biochemical failure after radiation or surgery depends upon the subsequent therapy considered. If salvage surgery, radiation or cryotherapy is considered, then bone scanning seems prudent.

RADIOIMMUNOSCINTOGRAPHY

The advent of monoclonal antibody (MAB) technology has permitted the development of radiolabelled tumour reactive probes that can be used in conjunction with gamma camera imaging equipment. This technology is compromised by the facts that truly tumour-specific antigens do not exist and that all target antigens of practical relevance are also expressed, to some degree, in other non-malignant and malignant tissues. Isotopes may be complexed to MABs against prostatic acid phosphatase and PSA. Although preliminary studies using prostatic acid phosphatase were promising[117,118], these have largely been abandoned because of low specificity and sensitivity[119]. The CYT-356 antibody is a murine immunoglobulin G MAB to a glycoprotein antigen originally described as on the membrane of benign and malignant prostatic epithelium[120]. It can be bound to an indium isotope and the radioimmuno-conjugate, known as capromab pendetide, and is now commercially available. Its use has been reported as a staging modality in newly diagnosed patients who have prostate cancer and in treated patients who have biochemical failure. In 19 newly diagnosed patients such imaging was carried out before pelvic LND: eight of these patients had nodal metastases. Radioimmunological scanning was positive at a site that corresponded to the metastases

in four, a sensitivity of 50%, compared with a sensitivity for CT and MRI of 12.5%[121]. Manyak and Javitt[122] reported somewhat better results for lymph node detection in 152 evaluable radical prostatectomy candidates with high-risk disease (Gleason score >7 with PSA >20 ng/ml; clinical T3 disease with Gleason score >6; elevated PSA with equivocal CT or MRI, Gleason score >8). Sixty-four patients had lymph node metastasis at surgery; 40 of these had positive scans, 38 of which were positive on the side with positive pathology, a sensitivity, if one does not count the two positive scans on the contralateral side, of 59%. Only 63 of 88 patients who have no lymph node metastases had negative scans.

Radioimmunoscintography has the potential to provide information about site of recurrence in patients who have biochemical failure after definitive treatment. This could greatly influence treatment choice. Levesque et al.[123] claim that the indium CYT-356 scan helps to localize PSA detected recurrent disease and guides treatment after radical prostatectomy. They base this conclusion on studies on 48 such patients who were scanned. Only three (6%) had activity in the prostatic fossa alone, 73% had activity beyond the fossa – 65% in the pelvic lymph nodes and 23% in abdominal and extrapelvic retroperitoneal lymph nodes. Twelve patients had radiation, which was deemed successful in two of five patients who had scans positive outside the field of radiation and in five of seven patients who had no activity beyond the irradiated field. However, the follow-up was short (17 months for responders, 14 months for non-responders, range 5–31 months), and the non-responders had a generally higher Gleason score, surgical stage and pre-operative PSA value.

Manyak and Javitt[122] report the following sources for misinterpretation of the radiolabelled MAB scan: asymmetrical pelvic vasculature, radionuclide excretion in the gastrointestinal tract or bladder, asymmetry in normal bone marrow and non-specific localization in scar or inflammation. Repeat scans 72–120 hours after injection are recommended in an attempt to avoid these pitfalls. It has been reported that the epitope of the PSMA, which is recognized by the CYT-356 antibody, is located intracellularly and concluded that recognition of living tumours by this antibody may be dependent upon the presence of dead cells at the tumour site that exclusively express the intracellular epitope, thus limiting the sensitivity of such imaging[123].

Although promising in potential, radioimmunoscintography needs further study before being considered for routine inclusion in the evaluation of patients who have newly diagnosed or recurrent disease.

CONCLUSIONS

Carcinoma of the prostate is an insidious progressive disease. Unless early detection strategies are employed, many patients present with cancer that has already spread beyond the confines of the gland and is therefore usually incurable. Early detection

by a combination of DRE and PSA testing has been shown to increase the yield of cancers confined to the prostate, but as yet, there has been no definite confirmation that this in itself reduces the disease-specific mortality.

Accurate diagnosis and staging is crucial for the selection of the most appropriate treatment modality (**8.22**). Digital rectal examination and PSA provide inexact indications of the local stage. On TRUS biopsy the number and percentage of the cores infiltrated and the tumour grade of the biopsies are useful ancillary features, which when

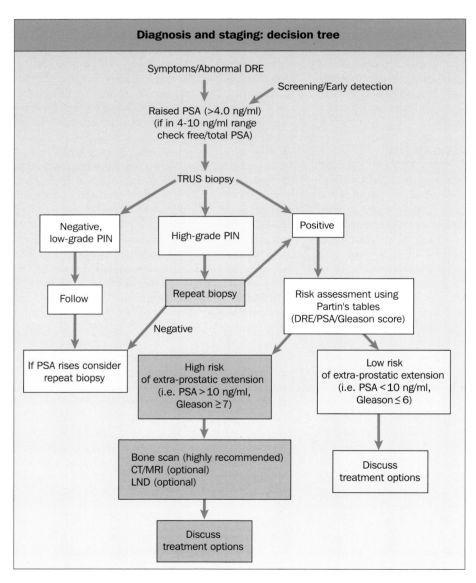

8.22 Prostate cancer diagnosis and staging: decision tree. PIN, prostatic intraepithelial neoplasia.

evaluated together with the serum PSA value and clinical stage, provide an estimate of the probability of prostatic extension in the individual patient. RT-PCR technology has not proven as helpful as first anticipated, but in the future artificial intelligence with multivariate analysis of a large number of parameters (neural networks) seems to hold the prospect for improving the accuracy of staging.

Computed tomography and MRI have proved disappointing as precise staging studies but may be helpful in selected cases. Bone scanning is now only recommended routinely for those who have PSA values higher than 10 ng/ml, unless other specific indications exist such as a high Gleason score, elevated acid phosphatase or skeletal symptoms, because it is almost always negative in these patients.

Immunoscintigraphy is currently in its infancy but holds some promise for the future. The Prostascint scan may be helpful, but needs further evaluation. Lymph node sampling by laparoscopy or minilaparotomy may be considered for those relatively few patients who have either poorly differentiated bilateral tumours and/or PSA values higher than 20 ng/ml, who by virtue of their life expectancy are otherwise candidates for curative therapy.

The challenge for the future is to identify with greater precision those patients who have apparently localized disease who, in fact, have extraprostatic extension. Pre-operative identification of this subgroup will not only improve the results of radical therapy, but also reduce the numbers of patients undergoing non-curative therapy. For these individuals, alternative strategies focused on managing their disseminated disease are more appropriate.

REFERENCES

1 Brawer MK, Beatie J, Wener MH, Vessella RL, Preston SD, Lange PH. Screening for prostatic carcinoma with prostate-specific antigen: results of the second year. *J Urol* 1993;**150**:106–109.

2 Smith DS, Catalona WJ. Interexaminer variability of digital rectal examination in detecting prostate cancer. *Urology* 1995;**45**:70–74.

3 Angulo J, Montie J, Buckowsky T, *et al*. Interobserver consistency of digital rectal examination in clinical staging of localised prostate carcinoma. *Urol Oncol* 1995;**1**:199–205.

4 Kenny B, Read A, Naylor A, Greengrass P, Carter A, Wyllie M. Effect of alpha-1 adrenoceptor antagonists on prostatic pressure and blood pressure in the anaesthetised dog. *Urology* 1994;**44**:52–55.

5 Oesterling JE. Prostate-specific antigen. A critical assessment of the most useful tumor marker for adenocarcinoma of the prostate. Review article. *J Urol* 1991;**145**:907–923.

6 Catalona WJ, Smith DS, Ratliff TL, *et al*. Measurement of prostate-specific antigen in serum as a screening test for prostate cancer. *N Engl J Med* 1991;**324**:1156.

7 Polascik TJ, Oesterling JE, Partin AW. Prostate-specific antigen: a decade of discovery – what have we learned and where are we going? *J Urol* 1999:**162**:293–306.

8 Lange PH, Ercole CJ, Lightner DJ, Fraley EE, Vessella R. The value of serum prostate-specific antigen determinations before and after radical prostatectomy. *J Urol* 1989;**141**:873–879.

9 Chybowski FM, Larson-Keller JJ, Bergstralh EJ, *et al*. Predicting radionuclide bone scan findings in patients with newly diagnosed, untreated prostate cancer. Prostate-specific antigen is superior to all other clinical parameters. *J Urol* 1991;**145**:313.

10 D'Amico AV, Whittington R, Schultz D, *et al*. Outcome based staging for clinically localized adenocarcinoma of the prostate. *J Urol* 1997;**158**:1422–1426.

11 D'Amico AV, Whittington R, Malkowicz SB, *et al*. A multivariate analysis of clinical and pathological factors that predict for prostate-specific antigen failure after radical prostatectomy for prostate cancer. *J Urol* 1995;**154**:131–138.

12 McCormack RT, Rittenhouse HG, Finlay JA, *et al*. Molecular forms of prostate-specific antigen and the human kallikrein gene family. A new era. *Urology* 1995;**45**:729–744.

13 Murphy GP, Holmes EH, Boynton AL, *et al*. Comparison of prostate-specific antigen, prostate specific membrane antigen, and LNCaP-based enzyme-linked immunosorbent assays in prostatic cancer patients and patients with benign prostatic enlargement. *Prostate* 1994;**26**:164–168.

14 Chodak GW, Keller P, Schoenberg HW. Assessment of screening for prostate cancer using digital rectal examination. *J Mol* 1989;**141**:1136.

15 Scardino PT. Early detection of prostate cancer. *Urol Clin North Am* 1989;**16**:635.

16 Peters PC. Staging, clinical manifestations and indications for intervention in prostate cancer. In. Lepor H, Lawson RK, eds. *Prostate Diseases*. Philadelphia: WB Saunders; 1993:269.

17 Smith BR, Middleton RG. Prostate-specific antigen: correlation with pathological staging. *J Urol* 1993;**149**:262A.

18 Pannek J, Subong ENP, Jones KA, *et al*. The role of free/total prostate-specific antigen ratio in the prediction of final pathologic stage for men with clinically localized prostate cancer. *Urology* 1996;**48(6A)**:51.

19 Badalament RA, Miller MC, Peller PA, *et al*. An algorithm of predicting nonorgan-confined prostate

cancer using the results obtained from sextant core biopsy with PSA level. *J Urol* 1996;**156**:1375.

20 McNeal JE, Villers AA, Redwine EA, *et al.* Histologic differentiation, cancer volume and pelvic lymph node metastasis in adenocarcinoma of the prostate. *Cancer* 1990;**66**:220–225.

21 Epstein JI. The diagnosis and reporting of adenocarcinoma of the prostate in core needle biopsy specimens. *Cancer* 1996;**78**:350.

22 Narayan P, Gejendran V, Taylor SK, *et al.* The role of transrectal ultrasound guided biopsy based on staging, preoperative serum prostate-specific antigen, and biopsy Gleason score in production of final pathological diagnosis in prostate cancer. *Urology* 1995;**46**:250.

23 Ackerman DA, Barry JM, Wickland RA, Olson N, Lowe BA. Analysis of risk factors associated with prostate cancer extension to the surgical margin and pelvic node metastasis at radical prostatectomy. *J Urol* 1993;**150**:1845.

24 Hammer P, Huland H, Sparenberg A. Digital rectal examination imaging and systemic sextant biopsy in identifying operable lymph node negative prostatic carcinoma. *Eur Urol* 1992;**22**:281.

25 Bostwick DG, Qian J, Bergstraili E, *et al.* Prediction of capsular perforation and seminal vesicle invasion in prostate cancer. *J Urol* 1996;**155**:1361.

26 Daniels GF, McNeal JE, Stamey TA. Predictive value of contralateral biopsies in unilaterally palpable prostate cancer. *J Urol* 1992;**141**:870.

27 Villers AA, McNeal JE, Redwine EA, *et al.* Pathogenesis and biological significance of seminal vesicle invasion in prostatic adenocarcinoma. *J Urol* 1990;**143**:1883.

28 Stamey TA, McNeal JE. Adenocarcinoma of the prostate. In: Walsh PC, Retik AB, Stamey TA, Vaughn ED, eds. *Campbell's Urology*, 6th edition. Philadelphia: WB Saunders; 1992:1159.

29 Oesterling JE, Chan DW, Epstein JI, *et al.* Prostate-specific antigen in the preoperative and postoperative evaluation of localized prostatic cancer treated with radical prostatectomy. *J Urol* 1988;**139**:766.

30 Kleer E, Larson-Keller JJ, Zincke H, Oesterling JE. Ability of pre-operative serum prostate-specific antigen value to predict pathologic state and DNA ploidy. *Urology* 1993;**41**:207.

31 Blackwell KL, Bostwick DG, Myers RP, Zincke H, Oesterling JE. Combining prostate-specific antigen with cancer and gland volume to predict more reliably pathological state. The influence of prostate-specific antigen cancer density. *J Urol* 1994;**151**:1565.

32 Bluestein DL, Bostwick DG, Bergstralh EJ, Oesterling JE. Eliminating the need for bilateral pelvic lymphadenectomy in select patients with prostate cancer. *J Urol* 1994;**151**:1315.

33 Sands ME, Zagars GK, Poilack A, Von Eschenbach AC. Serum prostate-specific antigen, clinical stage, pathologic grade, and the incidence of nodal metastases in prostate cancer. *Urology* 1994;**44**:215.

34 Narayan P, Fournier G, Gajendran V, *et al.* Utility of preoperative serum prostate-specific antigen concentration and biopsy Gleason score in predicting risk of pelvic lymph node metastases in prostate cancer. *Urology* 1994;**44**:519.

35 Rogers E, Gurpinar T, Dillioglugil O, *et al.* The role of digital rectal examination, biopsy Gleason sum, and prostate-specific antigen in selecting patients who require pelvic lymph node dissections for prostate cancer. *Br J Urol* 1996;**78**:419.

36 Kattan MN, Stapleton AMF, Wheeler TM, Scardino PT. Evaluation of a nomogram for predicting pathological state of men with clinically localized prostate cancer. *Cancer* 1996;**79**:528.

37 Partin AW, Yoo J, Carter HB, *et al.* The use of prostate-specific antigen, clinical stage and Gleason score to predict pathological stage in men with localized prostate cancer. *J Urol* 1993;**50**:110.

38 Partin AW, Kattan MW, Subong EN, *et al.* Combination of prostate-specific antigen, clinical stage and Gleason score to predict pathological stage of localized prostate cancer. A multi-institutional update. *JAMA* 1997;**277**:1445.

39 Snow PB, Smith DS, Catalona WJ. Artificial neural networks in the diagnosis and prognosis of prostate cancer: a pilot study. *J Urol* 1994;**152**:1223.

40 Douglas TH, Moul JW. Applications of neural networks in urologic oncology. *Semin Urol Oncol* 1998;**16**:35.

41 Naguib RN, Robinson MC, Neal DE, Hamdy FC. Neural network analysis of combined conventional and experimental prognostic markers in prostate cancer: a pilot study. *Br J Cancer* 1998;**78**:246.

42 Tewari A, Narayan P. Novel staging tools for localized prostate cancer: a pilot study using genetic adaptive neural networks. *J Urol* 1998;**160**:430.

43 Bostwick DG. Practical clinical application of predictive factors in prostate cancer. A review with an emphasis on quantitative methods in tissue specimens. *Analytic Quant Cytol Histol* 1998;**20**:323.

44 Kirby RS. Pre-treatment staging of prostate cancer. recent advances and future prospects. *Pr Cancer Pr Dis* 1997;**1**:2–10.

45 Brawer MK. Quantitative microvessel density; a staging and prognostic marker for human prostatic carcinoma. *Cancer* 1996;**78**:345–349.

46 Weidner N, Carroll PR, Flax J, Blumenfeld W, Folkman J. Tumour angiogenesis correlates with metastasis in invasive prostate carcinoma. *Hum Pathol* 1993;**143**:401–409.

47 Weidner N. Tumour angiogenesis. Review of current applications in tumour prognostication. *Semin Diagn Pathol* 1993;**10**:302–331.

48 Bigler SA, Deering RE, Brawer MK. Comparison of microscopic vascularity in benign and malignant prostate tissue. *Hum Pathol* 1993;**24**:220–226.

49 Brawer MK, Deering RE, Brown M, Preston SD, Bigler SA. Predictors of pathologic stage in prostatic carcinoma. *Cancer* 1994;**73**:678–687.

50 Weidner N, Folkman J. Tumoral vascularity as a prognostic factor in cancer. In: DeVita VT, Hellman S, Rosenberg SA, eds. *Important Advances in Oncology.* Philadelphia: Lippincott-Raven; 1996:167–190.

51 Bostwick DG, Wheeler TM, Blute M, *et al.* Optimized microvessel density analysis improves prediction of cancer stage from prostate needle biopsies. *Urology* 1996;**48**:47–57.

52 Siegal JA, Ye E, Brawer MK. Topography of neovascularity in human prostate carcinoma. *Cancer* 1995;**75**:2545–2551.

53 Mydlo JH, Kral JG, Volpe M, Axotis C, Macchia RJ, Pertschuk LP. An analysis of microvessel density, androgen receptor, p53 and HER-2/neu expression and Gleason score in prostate cancer: preliminary results and therapeutic implications. *Eur Urol* 1998;**34**:426–432.

54 Borre M, Offersen BV, Nerstrom B, Overgaard J. Microvessel density predicts survival in prostate cancer patients subjected to watchful waiting. *Br J Cancer* 1998;**78**(7):940–944.

55 Gettman MT, Bergstralh EJ, Blute M, Zinncke H, Bostwick DG. Prediction of patient outcome in pathologic stage T2 adenocarcinoma of the prostate: lack of significance for microvessel density analysis. *Urology* 1998;**51**:79–85.

56 Rubin MA, Buyyounouski M, Bagiella E, *et al.* Microvessel density in prostate cancer: lack of correlation with tumour grade, pathologic stage and clinical outcome. *Urology* 1999;**53**:542–547.

57 Katz AE, Olsson C, Raffo A, *et al.* Molecular staging of prostate cancer with the use of an enhanced reverse transcriptase-PCR assay. *Urology* 1994;**43**:765–775.

58 Cama C, Olsson C, Raffo A, *et al.* Molecular staging of prostate cancer II. A comparison of the application of an enhanced reverse transcriptase polymerase chain reaction assay for prostate-specific antigen and prostate specific membrane antigen. *J Urol* 1995;**153**:1373–1378.

59 Olssen CA, De Vried G, Raffo GM, *et al.* Pre-operative reverse transcriptase polymerase chain reaction for prostate-specific antigen predicts treatment failure. *J Urol* 1996;**155**:1557.

60 Sokoloff MH, Tso CL, Kaboo R, *et al.* Quantitative PCR does not improve pre-operative prostate cancer staging: clinicopathological molecular analysis of 121 patients. *J Urol* 1996;**156**:1560.

61 Ignatoff JM, Oefelein MG, Watkin W, *et al.* RSA PCR-RT assay in pre-operative staging of prostate cancer. *J Urol* 1997;**158**:1870.

62 Ellis WJ, Vessella RL, Coney E, *et al.* The value of a RT-PCR assay in pre-operative staging and follow-up of patients with prostate cancer. *J Urol* 1998;**159**:1134.

63 Dumas F, Eschwege P, Le Maine V, *et al.* Blood prostatic epithelial cells during radical surgery and prostatic transurethral resection. *J Urol* 1997;**157**:394A:1543.

64 Seiden MV, Kantoff PW, Krithivas K, *et al.* Detection of circulating tumor cells in men with localized prostate cancer. *J Clin Oncol* 1994;**12**:2634.

65 Ghossein RA, Scher HI, Gerals WL, *et al.* Detection of circulating tumour cells in patients with localized and metastatic prostate carcinoma: clinical implications. *J Clin Oncol* 1995;**13**:1195.

66 Israeli R, Miller WH Jr, Su SL. Sensitive rested RT-PCR detection of circulating tumor cells: comparison of PSMA and PSA assays. *Cancer Res* 1994;**54**:6306.

67 de Cremoux P, Ravery V, Podgomiak MP. Value of the pre-operative detection of PSA positive circulating cells by rested RT-PCR in patients submitted to radical prostatectomy. *Eur Urol* 1997;**32**:69.

68 Oetelein M, Kaul K, Herz B, *et al.* Molecular detection of prostate epithelial cells from the surgical field and peripheral circulation during radical prostatectomy. *J Urol* 1996;**155**:238.

69 Oetelein M, Ignatoff JM, Clemens JQ, *et al.* Clinical and molecular follow-up after radical retropubic prostatectomy. *J Urol* 1999;**162**:307–311.

70 Rifkin M, Sudakoff G, Alexander A. Prostate. Techniques, results and potential applications of colour Doppler US scanning. *Radiology* 1993;**186**:509–513.

71 Ferguson JK, Bostwick DG, Suman V, Zincke H, Oesterling JE. Prostate-specific antigen detected prostate cancer. Pathological characteristics of ultrasound visible versus ultrasound invisible tumours. *Eur Urol* 1995;**27**:8–12.

72 Rifkin M, Choi H. Implications of small, peripheral hypoechoic lesions in endorectal US of the prostate. *Radiology* 1998;**166**:619–622.

73 Ohori M, Egawa S, Shinohara K, *et al.* Detection of microscopic extracapsular extension prior to radical prostatectomy for clinically localized prostate cancer. *Br J Urol* 1994;**74**:72–79.

74 Narayan P, Jajodia P, Stein R. Core biopsy instrument in the diagnosis of prostate cancer superior accuracy to fine needle aspiration. *J Urol* 1991;**145**:795–799.

75 Brawer MK, Deering RE, Brown M, Preston SD, Bigler SA. Predictors of pathologic stage in prostatic carcinoma. The role of neovascularity. *Cancer* 1994;**73**:678–687.

76 Aihara M, Wheeler TM, Ohori M, Scardino PT. Heterogeneity of prostate cancer in radical prostatectomy specimens. *Urology* 1994;**43**:60–67.

77 Haggman M, Norberg M, de la Torre M, Fritiofsson A, Busch C. Characterization of localized prostatic cancer: distribution, and pT-staging in radical prostatectomy specimens. *Scand J Urol Nephrol* 1993;**27**:7–13.

78 Donahue RE, Miller GJ. Adenocarcinoma of the prostate. Biopsy to whole mount. Denver VA experience. *Urol Clin North Am* 1991;**18**:449–452.

79 True LO. Surgical pathology examination of the prostate gland. Practice survey by American Society of Clinical Pathologists. *Am J Clin Pathol* 1994;**10**:572–579.

80 Henson DE, Hutter RVP, Farrow GM. Practice protocol for the examination of specimens removed from patients with carcinoma of the prostate gland. A publication of the Cancer Committee. College of

American Pathologists. *Arch Pathol Lab Med* 1994;**118**:779–783.

81 Amin MB, Grignon D, Bostwick D, *et al.* Recommendations for reporting resected prostatic carcinomas. *Hum Pathol* 1996;**27**:321–323.

82 Sakr WA, Wheeler TM, Blute M, *et al.* Staging and reporting of prostate cancer – sampling of the radical prostatectomy specimen. *Cancer* 1996;**78**:366–368.

83 Bostwick DG, Cupp MR, Oesterling JE. Tumor volume in prostate cancer. Correlation of needle biopsy and radical prostatectomy findings. *Mod Pathol* 1993;**6(Abstract)**:57A.

84 Egan AJM, Bostwick DG. Prediction of extraprostatic expansion of prostate cancer based on needle biopsy findings. *Am J Surg Pathol* 1997;**21**:1496–1500.

85 Epstein JL, Carmichael M, Pizov G, Walsh PC. Influence of capsular penetration on progression following radical prostatectomy: a study of 196 cases with long-term follow-up. *J Urol* 1993;**150**:135–141.

86 Muru M, Ultsumoniya T, Kattan MW. Significance of perineural invasion in addition to other pathological features in the prediction of progression of prostate cancer. *J Urol* 2000;**163**:321–322.

87 McNeal JE, Viller M, Redwine EA, Freiha FS, Stamey TA. Capsular penetration in prostate cancer. Significance for natural history and treatment. *Am J Surg Pathol* 1990;**14**:240–247.

88 Epstein JI, Partin AW, Suavageot J, Walsh PC. Prediction of progression following radical prostatectomy: a multivariate analysis of 721 men with long-term follow-up. *Am J Surg Pathol* 1996;**20**:286–292.

89 Paulson DF, Moul JW, Walther PJ. Radical prostatectomy for clinical state T1–2N0M0 prostatic adenocarcinoma: long-term results. *J Urol* 1990;**144**:1180–1184.

90 Epstein JI, Carmichael J, Partin AW, Walsh PC. Is tumor volume an independent predictor of progression following radical prostatectomy? A multivariate analysis of 185 clinical stage B adenocarcinoma of the prostate with 5 years of follow-up. *J Urol* 1993;**194**:1478–1485.

91 Ayala AG, Ro JY, Babaian R, Troncoso P, Grignon DJ. The prostatic capsule: does it exist? Its importance in the staging and treatment of prostatic carcinoma. *Am J Surg Pathol* 1989;**13**:21–27.

92 Babaian R, Troncoso P, Bhadkamkar VA, Johnston DA. Pathologic category specific modeling to predict biochemical failure in men undergoing radical prostatectomy. *J Urol* (in press)

93 McNeal JE, Villers AA, Redwine EA, Freiha FS, Stamey TA. Histologic differentiation, cancer volume, and pelvic lymph node metastasis in adenocarcinoma of the prostate. *Cancer* 1990;**66**:1225–1233.

94 Stamey TA, McNeal JE, Yemoto CM, Bronislava MS, Johnstone IM. Biological determinants of cancer progression in men with prostate cancer. *JAMA* 1999;**281**:1395–1400.

95 Wymenga LFA, Duisterwinkel FJ, Groenier K, Mensink HJA. Ultrasound-guided seminal vesicle biopsies in prostate cancer. *Prostate Cancer and Prostatic Diseases* 2000; (in press).

96 White S, Hricak H, Forstner M, *et al.* Prostate cancer: effect of post biopsy hemorrhage on interpretation of MR images. *Radiology* 1995;**195**:339–342.

97 Rifkin MD, Zerhouni EA, Gatsonis CA, *et al.* Comparison of magnetic resonance imaging and ultrasonography in staging early prostate cancer. Results of a multi-institutional cooperative trial. *N Engl J Med* 1990;**323**:621–625.

98 Bernstein MR, Wein AJ, Siegelman ES, Tomaszewski JE, Malkowitz SB. Lack of correlation of clinical and pathologic staging of capsular involvement in prostate cancer using endorectal coil magnetic resonance imaging. *J Pelvic Surg* 1999;**4**:203–207.

99 Forman H, Heiken J, Brink J, Glazer H, Fox L, McClennan B. CT screening for comorbid disease in patients with prostatic carcinoma. Is it cost-effective? *AJR Am J Roentgenol* 1994;**162**:1125–1128.

100 Pisansky T, Zinke H, Suman V, Bostwick D, Earle J, Oesterling J. Correlation of pretherapy prostate cancer characteristics with histologic findings from pelvic lymphadenectomy specimens. *Int J Radiation Biol Phys* 1996;**34**:33–39.

101 Edelstein R, Zeitman A, Morenas A, *et al.* Implications of prostate micrometastases in pelvic lymph nodes. An archival tissue study. *Urology* 1996;**47**:370–375.

102 Kirby R, Christmas T, Brawer M. Tumour markers in prostate cancer. In: Kirby R, Christmas T, Brawer M, eds. *Prostate Cancer*. London: Mosby; 1996:55–64.

103 Wirth MP, Frohmuller HGW. Prostate-specific antigen and prostatic acid phosphatase in the detection of early prostate cancer and in the prediction of regional lymph node metastases. *Eur Urol* 1992;**21**:263–268.

104 Lee CT, Oesterling JE. Using prostate-specific antigen to eliminate the staging radionuclide bone scan. *Urol Clin North Am* 1997;**24(2)**:389–394.

105 Gleave ME, Coupland D, Drachenberg D, *et al.* Ability of serum prostate-specific antigen levels to predict normal bone scans in patients with newly diagnosed prostate cancer. *Urology* 1996;**46**:708.

106 Levran Z, Gonzalez JA, Dickno AC, *et al.* Are pelvic computer tomography bone scan and pelvic lymphadenectomy necessary in the staging of prostate cancer? *Br J Urol* 1995;**75**:778.

107 Middleton RG, Thompson IM, Austerfeld MS, *et al.* Report on the management of clinically localised prostate cancer. Baltimore MD: American Urologic Association; 1995:1–49.

108 Baker LH, Hanks G, Gersherson D, *et al.* NCCN Prostate cancer guidelines. The National Comprehensive Cancer Network. *Oncology* 1996;**10(Suppl)**:265.

109 Richie JP, Murphy GP, Walther P, *et al.* Prostate cancer surgical practice guidelines. Oncology 1997;**11(6)**:907–912.

110 O'Dowd GJ, Ventri RW, Orzco R, *et al.* Update on the appropriate staging evaluation for newly diagnosed prostate cancer. *J Urol* 1997;**158**:687–698.

111 Manyak MJ. Clinical applications of radioimmuno-scintography with prostate specific antibodies for prostate cancer. *Cancer Control* 1998;**5**:493–499.

112 Plawker MW, Fleisher JM, Vaprek EM, Macchia RJ. Current trends in prostate cancer diagnosis and staging among US urologists. *J Urol* 1997;**158**:1853–1858.

113 Perotti M, Fair WR. Prostate cancer staging in the newly diagnosed patient. Houston: American Urological Association Office of Education; AUA Update Series 1997;**16**(30):234–239.

114 Jorgensen T, Muller C, Kaalhus O, Daniellsen H, Tveter K. Extent of disease based on bone scan. Important prognostic indicator for patients with metastatic prostate cancer. *Eur Urol* 1995;**28**:40–46.

115 Johnstone PAS, Tarman GJ, Riffenburgh R, *et al.* Yield of imaging and scintigraphy assessing biochemical failure in prostate cancer patients. *Urol Oncol* 1997;**3**:108–112.

116 Miller PD, Eardley I, Kirby RS. Prostate-specific antigen and bone scan correlation in staging and monitoring of patients with prostate cancer. *Br J Urol* 1992;**70**:295–298.

117 Vikko P, Heikkila I, Kontturi M. Radioimaging of the prostate and metastases of prostatic carcinoma with 99m Tc labeled prostatic acid phosphatase specific antibodies and their FAB fragments. *Ann Clin Res* 1984;**32**:723–727.

118 Leroy T, Teillac P, Rain JDE. Radioimmunodetection of lymph node invasion in prostatic cancer. The use of iodine 123 (^{123}I)-labelled monoclonal anti-prostatic acid phosphatase (PAP) 227 AF (ab')2 antibody fragments *in vivo*. *Cancer* 1989;**64**:1–5.

119 Ahonen A, Kairemo K, Karnani PE. Radioimmunodetection of prostatic cancer by ^{111}In-labelled monoclonal antibody against prostatic acid phosphatase. *Acta Oncol* 1993;**32**:723–727.

120 Horoszewicz JS, Kawinski E, Murphy GP. Monoclonal antibodies to a new antigenic marker in epithelial prostatic cells and serum of prostatic cancer patients. *Anticancer Res* 1987;**7**:927–935.

121 Babaian RJ, Sayer J, Podoloff DA, *et al.* Radioimmunoscintography of pelvic lymph nodes with III indium-labelled monoclonal antibody CTT-356. *J Urol* 1994;**152**:1954–1955.

122 Manyak MJ, Javitt MC. The role of computerized tomography, magnetic resonance imaging, bone scan and monoclonal antibody nuclear scan for prognosis prediction in prostate cancer. *Semin Urol Oncol* 1998;**16**:145–152.

123 Levesque PE, Nieh PT, Zinman N, *et al.* Radiolabeled monoclonal indium 111-labeled CYT-356 localizes extraprostatic recurrent carcinoma after prostatectomy. *Urology* 1998;**51**:978–984.

Chapter 9

Treatment of localized prostate cancer: radical prostatectomy and radiation therapy

The treatment of clinically localized adenocarcinoma of the prostate has undergone considerable evolution and refinement over the 90 years that have passed since Hugh Hampton Young developed the radical perineal prostatectomy (**Table 9.1**). Factors such as downward stage migration in the clinical presentation due to prostate-specific antigen (PSA) testing, the development of and subsequent improvements in radiation delivery to the prostate, as well as modifications in surgical technique associated with decreased morbidity, have all contributed towards enhancement in treatment approaches for confined prostate cancer.

Implicit within the concept of treatment of clinically localized cancer is the ability to identify such cancers at a stage where effective therapy is both possible and necessary.

The determination of a localized malignancy (T1–T3) is dependent upon accurate staging techniques. As discussed in the chapter on staging, one of the major problems in prostate cancer is our inability to define the clinical stage with precision. Significant upstaging and, to a lesser degree, downstaging of neoplasms in men subjected to radical prostatectomy have consistently demonstrated the inadequacy of current staging modalities[1–7]. Currently, urologists use digital rectal examination (DRE), serum acid phosphatase and prostate-specific antigen and transrectal ultrasound techniques, as well as other methods including computed tomography (CT), magnetic resonance imaging and, more recently, endorectal coil magnetic resonance imaging, to assist in arriving at what is admittedly only an estimate of the clinical stage (see Chapter 8).

The use of prostate-specific antigen in combination with clinical stage and Gleason score on biopsy has been shown in a multi-institutional study involving 4133 men to improve the ability to predict pathological stage as compared to each variable independently[8]. These authors have provided nomograms to predict pathological stage (see Chapter 8).

The use of tissue-derived parameters to augment staging studies, including tumour grade, DNA ploidy and investigational studies of neovascularity, expression of oncogenes and tumour suppressor genes, as well as growth factors, is discussed more fully in the chapters on molecular biology and pathology.

With the increasing worldwide interest in early detection and screening, there has been a pronounced movement towards a more favourable stage at presentation (both between stages in general, and within given stages), which is most marked in the USA. Instead of the bulky T3/T4 cancers with gross capsular penetration and extension into the pelvic sidewall or seminal vesicles, most modern radical prostatectomy series currently describe only minimal, microscopic capsular penetration or positive margins in patients who are pathologically upstaged. Thus, it is not always appropriate to apply the lessons of historical series to current patient care.

Table 9.1 Milestones in the treatment of prostate cancer

Year	Author	Milestone
1904	Young	Development of radical prostatectomy
1910	Paschkis, Tittinger	Intraurethral radium
1934	Widmann	External beam radiation
1941	Huggins, Hodges	Hormonal ablation
1979	Wang	Characterization of PSA
1979	Reiner, Walsh	Anatomical radical prostatectomy
1982	Walsh, Donker	Nerve sparing radical prostatectomy
1987	Labrie	Maximal androgen blockade

The goal of treatment of clinically localized prostate cancer is cure; that is to say, as suggested by a recent prostate cancer consensus meeting in Antwerp, Belgium[9], 'affording the patient the best chance of dying of something else'. A number of factors need to be considered when deciding whether a patient is suitable for therapy with curative intent. Perhaps of greatest significance is that the patient should have at least a ten-year life expectancy. Thus, an accurate assessment of intercurrent disease, as well as other risk factors for longevity, must be conducted. As the majority of men with clinically localized prostate cancer will have minimal impact from their disease for several years at least, it obviously makes little sense to subject an individual to the morbidity of locally directed therapy if they have a limited life expectancy.

The treatment options (**Table 9.2**) include watchful waiting or expectant management, radical prostatectomy, radiation therapy delivered by either external or brachytherapy approaches, androgen deprivation and, more recently, cryotherapeutic ablation. Neo-adjuvant therapies offer the promise of prostate gland volume reduction. Results with abarelix (a GnRH antagonist) showed a median 35% decrease in gland volume before brachytherapy or radiation therapy[10]. With all these alternative treatment modalities, the concern is lack of adequate long-term randomized trials to compare and contrast the merits of one therapy with another. In the absence of the results of such studies, it is exceedingly difficult to offer answers as to which treatment modality is optimal for a given individual.

Another difficulty in evaluating the different treatment modalities is the problem inherent in defining what is 'cure'. **Table 9.3** illustrates a

Table 9.3 Possible definitions of cure

Death from non-prostatic cause
Absence of disseminated disease
Absence of local/regional disease
Negative prostate or prostatic bed biopsy
Normal rectal examination
Non-detectable serum PSA

hierarchical schema of the evidence of failure of cure in prostate cancer. Given that the goal of treatment of clinically localized prostate cancer is to afford the opportunity of the patient to die of something else, one might conclude that patients are 'cured' if this is achieved.

However, even in this simplistic approach, confusion arises as it is often difficult to state definitively whether a patient with prostate cancer actually died of his disease. Given the age of the patients at risk with significant intercurrent illness, competing causes of mortality must always be considered in the aetiology of a patient's demise. Even in cases of clearcut progression of disease, one must consider whether 'failed' local therapy actually afforded improvement in the patient's quality and quantity of life, at least for a time.

This concept is certainly biased by the development of a valuable marker of progression of prostate cancer – prostate-specific antigen (PSA). This analyte, particularly in men following radical prostatectomy, affords absolute and unequivocal evidence of progression in that, if the PSA does fall to the non-detectable level, then there is evidence of persistent disease, and if PSA falls but subsequently becomes detectable at ever higher levels, there is progression. PSA is an exquisitely sensitive marker of progression, and is generally a harbinger of subsequent clinical disease. One can therefore rely on this simple assay to select patients for further evaluation of potential of progression, including radionucleotide bone scan for bony metastases, upper tract studies to assess hydronephrosis, serum creatinine, and full blood count to assess systemic illness, and so forth.

However, whether this biochemical evidence of progression actually indicates a deterioration in the patients' quality and quantity of life is not known. Certainly, a man who has a detectable level of PSA 12 years after radical prostatectomy has evidence of persistent disease. If he succumbs to a myocardial

Table 9.2 Localized prostate cancer: therapeutic options

Watchful waiting
Transurethral resection
Radical prostatectomy
External-beam radiation therapy
Brachytherapy
Cryotherapy
Androgen deprivation
Laser combination therapy
Interstitial laser therapy

infarction, it would seem that his persistent disease contributed little to his demise. Thus one could argue in pragmatic terms that he was 'cured'.

PSA allows us to monitor patients following radical prostatectomy with greater reliability. Its use after radiation therapy remains somewhat confusing, however, but it seems highly likely that progressive elevation of PSA as well as failure to achieve a significant nadir after definitive radiation therapy are ominous prognostic indicators.

In general, with either of these treatment approaches, PSA monitoring in conjunction with history and physical examination provides the most efficient and economical approach to following patients after therapy. Nonetheless, it has to be conceded that patients run a risk of becoming obsessed with their PSA result, regardless of whether a PSA rise is in fact accompanied by symptoms.

One of the major controversies in the treatment of prostate cancer is between radical prostatectomy and radiation therapy. However, only one study has attempted to look at this in a prospective fashion and this had several methodologic problems[11]. Although this study did show a slightly improved outcome in men randomized to radical prostatectomy more contemporary series have questioned this. Recently, Kupelian demonstrated that at 5-year follow-up of two comparable but not randomized cohorts of men biochemical reoccurrence rate was similar in both groups[12]. It is often stated that we must wait for a prospective randomized trial to resolve what is the best treatment modality. It is unlikely that a major trial comparing radiation therapy (either by external beam or brachytherapy) versus radical prostatectomy will ever be completed. Therefore one is generally left with quality of life issues versus perhaps slightly greater biochemical cure rates in making treatment decisions between the modalities.

Therefore one is left with a comparison of series of radical prostatectomy versus radiation therapy. In this regard it is quite clear that historical series recorded in general less aggressive malignancies being treated with surgery and the radiation cohort had more extensive disease. The evidence for this stems from the Massachusetts General Hospital series[13]. In an example, 54% of the men who had T2b/T2c cancer had radiation therapy compared with 41% of those undergoing radical prostatectomy. This and other biases make such comparisons unreliable.

RADICAL PROSTATECTOMY

Radical prostatectomy has been recommended by some for almost all stages of prostate cancer. Affording cure is the goal in localized disease, whereas efforts to provide a reduction in local symptoms of progression is the intent in patients with established, advanced disease. Radical prostatectomy is widely used today only in men in whom it is likely to afford cure – in effect, only in those in whom it is felt that the malignancy is completely extirpable by surgery. This, in general, applies to those men with a stage T1 or T2 disease with low-to-moderate grade pathology and a life expectancy of more than 10 years. Cure may be achieved in some patients with minimal T3 disease, and perhaps a very few with minimal lymph node metastases. **Table 9.4** depicts the criteria for the selection of patients for radical prostatectomy.

Patients undergoing radical retropubic prostatectomy should be evaluated with a careful history and physical examination, with care being taken to detect comorbidity due to underlying cardiovascular and pulmonary disease. Chest x-ray and electrocardiography, along with urinalysis, serum creatinine and complete blood count, are obtained. Some surgeons now ask the patients to donate 2–3 units of autologous blood prior to the procedure. A cleansing enema and systemic antimicrobial prophylaxis are often used.

The goal of radical prostatectomy, whether by the retropubic or perineal approach, is to achieve complete excision of the prostate, seminal vesicles and adjacent tissue. The caudal and cephalad margins include the membranous urethra and the bladder neck. The posterior margin is Denonvillier's fascia, and anteriorly is the fibroadipose tissue of the cave of Retzius. Laterally, the boundary is the prostatic plexus medial to the neurovascular bundle if a nerve-sparing approach is performed. Radical retropubic prostatectomy can now be

Table 9.4 Criteria for radical prostatectomy
Histological evidence of prostate cancer
Clinically localized stage T1–T2
10-year or more life expectancy
Absence of surgical contraindication
Adequate informed consent

reliably accomplished in less than 2–3 hours with minimal morbidity. The patient is placed on the operating table with 10–20° of break at its midpoint to increase the distance between the pubis and xiphisternum. A 20F urethral catheter is passed and balloon inflated. A lower-midline or lower-transverse abdominal incision is made and the dissection kept extraperitoneal. Bilateral, internal iliac node dissections are generally performed, but frozen section histology is no longer generally obtained (unless there is reasonable degree of suspicion that they may be positive, i.e. PSA >10 ng/ml). After division of the endopelvic fascia, attention is then paid to the division of the avascular pubo-prostatic ligaments close to the pubis (**9.1**), and to securing the dorsal venous complex. If this is accomplished successfully, blood loss from the entire procedure rarely exceeds 700 ml. After 'bunching' the structure with a long-handled Babcock retractor (**9.2**), a strong absorbable ligature or suture may be passed around the dorsal vein complex, which is then divided to expose the urethra, as it enters the apex of the prostate. Careful dissection in this location using a Gil-Vernet renal retractor increases the length of urethra for subsequent anastomosis to the bladder neck. The urethra and the catheter it contains are then divided sharply, with careful attention being paid to the avoidance of the neuro-vascular bundles, which are located dorsolaterally (but very close to the apex of the prostate) at this point. The proximal end of the catheter may then be used as a retractor to facilitate the 'peeling back'

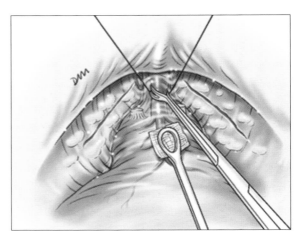

9.2 The dorsal venous complex is 'bunched' with a long-handled Babcock retractor and ligated.

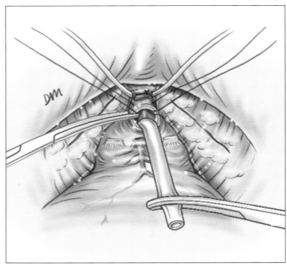

9.3 The anterior aspect of the urethra is sharply divided, the catheter cut, and its proximal end used as a retractor. The posterior portion is then divided.

of the prostate with the division of the rest of the urethra (**9.3**), and the stepwise securement and division of the lateral vascular pedicles, keeping close to the prostate to preserve the internally placed neurovascular bundles (**9.4**). The seminal vesicles and ampullary portions of both vasa come into view, and may be dissected out via this inferior approach. The ampullary portions of both vasa are divided, and the seminal vesicles freed (**9.5**). A small artery supplies the medial side of each seminal

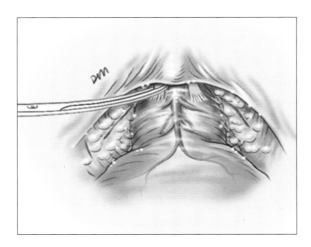

9.1 The puboprostatic ligaments are divided near to the pubis after the endopelvic fascia has been incised.

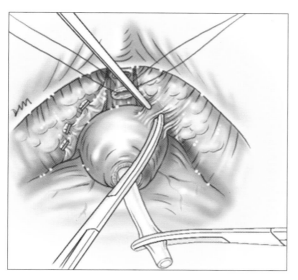

9.4 The lateral pedicles containing vessels are clipped and divided close to the prostate, thus preserving the neuro-vascular bundles.

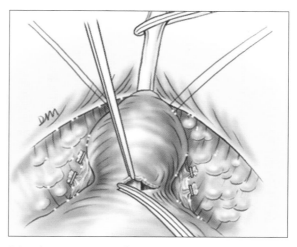

9.6 The prostate is carefully dissected away from the bladder neck.

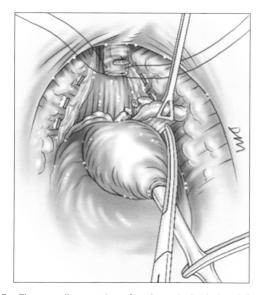

9.5 The ampullary portion of each vas is divided and the seminal vesicles dissected free, their apical vessels having been clipped.

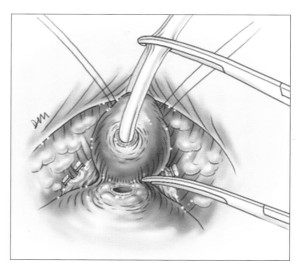

9.7 The catheter can be used as a 'loop retractor' to help the separation of the prostate from the trigone.

vesicle. This should be secured before its division. The prostate is then carefully dissected away from the bladder neck, using a bladder-neck sparing technique (**9.6**). The catheter is sometimes used as a loop retractor to facilitate dissection of the junction of the trigone and the prostate (**9.7**), and the specimen together with the seminal vesicles are removed. After eversion of the bladder mucosa to prevent anastomotic stricture an anastomosis is created between the bladder neck and urethra over a 18 or 20F urethral catheter using from six to seven absorbable Vicryl or Dexon sutures (**9.8**). A tube wound drain is inserted and the wound closed in layers.

Early post-operative mobilization is encouraged, free fluids and subcutaneous heparin started the first post-operative day, and most patients leave hospital within 3–5 days. The urethral catheter is retained

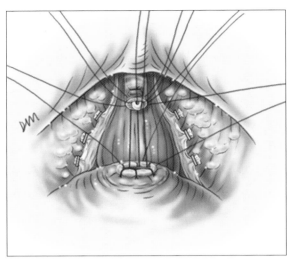

9.8 An anastomosis is created with 4–7 absorbable sutures between the bladder neck with its everted mucosa and urethra.

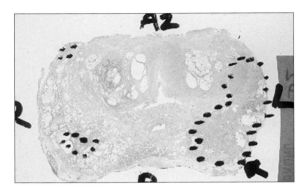

9.9 A whole mount specimen showing a sizable tumour in the left peripheral zone and a smaller cancer in the right peripheral zone as well as one anteriorly. All cancers were specimen confined and the patient remains disease free.

Table 9.5 Advantages and disadvantages of radical prostatectomy	
Advantages	**Disadvantages**
Cure if pathologically confined	Major operation
Definitive staging	Potential mortality
Treatment of symptomatic BPH	Potential morbidity including:
Decreased patient anxiety in follow-up	impotence, incontinence,
Ease of monitoring for persistent disease	rectal injury, urethral stricture, bleeding
	May not be necessary

for 2 weeks and on its removal, most patients are fully continent within a few days. Some suffer stress leakage for longer but this rapidly resolves.

Table 9.5 demonstrates the advantages and disadvantages of radical prostatectomy. Clearly the greatest advantage of this treatment is that, if indeed the cancer is 'specimen confined', the patient may be generally assured of cure (**9.9**). This allays significant anxiety in the post-operative period – a factor of considerable importance in this neoplasm given the long natural history. Significant advances in surgical technique, pioneered by Walsh and asso-

ciates at Johns Hopkins, Baltimore, USA, have made the operation considerably safer, with reduction of blood loss and decrease in significant urinary incontinence[14,15]. Moreover, when a nerve-sparing approach is elected, preservation of potency in at least a proportion of younger men may be achieved[16–19]. Finally, radical prostatectomy affords the benefit of definitive treatment of bladder-outlet obstruction owing to benign prostatic hyperplasia – a condition very frequently co-affecting patients diagnosed with carcinoma.

There are, however, several disadvantages to radical prostatectomy. This is still a not inconsiderable operation, with potential for morbidity and indeed very occasional mortality. The latter has been shown to be low in a large US series (**Table 9.6**). However, more widespread application of this surgical procedure has resulted in reports of higher mortality rates[20].

With greater experience, the rate of complications following radical prostatectomy has been decreasing. A recent compilation of the St Louis University experience is shown in **Table 9.7**[21].

Damage to surrounding structures, namely the ureter and rectum, may occur during the surgical procedure. However, in general, if these are recognized and repaired, with the judicious employment of an omental wrap during the operative procedure, there are few long-term side-effects.

Major long-term complications include urethral strictures, incontinence and erectile dysfunction. The frequency of urethral or bladder neck stricture is about 2–5% or less and, in general, is relatively

Table 9.6 Pelvic lymphadenectomy and radical retropubic prostatectomy operative mortality rate 1982–1992

Institution	Dates	Total no. patients	No. of deaths	Mortality rate (%)
Baylor	1988–92	764	2	0.26
Washington University	1983–92	810	0	0
Johns Hopkins	1982–92	1300	2	0.15
Stanford	1984–92	700	0	0
Total		3574	4	0.11

After Scardino, presented at the American Urological Association Meeting, 1993, San Antonio

Table 9.7 Percentage of 1870 patients with postoperative complications excluding impotence and incontinence

	Number of patients	% (95% CI)
Anastomotic stricture	71	4 (2.9–4.7)
Thromboembolic	39	2 (1.4–2.7)
Inguinal hernia	25	1 (0.8–1.8)
Miscellaneous*	21	1 (0.6–1.6)
Infectious	15	0.8 (0.4–1.2)
Incisional hernia	11	0.6 (0.2–0.9)
Lymphatic	7	0.4 (0.1–0.6)
Neurological	5	0.3 (0.03–0.5)
Myocardial infarction	2	0.1 (0.0–0.2)
Total	196	10 (9–11.8)
Death	0	0 (nonapplicable)

*Includes 6 cases of Peyronie's disease, 5 unknown hernia, 1 cholecystitis, 1 catheter-related complication, 1 wound haematoma, 1 wound seroma, 1 rectal injury, 1 ureteral injury and 2 unrelated complications. (Data with permission from Catalona WJ, Carvalhal GF, Mager DE, Smith DS. Potency, continence and complication rates in 1870 consecutive radical retropubic prostatectomies. *J Urol* 1999; **162(2)**:433–438.)

easily handled. The treatment of problematic strictures, however, may sometimes render the patient incontinent.

Urinary incontinence has been reduced significantly by the development of an anatomical approach to radical retropubic prostatectomy. Nevertheless, incontinence still can and does occur and, in general, some minor incontinence may be expected to be seen in a significant number of patients. Major or total incontinence requiring the placement of an artificial urinary sphincter or, more recently, the injection of collagen (Bard Urologic, Covington, GA, USA) is now very unusual. Herr[22] evaluated the impact of urinary incontinence in men undergoing radical prostatectomy. He noted that whereas 74% dealt well with their morbidity with no limitations in activities, 26% were significantly bothered. A total of 64% of the men stated that if asked to decide on therapy again they would again choose surgery.

Erectile dysfunction previously occurred in virtually 100% of patients undergoing radical prostatectomy. The recognition of pelvic plexus innervation of the corpora cavernosa has allowed sparing of the nerves and the maintenance of erectile function in a significant percentage of men[16–19]. Use of the Cavermap™ intraoperative nerve-stimulating device facilitates nerve preservation and provides evidence of their continuity after removal of the prostate. Risk factors for failure of this approach include patient age, preoperative sexual function level, tumour stage, and, perhaps most importantly, the surgeon's experience. Sacrifice of the nerve ipsilateral to the clinically recognized cancer, while reducing somewhat the potency rate, still affords maintenance of erection in many individuals, with perhaps some decrease in the rate of positive margins, as compared with a bilateral nerve sparing approach.

Few data are available with regard to a definitive evaluation of sexual function prior to and after a radical retropubic prostatectomy. Such studies are certainly indicated for our greater understanding of the adequacy of erection, orgasm and sexual function in general in men so treated (see Chapter 15). The use of oral agents such as sildenafil (Viagra™) show promise in these men and is reported to be effective in around 42% of cases.

Other complications of radical prostatectomy may include thrombophlebitis and pulmonary emboli, development of a lymphocoele, anastomotic urinary leakage, and wound infection.

Radical prostatectomy may be performed by two alternative surgical approaches: either retropubic as described, or perineal. The perineal was the first approach to be used, and has certain advantages to the retropubic, including probably fewer complications in the post-operative period, particularly in patients with pulmonary disease. Decreased blood loss and ease of performing the vesico-urethral anastomosis are also claimed. One particular disadvantage of this technique is the inability to perform a pelvic lymph-node dissection. However, this may be provided by a prior pelvic lymphadenectomy achieved by either open or laparoscopic technique (see Chapter 8). Recently, Levy and Resnick[23] have described the use of radical perineal prostatectomy following laparoscopic pelvic lymphadenectomy as a viable option.

Technique of Radical Perineal Prostatectomy

The following description of radical perineal prostatectomy is based on the excellent and more complete reviews by Vernon E. Weldon in Das and Crawford's *Cancer of the Prostate* (Marcel Dekker, New York, 1993) and that of David F. Paulson in *Prostate Diseases* (WB Saunders, Philadelphia, 1993). The procedure is undertaken with the patient in the exaggerated lithotomy position. An inverted U-shaped incision is then made as shown in **9.10**. Deepening of this incision is accomplished by careful transection of the central muscles of the perineum which connect the external anal sphincter to the transverse perineal and bulbar spongiosus muscles at the perineal body. The rectal sphincter can then be visualized as a muscular arch overlying the rectum. Dissection beneath this musculature reveals the pale anterior rectal fascia which serves as a guide to the prostate.

At this point, or a little earlier, it is helpful to insert a prostatic tractor retrogradely into the bladder. The Loseley curved tractor is often easier to insert

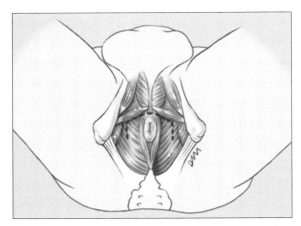

9.10 The anatomical structures underlying the U-shaped perineal incision (dotted line) for radical perineal prostatectomy. (Reprinted from Weldon[88] by courtesy of Marcel Dekker, Inc.)

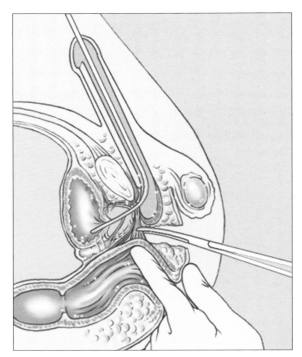

9.11 A curved urethral tractor puts the rectourethralis muscle on the stretch. (Reprinted from Weldon[88] by courtesy of Marcel Dekker, Inc.)

than the Young's straight prostatic tractor. If there is difficulty inserting either of these devices then a urethral catheter or urethral sound may be used (**9.11**). Identification of the rectourethralis muscle is assisted by placing it under tension. The rectum is tented upwards by the muscle, and therefore division of these muscle fibres permits posterior displacement of the rectum. At this stage identification of the rectum can be facilitated by the insertion of a finger in it, a manoeuvre that may prevent inadvertant damage to the structure. Blunt dissection then permits the exposure of the lateral anterior margins of the prostate. The overlying prostatic fascia appears white and glistening and should usually be removed intact with the specimen. If, however, a potency preserving prostatectomy is intended, this structure can be divided in the midline so that the periprostatic neurovascular plexi can be preserved on one or both sides. However, visualization of the neuromuscular bundle is more difficult using this approach.

The membranous urethra is then exposed at the prostatic apex and gently freed from its surrounding tissues and encircled using a right-angled clamp. The dorsal wall of the membranous urethra is transected sharply just at its junction with the prostatic apex (**9.12**). The incision is then carried down to the prostatic tractor or catheter which is removed, and the ventral urethral wall is transected.

At this stage, a short straight prostatic tractor is passed through the prostatic urethra into the bladder and the blades extended. The presence of this device helps to mobilize the prostate and facilitates dissection and division of the lateral pedicles close to the gland (**9.13**). The lateral prostatic fascia usually contains several large vessels, and it is often helpful to place haemostatic clips systematically

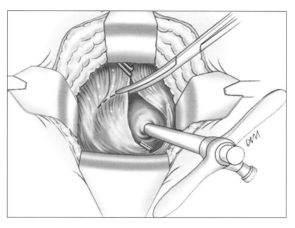

9.13   A short, straight prostatic tractor helps to mobilize the prostate and facilitates division of the lateral pedicles close to the gland. (Reprinted from Weldon[88] by courtesy of Marcel Dekker, Inc.)

along these fascial sheaths and transect beneath the clips. Rotation of the straight prostatic tractor contralaterally exposes the remaining lateral prostatic fascia which can then be transected up to the level of the bladder neck. Anterior bladder neck transection can then be accomplished with careful preservation of the circular detrusor fibres which may be separated by careful dissection from the prostate, exposing the bladder neck mucosa. At this stage, it is often helpful to withdraw the Young's straight prostatic tractor and replace it with a Foley catheter, which can be passed through the prostatic urethra and brought out as a loop superiorly through the line of the incision between the prostate and the bladder neck. Traction on this catheter permits the prostate to be displaced posteriorly and defines the line of cleavage between the bladder neck and the prostate.

The posterior vesical neck musculature can then be divided sharply in the midline down to the anterior fascia overlying the ampulla of the vasa differentia and seminal vesicles. As in radical retropubic prostatectomy, the posterior bladder neck muscle is often found to be quite thick and this dissection therefore needs to be continued deeper than is often anticipated. In both radical retropubic and perineal prostatectomy, dissection in the wrong plane runs a risk of inadvertent injury to the ureters. In the circumstance of the plane of transection being unclear, it is often safer to delay this dissection until the time of division of the vascular pedicles when the seminal

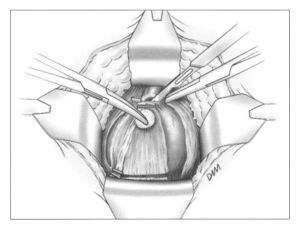

9.12   The posterior aspect of the urethra is divided under direct vision at the apex of the prostate. (Reprinted from Weldon[88] by courtesy of Marcel Dekker, Inc.)

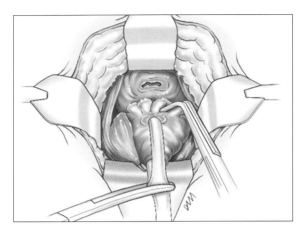

9.14 The seminal vesicles and ampullary portions of the vasa are dissected free and the vasa divided. (Reprinted from Weldon[88] by courtesy of Marcel Dekker, Inc.)

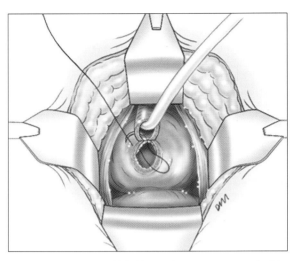

9.15 The urethra and bladder neck are anastomosed with interrupted sutures over a catheter. (Reprinted from Weldon[88] by courtesy of Marcel Dekker, Inc.)

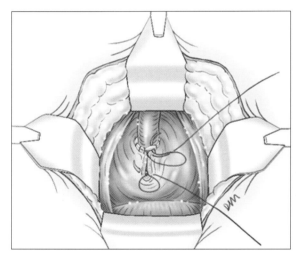

9.16 The anastomosis is completed with a closure of the bladder neck itself. (Reprinted from Weldon[88] by courtesy of Marcel Dekker, Inc.)

vesicles, ampullary portions of the vasa and the plane of the genital fascia are easier to visualize (**9.14**). At this stage the prostate and seminal vesicles remain secured posterio-laterally by the vascular pedicles, but entire gland is free from the bladder.

The vascular pedicles can be isolated at 5 and 7 o'clock, and controlled either by surgical clips or by the careful insertion of absorbable sutures. After division of these pedicles bilaterally, the specimen is then held only by the seminal vesicles and the vasa deferentia. The vasa deferentia may be clipped and divided. Often small blood vessels are found at the apex of the seminal vesicles and these should be controlled either by diathermy or by the use of clips before the entire specimen is removed and sent for pathological examination.

Once reasonable haemostasis has been accomplished, reconstruction of the bladder neck is often necessary. The anterior bladder neck is then anastomosed to the membranous urethra using 4 to 7 absorbable sutures over a 20 or 22F silicone Foley catheter (**9.15**). Further sutures may be inserted into the bladder neck as this anastomosis is accomplished so that the bladder neck is snug around the catheter. The wound is then closed in layers with a corrugated drain left down to the anastomosis, and the U-shaped skin incision repaired using either an interrupted or a subcuticular absorbable suture (**9.16**). Early postoperative mobilization is encouraged and the catheter generally retained for a period of about two weeks, but the patient is usually able to leave hospital within 72 hours of surgery.

Efficacy of Radical Prostatectomy

Most urologists today favour retropubic rather than perineal radical prostatectomy. This is largely due to the familiarity with the retropubic anatomy, but also because this approach affords the opportunity for wider excision of adjacent tissue in patients who may have extension of their neoplasm through the capsule. Moreover, a pelvic lymphadenectomy may be readily performed, rapidly, and with minimal morbidity through the same incision. This provides definitive staging and inherent prognostic information, but the therapeutic benefit of lymphadenectomy itself has never been demonstrated.

As noted, it is difficult to make meaningful conclusions about the outcome of treatment owing to a number of factors. The significant competing mortalities, along with the variable natural history of prostatic carcinoma, mandate long-term follow-up prior to making definitive conclusions with regard to cure. Several studies of long-term follow-up are available (**Table 9.8**), demonstrating excellent overall mortality which compares favourably to age-matched controls without prostatic carcinoma.

It should be emphasized that these earlier series involved profiles different from those of patients generally operated on today. Significant stage migration, improvements in staging techniques and more accurate grading strategies now allow more appropriate selection of patients for radical prostatectomy than in the historical series. In many of the older series, radionucleotide bone scans were not performed and, as the majority of these patients underwent perineal prostatectomy, definitive nodal staging afforded by pelvic lymphadenectomy was not provided. It would seem likely that, owing to these differences, and the important influence of PSA measurement plus improved surgical techniques, more contemporary series will provide even better disease-free survival outcomes.

The reduction in morbidity afforded by the anatomical approach to radical prostatectomy has resulted in some surgeons extending the indication to men with clinical T3 disease. There has also been renewed interest in upfront (neoadjuvant) hormonal-deprivation therapy to shrink and hopefully downstage the tumour in patients with extra-prostatic extension of disease before radical prostatectomy. While definitive answers cannot be provided, Labrie *et al.* demonstrated significant reduction in positive margins in men receiving three months of an antiandrogen plus a luteinizing hormone-releasing hormone (LHRH) agonist prior to radical prostatectomy, when compared to men undergoing immediate surgery without hormone therapy[24]. Other studies, while demonstrating significant reduction in serum PSA and tumour size, have rarely shown genuine downstaging to organ-confined disease. Randomized trials applying neoadjuvant hormonal manipulation are underway in the USA and in Europe, but none to date have shown either improvement in time to PSA relapse or enhanced survival.

The cost as well as morbidity of radical prostatectomy has been shown to be reduced by using clinical pathways that standardize the treatment. First reported by Koch and associates[25] and echoed by Litwin *et al.*[26], these pathways include refinement in pre-operative care, operative technique, anaesthetic use and post-operative pain management. These have been associated with a significant decrease in hospital stay to approximately 2.4 days post-operatively and a dramatic decrease in hospital costs.

The inadequacies of current pre-operative staging procedures noted above have resulted in considerable pathological upstaging (**9.15**) in men undergoing radical prostatectomy to capsular penetration or beyond. **Table 9.9** demonstrates the incidence of this in several series.

The identification of pathological upstaging (capsular extension, positive margins, seminal vesicle extension, etc.) is certainly intrinsically related to the thoroughness of the pathological examination of the surgical specimen. Even with rigorous step sectioning, the detection of cancer cells dotted with ink on the margin of the specimen may not provide definitive evidence that residual neoplasm is left within the patient. In this regard, post-operative serum PSA is particularly helpful. An 'iatrogenic' margin owing to traumatic denuding of the prostatic capsule may result in a false positive margin. Each laboratory must determine their lower limit of detectability of serum PSA and, in general, one should not make therapeutic decisions until a trend of increasing PSA above this nadir level is noted.

Table 9.8 Radical prostatectomy 15-year NED and survival				
Author	Clinical stage	Patho-logical stage	No.	15-year NED/survival
Jewett[48]	B1	B–C2	86	28 (33)
	B1	C3	17	0
Elder[7]	B2	B	14	7 (50)
	B2	C2–3	32	4 (13)
Gibbons[6]	B1	B,C	43	26 (61)
	B2	B,C	9	3 (33)

NED, No evidence of disease

Table 9.9 Incidence of extracapsular disease after radical prostatectomy			
Author	Clinical stage	No.	No. upstaged (%)
Lange and Narayah[1]	A2	6	3 (50)
Boxer, Kaufman and Goodwin[2]	A	35	8 (23)
Catalona and Stein[3]	A2	9	1 (11)
Veenema, Gursel and Lattimer[4]	A,B	159	66 (42)
Jewett[5]	B1	103	26 (25)
Catalona and Stein[3]	B1	48	8 (17)
Gibbons et al.[6]	B	143	46 (31)
Lange and Narayah[1]	B2	25	15 (60)
Catalona and Stein[3]	B2	23	9 (39)
Elder, Jewett and Walsh[7]	B2	53	35 (66)

The concept of neoadjuvant hormonal therapy before definitive treatment of localized prostate carcinoma has been around since the 1940s[27,28]. Additional studies were initiated later in that decade[29,30]; however, clear evidence of improved outcome was lacking. In 1969, Scott and Boyd[31] reported on 25 years of experience with androgen ablation before radical prostatectomy. These authors reported impressive 10- and 15-year survival rates for men with T3 disease. However, as most patients continued androgen suppression following surgery, definitive conclusions could not be made.

Owing to the development of reversible castration (LHRH analogues and antiandrogens) neoadjuvant hormonal therapy enjoyed a resurgence (Table 9.10). Most authors have demonstrated a significant decrease in positive margin rate following androgen suppression in randomized trials. However, difficulty in making an accurate pathologic determination in men subjected to androgen ablation may render some of these impressive results spurious. Phenotypic changes of androgen suppression are recognized by expert pathologists and include pyknosis, cell atrophy, vacuolization of cancer cells and increase in stromal epithelial ratio. Identification of persistent carcinoma, particularly at the margin can be difficult. Cytokeratin staining[32] as well as staining with PSA and prostatic acid phosphatase (PAP) may help in this often difficult pathological interpretation. Although the majority of studies

Table 9.10 Overview of randomized phase III studies				
		Positive margin (%)		
Study	No. of patients	Neoadjuvant therapy	RP	p
Labrie et al.[24]	142	13	38	<0.01
Van Poppel et al.[89]	127	PSL 32	PSL 43	NG
		API 31	API 27	NG
		BAS 18	BAS 10	NG
Soloway et al.[34]	282	18	48	<0.01
Goldenberg et al.[90]	213	28	65	<0.01
Witjes et al.[33]	354	27	46	<0.01

API, apical; BAS, basal; NG, not given; PSL, posterolateral; RP, radical prostatectomy.

have shown significant downstaging and shrinkage of the prostate as well as the tumour, and significant reduction in serum PSA, the definitive answer of whether adjuvant therapy will resolve and improve cancer-specific survival remains lacking. Several phase 3 randomized trials including the European Organization for Research and Treatment of Cancer (EORTC) neoadjuvant study group trial[33] and a similar trial headed by Soloway[34] are underway. Both studies have completed accrual. There has been significant pathological downstaging. However, no difference in biochemical failure rate has been reported between men receiving new neoadjuvant therapy compared with those who did not.

The use of the PSA as an intermediate endpoint may not provide the definitive answer and we wait the completion of these trials for evidence of clinical failure as well as prostate cancer death. This will provide conclusive evidence of the merit or lack of merit of neoadjuvant hormonal therapy. As will be seen subsequently, neoadjuvant hormonal therapy has, however, been shown to be highly efficacious in decreasing the rate of failure in men treated with definitive radiation therapy.

In the face of detectable serum PSA post-operatively, the next step should be an attempt at determining whether this is owing to residual local disease or whether it represents systemic carcinoma. Review of the pathological report may help in this regard, and, if a positive margin is noted this suggests that there may be local disease; however, this certainly does not exclude disseminated cancer. Men who have positive seminal vesicles and parti-cularly those with positive pelvic lymph nodes may, in general, be assumed to have disseminated disease. A radionucleotide bone scan in this setting is imperative and, if a pre-operative scan was obtained, the prior study must be carefully compared to the subsequent examination. Magnetic resonance or plain x-ray imaging of equivocal bone scan findings may improve specificity. Pelvic imaging studies in this setting have in general been unsatisfactory in detecting low levels of persistent clinical disease. Some authorities[35] have reported on digitally guided biopsy of the region of the vesical–urethral anastomosis to define pelvic disease persistence. The use of transrectal ultrasound alone has in general been disappointing in the demonstration of residual neoplasm[36]. In this respect the Prostascint scan[37], which is a radiolabelled scan based upon immuno-scintigraphy to prostate specific membrane antigen (PSMA) can be of value, although false positives may occur.

The significance of biochemical failure in radical prostatectomy remains unclear. For example, in the UCLA experience 33% of the patients had a biochemical relapse, defined as a serum PSA greater than 0.4 ng/ml, but only 10% of the patients had a clinically detectable relapse[38]. The rate of PSA rise after operation may be an important predictor of who will develop clinical recurrence[39]. If the doubling time is less than 6 months, clinical recurrence is detected in 20–35% of patients. In contrast, if the PSA doubles over more than 18 months only 15% of men had clinical recurrence.

Table 9.11 describes the incidence of clinical

Table 9.11 Local recurrence after radical prostatectomy alone				
Author	No. patients	Pathological stage	Recurrence (%)	Follow-up (years)
Culp[91]	123	B	26	1–14
Walsh and Jewett[92]	57	B	12	15
Tomlinson, Currie and Boyce[93]	24	C	8	2–14
Robey and Schellhammer[94]	13	C	31	15
Gibbons et al.[6]	51	B + C	10	15
Middleton et al.[95]	22	C	9	5
Catalona, Miller and Kavoussi[96]	9	C	11	6 Mean
Zincke, Utz and Taylor[97]	47	C,D1	28	4.9 Mean
Catalona, Miller and Kavoussi[96]	12	D1	25	7.5 Mean
Steinberg et al.[98]	64	D1	11	3.8 Mean

	Table 9.12 Adjuvant radiation therapy following radical prostatectomy				
Author	Pathological stage	No.	Local recurrence (%)	% 5 years disease free	Follow-up (years)
Rosenberg et al.[99]	B	34	3	88	3.3 Mean
Gibbons et al.[6]	C	22	5	71	9 Mean
Bahnson, Garnett and Grayhack[100]	C	14	0	75	5.3 Mean
Rosenberg et al.[99]	C	25	8.0	80	3.3 Mean
Ray, Bagshaw and Freiha[101]	C	13	23	57	5–15
Jacobson, Simith and Stewart[102]	C	26	0	69	5
Lange et al.[103]	C2,C3	35	3	80	4.2 Median
Pilepich, Walz and Baglan[104]	C,D1	18	0	50	3.4 Median
Forman et al.[105]	C,D1	16	0		4 Median
Bahnson, Garnett and Grayhack[100]	D1	6	17	41	5.3 Median
Rosenberg et al.[99]	D1	12	8	92	3.3 Mean
Lange et al.[103]	D1	36	3	69	4 Median

evidence of local recurrence after radical prostatectomy. If it is felt that the patient is at risk for local recurrence owing to the pathological stage, particularly if PSA is detectable following radical prostatectomy, many authorities recommend adjuvant radiation therapy.

Table 9.12 illustrates several reports demonstrating a significantly decreased local recurrence rate in men treated with adjuvant radiation therapy. While most studies have observed this, the absence of the randomized prospective data makes attempts at definitive conclusions impossible. Long-term follow-up with regard to cancer-specific and all-cause mortality in patients receiving adjuvant therapy is also lacking. Currently, trials evaluating both adjuvant hormonal therapy and radiation therapy in this setting are underway.

Adjuvant radiation therapy certainly contributes somewhat to morbidity. However, it is generally well-tolerated if it is delayed until the maximum return of urinary incontinence, if a limited pelvic lymphadenectomy has been performed, and if modern radiation therapy techniques are applied.

The results of adjuvant therapy with regard to serum PSA are somewhat controversial. Lange et al.[35] noted that approximately 30% of patients had their PSA fall to the non-detectable region. Link et al.[40] corroborated this early reduction in PSA, but noted that in the majority, the PSA had again begun to rise within a year. More recently, Andriole et al.[36] have reported the use of the 5 alpha-reductase inhibitor, finasteride, to delay any subsequent PSA rise in margin-positive patients after radical prostatectomy.

The use of adjuvant hormonal androgen ablation in patients undergoing radical prostatectomy who are seen to have advanced disease is controversial. The group from the Mayo Clinic[41] has demonstrated impressive outcomes in patients with pelvic lymph-node metastasis undergoing radical prostatectomy who receive adjuvant hormonal manipulation. It is unknown whether these patients derived benefit from the surgical procedure itself or only from the hormonal manipulation. Further investigation in this arena is certainly necessary before definitive conclusions are possible. Randomized trials evaluating this modality are also underway, including the CAPRI study, which has randomized a large cohort of patients to either Casodex™ (bicalutamide) or placebo.

In summary, radical prostatectomy by the retropubic or perineal route is now felt by many to afford the best opportunity single modality for cure in men with localized prostatic carcinoma. Considerable progress has been made towards the reduction of morbidity and this, coupled with an increasing incidence of diagnosis in patients with a more favourable pathological stage, has resulted in considerable enthusiasm for radical prostatectomy. The definitive answer as to whether radical prostatectomy actually results in a reduction in cancer-related mortality awaits the conclusion of ongoing trials that randomize men to radical prostatectomy versus watchful waiting. A Swedish study is in progress. The Prostate Intervention and Observation Trial (PIVOT) in the US will randomize 1050 men to radical prostatectomy versus observation, and will use all causes of mortality as the definitive endpoint. In the absence of the definitive answers that these studies will provide, it seems reasonable to offer radical prostatectomy to fitter, younger men with clinically localized prostate cancer and at least a 10-year life expectancy, provided that the patients are carefully counselled about the risks and benefits and have all other options explained to them.

RADIATION THERAPY

Radiation therapy provides an alternative, definitive treatment approach to clinically localized prostatic carcinoma. Radiation therapy has undergone considerable evolution since Paschkis first used cystoscopically applied radium sources to treat prostate cancer. Although various applications of radiation energy were applied to the prostate, followed by cobalt-beam external-radiation therapy, it was the application of the radiation energy derived from linear accelerator by Bagshaw and colleagues at Stanford that changed the course of definitive radiation.

In general, patients being considered for radiation therapy of the prostate should have similar criteria to those undergoing radical prostatectomy (**Table 9.13**). Significant bladder or rectal dysfunction may preclude such treatment approaches.

Problems with pre-operative surgical staging extend to patients being considered for radiation therapy. The issue, however, is intensified somewhat in the radiation therapy series because, in general, definitive pelvic-node staging is not provided as these patients rarely undergo lymphadenectomy. Moreover, patients treated with radiation therapy do not have the benefit of having definitive pathological staging.

Table 9.14 illustrates the advantages and disadvantages of this treatment approach. A significant benefit in patients selecting external-beam radiation therapy is the absence of the surgical procedure. The absence of a major operation allows this treatment approach to be added in patients with a less favourable, general medical condition. However, the benefit of treatment of localized prostate cancer and the potential risks must be carefully compared

Table 9.13 Criteria for radiation therapy

Histological evidence of prostate cancer
Clinically localized disease*
Sufficient life expectancy to render cure worthwhile
Absence of lower urinary-tract disorder
Absence of colorectal disease
Absence of recent or pending TURP
Adequate informed consent

* Some investigators may extend to T3–T4

Table 9.14 Advantages and disadvantages of radiation therapy

Advantages	Disadvantages
Potential cure	Prolonged treatment (EBRT)
Avoid surgery	Difficulty assessing cure
	Patient anxiety in follow-up
	No definitive staging
	No effect on BPH
	Potential mortality
	Potential morbidity including:
	rectal injury,
	bladder damage,
	incontinence,
	impotence,
	haematuria
	May not be necessary

EBRT, External-beam radiotherapy

with the patients' overall longevity. Disadvantages of radiation therapy include significant morbidity, including bladder and bowel injury (a small minority of patients requiring major surgical intervention for treatment of complications)[42], the time involved with a prolonged treatment course, a high incidence of persistent disease as evidenced by PSA and/or post-radiation positive biopsies, and the potential at least for the development of subsequent primary prostate carcinomas. Furthermore, the anxiety associated with the unknown status of a potentially persistent carcinoma exists in men so treated.

Partial urinary incontinence has been reported to occur in approximately 2% of patients undergoing external-beam radiation therapy, and total urinary incontinence in 1–3% of patients has been reported in large series[43–45]. A major potential complication – that of sufficient rectal injury to demand construction of a colostomy – has been reported in up to 3% of patients undergoing external-beam radiation therapy[45].

A compilation of complications of external beam radiation therapy is shown in **Table 19.14**.

In properly selected patients, external-beam radiation therapy affords a 15-year overall survival, similar to that observed in patients treated with radical prostatectomy. For example, Hanks[46] compared the survival in 3 series comprised of 134 patients receiving external-beam radiation therapy by the Stanford group[47], with 195 patients treated at Virginia Mason Medical Center[48], and with 57 treated at the Johns Hopkins Medical Center with radical prostatectomy[49]. The 15-year overall survivals were 52%, 57% and 51% respectively. Impressive results have extended to even more advanced cases (clinical stage C, T3–T4). For example, Perez et al.[27] found 5-year NED (no evidence of disease) survival rates of 54%. Zagars et al.[50] noted 15-year disease-free survival rates of 40% in such patients.

Perhaps even more enlightening is the compilation reported by Epstein[51], which is shown in **Table 9.15**. These series are noteworthy in that all patients underwent staging pelvic lymphadenectomy in conjunction with radical prostatectomy, or prior to external-beam radiation therapy.

Advances in external-beam radiation therapy have occurred in several arenas, most importantly in the appropriate selection of patients to receive such therapy. In particular, the use of neoadjuvant hormonal downstaging using an LHRH analogue in combination with an antiandrogen, has been shown to improve overall survival rates compared with the use of external beam radiation therapy alone. Moreover, recently conformal approaches have resulted in decreasing radiation doses to surrounding tissue, such as the bladder and rectum, with the potential for reduction in morbidity[52,53]. One difficulty in looking at the historical external-beam radiation series is the possibility that relatively inaccurate pelvic imaging techniques used in the determination of the radiation portals may have resulted in significant underdosing or actually missing portions of the prostate[54,55].

The goal of radiation therapy is to achieve the highest tumour dose while at the same time mini-

Table 9.15 Patterns of failure (%) after radiation therapy or surgery, stage B prostate cancer

Reference	68*	57**	11
Treatment method	EBRT	RP	RP
Any recurrence			
5-year	15	10	11
10-year	33	50	–
Local recurrence			
5-year	4	7	4
10-year	14	4	–
Cause-specific survival			
5-year	4	3	3
10-year	14	17	–
Survival			
5-year	87	94	93
10-year	63	67	–

EBRT, External-beam radiotherapy
RP, Radical prostatectomy
*Actuarial
**Absolute, lost patients eliminated

mizing radiation injury to the surrounding normal tissue. The major advances in prostate radiation therapy have been efforts to extend this.

Outcome After Radiotherapy

The evaluation of patients following radiation therapy of the prostate includes those tests useful for the patients after radical prostatectomy. However, in this setting, PSA is less well characterized, in that detectable serum levels of PSA are usually identified following radiation therapy. While several reports[56–60] have correlated the absence of progression with the nadir of PSA, the definitive identification of the nadir level and the duration of the nadir associated with improved prognosis have not been adequately determined.

One additional approach to the evaluation of patients following radiation therapy of the prostate is the ability to perform prostate needle biopsies. A number of studies have demonstrated unsettlingly high rates of positive biopsies in this setting. For example, Freiha *et al.* noted that 68% of patients with stage B2 or C prostate cancer have positive biopsies[61]. They correlated the presence of a positive biopsy with clinical recurrence. Similar data have been provided by Scardino *et al.*[62], who reviewed post-radiation biopsy in 803 men undergoing pelvic lymphadenectomy, radioactive gold-seed implantation, along with external-beam radiation therapy. Of 124 patients who had 1 or more biopsies performed, 6–36 months following completion of radiation therapy 43 (35%) had positive biopsies. These authors demonstrated not only that the incidence of positive biopsy correlated directly with the clinical stage of the tumour, but that local and distant metastases were much more commonly found in those patients with a positive biopsy than those with negative biopsies. This article unequivocally demonstrates the prognostic significance of persistent carcinoma following definitive radiotherapy[62]. Kabalin *et al.*[63] in a review of 27 men, 18 months or more following radiation therapy, demonstrated positive biopsies in 25 (93%). Of note, 20 of the 22 patients with normal feeling prostates on rectal examination had residual carcinoma. Furthermore, 10 of 12 patients with a serum PSA less than 10.0 ng/ml had positive biopsies, and all men with a PSA greater than this (15) had persistent carcinoma.

In contrast, Kuban *et al.*[64] noted that only 18% of patients with in general more favourable clinical stage had positive biopsies. One concern in this regard is the often exceedingly difficult diagnostic dilemma that the pathologist is faced with in the determination of post-radiation biopsies. Immunohistochemistry with high molecular weight cytokeratin has been shown to be a helpful adjunct in this regard[65] (see Chapter 2).

Table 9.16 illustrates that local tumour control (which is arguably the best way to compare local treatment) rate for low-stage prostatic carcinoma is approximately equivalent across all treatment modalities, including radical prostatectomy, external-beam radiation therapy and brachytherapy. Obviously, significant differences in patient mix and the absence of randomized trials obviate the ability to adequately compare the efficacy of therapy. It is of note that the efficacy of implantation of radiation appears to fall behind that of external-beam radiation therapy for more advanced disease.

Recently, Stamey *et al.*[66] reported on 124 consecutive unselected patients who had serial PSA following definitive external-beam radiation therapy. After a follow-up of 32 months, 51% of the patients had increasing values, while 41% were stable. The series was updated with additional follow-up of 48 months on 113 patients, and a mean over follow-up of 6 years. Seventy-eight percent of men had precipitously increasing PSA. In 23 men (20%), stable PSA values of less than 1.7 and a mean follow-up of 9 years were reported; these men were deemed by these authorities to be 'cured'. No correlation between clinical stage and the PSA evidence of progression versus cure was noted.

Problems associated with the use of PSA to follow men after radiation therapy are considerable. The kinetics of PSA decrease is significantly different compared with men treated with surgery. Whereas after radical prostatectomy PSA drops at a precipitous rate associated with a half-life of 2–3 days, there is a much slower decline in PSA following radiation therapy. This undoubtedly results from the prolonged cell kill effect even after completion of the radiation, but also the fact that normal prostate tissue may remain, even if all tumour is lethally injured with radiation therapy. This normal tissue can certainly contribute to the serum PSA[67]. Because of these and other concerns the definition of PSA nadir that is asssociated with cure remains problematic. Zagars *et al.*[68], for example, showed that evidence of relapse or persistently rising PSA was found in 17% of men who had a nadir PSA less than 1.0 ng/ml compared with 71% for those who had a nadir greater than 4.0 ng/ml. Baseline PSA also predicted evidence of failure in this series. If the PSA was less than 4.0 ng/ml, the mean subsequent PSA nadir was 0.8 ng/ml. In contrast, if the initial PSA was greater than 30 ng/ml, post-radiation nadir mean was 5.4 ng/ml. Zietman *et al.*[13] stated that cure was unlikely if the nadir was greater than 1.0 ng/ml. The Wayne State University Group[69] demonstrated a 10% incidence of failure in men who had a nadir PSA following radiation of less than 1.0 ng/ml compared with 100% if the nadir was greater than 2.0 ng/ml.

Owing to the high failure rate after conventional external beam radiation therapy, a number of clinicians have tried to make radiation more effective. **Table 9.17** lists some of these approaches.

In an effort to increase radiation dose, both conformal radiation therapy and interstitial radiation

Table 9.16 Local tumour control following implantation versus external-beam radiation therapy versus prostatectomy

Treatment	Stage A	Stage B	Stage C	Follow-up (years)	Reference
Implant	91% (11)*	74% (32)	56% (32)	3–12	Kuban, El-Mahdi and Schellhammer[106]
	88% (41)		86% (57)	3–7	Kim and Bueschen[107]
	100% (20)			2+	Giles and Brady[108]
	100%[a]	83%	71%	3–13	Morton and Peschel[109]
	100% (3)	95% (38)	85% (13)	2–9	Delaney et al.[110]
	100% (6)	91% (69)	95% (19)	7–13	Reddy, Mebust and Weigel[111]
		68% (191)[b]	24% (87)	10	Fuks et al.[112]
		41% (324)[c]		10	Fuks et al.[112]
EBRT	97% (35)	87% (104)	74% (107)	3–12	Kuban, El-Mahdi and Schellhammer[106]
	93% (23)	62% (87)	63% (111)	10	Amdur et al.[43]
	88% (41)	83% (185)	72% (328)	3–16	Perez et al.[44]
	100% (9)	94% (78)	82% (20)	3–13	Morton and Peschel[109]
Surgery	80% (5)	90% (41)	25% (4)	5	Schellhammer[113]
		90% (52)		15–32	Gibbons et al.[114]
		73% (123)		1–15	Culp[91]

*, Numbers in parentheses represent the number of patients treated
[a], 141 total patients implanted in series. 18% excluded as 'inadequately treated'. Stage breakdown not provided
[b], Stage B1 (unilobar, < 2 cm)
[c], Stage B2 (unilobar, > 2 cm)
(Reproduced from Wallner[115] with permission of ONCOLOGY, Melville, NY.)

Table 9.17 Methods to improve local control with radiotherapy in cancer of the prostate[116]

Increased radiation dose	Conformal radiation Interstitial irradiation
Particle beam radiotherapy	Protons Neutrons
Combined-modality treatment with androgen deprivation	Neoadjuvant Adjuvant
Combined-modality treatment with total prostatectomy	

therapy (brachytherapy) have been widely adopted. Brachytherapy is discussed in Chapter 14. Conformal radiation therapy is an attempt to correct some of the problems associated with conventional radiation therapy planning. Using CT to develop an accurate model of the prostate itself as well as surrounding tissue, conformal radiation therapy more precisely localizes the radiation ports using multiple beam arrangements aligned with computer-aided devises to plan and deliver the radiation. It allows fairly precise, three-dimensional configuration of the radiation ports, which increases radiation to the prostate and minimizes radiation to the surrounding normal tissue. Roach et al.[70] demonstrated, for example, that the inferior margin of the prostate had been inaccurately defined in up to 25% of men if standard pelvic bone landmarks were used to delineate the apex.

Conformal radiation has been reported to improve the outcome, particularly with respect to the serum PSA. For example, Corn et al.[71] demonstrated that PSA normalization occurred in 96% of men treated with conformal radiation compared with 85% of those treated with standard therapy (4.0 ng/ml). Realizing more stringent criteria of the PSA less than 1.0 ng/ml conformal radiation achieved this in 75% of men versus 55% with standard radiation.

In addition to probable improvement in efficacy, treatment-related toxicity is reduced with conformal therapy. For example, Vijaykumar[72] demonstrated 30% decrease in acute bladder and rectal symptoms in men treated with conformal approaches. This is a direct result of a significant decrease in radiation dose to the bladder and rectum, which has been reported to be approximately 14% in two series[53,73]. With conformal radiation, abnormal tissue treated to the 90% isodose has been reported to be reduced by approximately 40% in bowel and bladder[74].

Unfortunately, the impact of radiation therapy on erectile dysfunction has not been improved with conformal approaches. In large series; between one- and two-thirds of men who are potent will maintain potency after radiation and the method of delivery does not impact the statistic[75–77]. Another approach to increasing the radiation dose is simply dose escalation. Hanks[78] demonstrated that 7-year local recurrence rate was directly related to dose: 7-year local recurrence rate was 36% for men who had doses of 60–64.9 Gy, 32% for those who had 65–69 Gy, and 24% for those men who received 70 Gy or greater. The importance of local control cannot be overstated. For example, in the Memorial Sloan-Kettering series, 20 year metastasis-free survival was 70% for those men who achieved local control compared with 13% for men who had local relapse[79].

Owing to the potential benefit of increasing doses, there has been increased interest in attempting to deliver ever increasing doses. Of course, the limitation will be toxicity.

Another approach to make radiation more effective has been the use of novel energy sources. Fast neutrons and protons have increased linear energy transfer and therefore potentially at least have increased tumor kill effect. In one study[80] photon radiation was combined with neutrons and compared with conventional photon therapy alone. Progression at 5-year follow-up was 38% in the conventional group. In contrast, only 7% of the patients who received neutrons plus protons failed. An additional study[81] showed a 5-year local regional failure rate of 11% for men treated with neutrons and

photons compared with 32% for men treated with photons alone. The corresponding PSA relapse rate was 17 versus 45%. However, in this study, the complication rate was significantly greater for the men receiving neutrons (24% grade 3 and 4 rectal toxicity compared with 8% in the photon group). In addition, owing to the expense required to deliver neutrons, only two centres in the USA are currently using this approach.

One of the most impressive advances in radiation therapy has been combined therapy using neo-adjuvant hormonal therapy. Effective hormonal ablation in combination with radiation therapy has both direct and indirect effects. Direct effects include a decrease in the cell cycle leading to inability of the tumour to repopulate during radiation therapy. In addition, apoptosis may be enhanced by a combination of radiation plus the androgen-deficient milieu relative to what is achieved with single modality therapy. The indirect effects include shrinkage of the tumour and the prostate itself, which may have advantages both in radiation delivery to the prostate relative to the surrounding normal tissue. Several trials have been reported showing the efficacy of a combination of androgen suppression and radiation therapy, which has largely adopted. This is becoming the standard approach by many radiation oncologists. The Radiation Therapy Oncology Group (RTOG) study 94–08 randomized men to radiation alone versus radiation followed by 4 months of total androgen blockade. This pilot study demonstrated eradication of tumour in 93% of men with a minimum of 2-year follow-up[82].

This study led to the RTOG 86–10, which was a phase 3 investigation in which men were randomized to radiation therapy alone versus neoadjuvant hormone therapy with goserelin acetate and flut-amide[83]. Five-year local progression was 46% in the combination group versus 71% in the radiation only series. A 34% rate of distant metastasis was found in the combination group compared with 41% in the monotherapy group. Five-year progression-free survival was 36 versus 15%, respectively. It should be noted that this study comprised men who had locally advanced disease.

The EORTC conducted an investigation that received an inordinate amount of attention.[84] This trial randomized men to radiation therapy alone versus radiation therapy plus goserelin and cypro-terone acetate, which was continued for 3 years. The local control rate was 95% for the combination group versus 75% for those who received radiation alone. The clinical disease-free survival was 85 and 44%, respectively. Most dramatic was the difference in metastases-free survival, which was 85% in the combined group versus 48% in those receiving radiation alone.

The largest series of cryosurgery has been that developed from the Allegheny Hospital[85,86]. Negative biopsy rates at 2 years have been reported to be 89.5%. The men have not undergone any previous therapy. Among those men who had clinical T3 or greater disease and who had been followed up for 21 or more months, 76% had a PSA less than 1.0 ng/ml and 55% less than 0.4 ng/ml; 78% had negative biopsies at 3 months. A number of investigators have adopted a double free cycle with cryosurgery and there has been a suggestion that this may result in better cancer control. Erectile dysfunction after cryosurgery has been reported in 41–86% of patients and incontinence in approximately 3% of men who have not had other previous procedures in the prostate.

Brachytherapy is a newly emerging treatment option and is the subject of Chapter 11.

CONCLUSIONS

The treatment of clinically localized prostatic adenocarcinoma has evolved, and continues to evolve owing to a variety of factors over the past few decades. Men to be considered for such therapy should have a life expectancy of at least 10 years, and be made well aware of the controversies surrounding aggressive management as opposed to watchful waiting. Available options for the treatment of such patients include radical prostatectomy, radiation therapy, and more recently cryosurgical ablation of the prostate.

Each therapy has significant advantages and disadvantages. The absence of definitive, prospective, randomized trials comparing one mode of therapy to another makes conclusive recommendations for an individual patient impossible[87]. It is therefore encumbent upon the clinician involved in counselling men with localized prostate cancer to most carefully assess the risk:benefit ratio for the individual patient in order to help him and his family decide upon the most appropriate therapeutic option.

REFERENCES

1 Lange P, Narayan P. Understaging and undergrading of prostate cancer: argument for postoperative radiation as adjuvant therapy. *Urology* 1983;**21**:113–118.

2 Boxer R, Kaufman J, Goodwin W. Radical prostatectomy for carcinoma of the prostate: 1951–1976. A review of 329 patients. *J Urol* 1977;**117**:208–213.

3 Catalona W, Stein A. Staging errors in clinically localized prostatic cancer. *J Urol* 1982;**127**:452–456.

4 Veenema R, Gursel E, Lattimer J. Radical retropubic prostatectomy for cancer: a 20-year experience. *J Urol* 1977;**117**:330–331.

5 Jewett H. The case for radical perineal prostatectomy. *J Urol* 1970;**103**:195–199.

6 Gibbons R, Cole B, Richardson R, *et al.* Adjuvant radiotherapy following radical prostatectomy: Results and complications. *J Urol* 1986;**135**:65–68.

7 Elder J, Jewett J, Walsh P. Radical perineal prostatectomy for clinical stage B2 carcinoma of the prostate. *J Urol* 1982;**127**:704–706.

8 Partin A, Kattan MW, Subong E, *et al.* Combination of prostate-specific antigen clinical stage and Gleason score to predict pathological stage of localized prostate cancer. *JAMA* 1997;**277**:1445–1451.

9 Denis LJ, Murphy GP, Schroder FH. Report of the consensus workshop on screening and global strategy for prostate cancer. *Cancer* 1995;**75**:1187–1207.

10 Garnick MB, Gittleman M, Steidle C, *et al.* Abarelix (PPI–149), a novel and potent GnRH antagonist, induces rapid and profound prostate gland volume reduction (PGVR) and androgen suppression before brachytherapy (BT) or radiation therapy (XRT). *J Urol* 1998;**159**:Ab850, 220.

11 Paulson D, Lin G, Hinshaw W, *et al.* Radical surgery versus radiotherapy for adenocarcinoma of the prostate. *J Urol* 1982;**128**(**3**):502–504.

12 Kupelian P. Beam or scalpel for prostate cancer? *Urol Times* 1997;**25**(**1**):28.

13 Zietman AL, Coen JJ, Shipley WV, Willett CG, Eferd JT. Radical radiation therapy in the management of prostatic adenocarcinoma: the initial PSA value as a predictor of treatment outcome. *J Urol* 1994;**151**:640–645.

14 Reiner W, Walsh P. An anatomical approach to the surgical management to the dorsal vein and Santorini's plexus during radical retropubic surgery. *J Urol* 1979;**121**:198–200.

15 Walsh PC. Radical retropubic prostatectomy with reduced morbidity: An anatomic approach. *NCI Monogr* 1988;**7**:133–137.

16 Lepor H, Gregerman M, Crosby R, *et al.* Precise localization of the autonomic nerves from the pelvic plexus to the corpora cavernosa: A detailed anatomical study of the adult male pelvis. *J Urol* 1985;**133**:207–212.

17 Walsh PC, Donker PJ. Impotence following radical prostatectomy: insight into etiology and prevention. *J Urol* 1982;**128**:492–497.

18 Quinlan D, Epstein J, Carter B, *et al.* Sexual function following radical prostatectomy: influence of preservation of neurovascular bundles. *J Urol* 1991;**145**:998–1002.

19 Catalona W, Basler J. Return of erections and urinary continence following radical retropubic prostatectomy. *J Urol* 1993;**150**:905–907.

20 Lu-Yao GL, McLerran D, Wasson J, *et al.* An assessment of radical prostatectomy. *JAMA* 1993;**269**:2633–2636.

21 Catalona WJ, Carvalhal GF, Mager DE, Smith DS. Potency, continence and complication rates in 1,870 consecutive radical retropubic prostatectomies. *J Urol* 1999;**162(2)**:433–438.

22 Herr HW. Quality of life of incontinent men after radical prostatectomy. *J Urol* 1994;**151**:652–654.

23 Levy DA, Resnick, MI. Laparoscopic pelvic lymphadenectomy and radical perineal prostatectomy: A viable alternative to radical retropubic prostatectomy. *J Urol* 1994;**151**:905–908.

24 Labrie F, Dupont A, Cusan L, *et al.* Downstaging of localized prostate cancer by neoadjuvant therapy with Flutamide and Lupron: the first controlled and randomized trial. *Clin Invest Med* 1993;**16**:499–509.

25 Koch MO, Smith JR. Clinical outcomes associated with the implementation of a cost-efficient programme for radical retropubic prostatectomy. *Br J Urol* 1995;**76**:28.

26 Litwin MS, Smith RB, Thind A, et al. Cost-efficient radical prostatectomy with a clinical care path. *J Urol* 1996;**155**:989.

27 Vallett BS. Radical perineal prostatectomy subsequent to bilateral orchiectomy. *Del Med J* 1944;**16**:19–20.

28 Colston JAC, Brendler J. Endocrine therapy in carcinoma of the prostate. *J Am Med Assoc* 1947;**134**:848–853.

29 Guttierez R. New horizons in the surgical management of carcinoma of the prostate gland. *Am J Surg* 1949;**78**:147–52.

30 Parlow AL, Acott WW. Hormone control therapy as a preparation for radical perineal prostatectomy in advanced carcinoma of the prostate. *NY J Med* 1949;**49**:629–634.

31 Scott WW, Boyd JL. Combined hormone control therapy and radical prostatectomy in the treatment of selected cases of advanced carcinoma of the prostate: a retrospective study based upon 25 years of experience. *J Urol* 1969;**101**:86–92.

32 Brawer MK, Peehl DM, Stemey TA, Bostwick DG. Keratin immunoreactivity in the benign and neoplastic human prostate. *Cancer Res* 1985;**45(8)**:3663–3667.

33 Witjes WPJ, Schulman CC, Debruyne FMJ, *et al.* Preliminary results of a prospective randomized study comparing radical prostatectomy versus radical prostatectomy associated with neoadjuvant hormonal combination therapy in T2–3N$_0$M$_0$ prostatic carcinoma. *Urology* 1997;**49(Suppl)**:65–9.

34 Soloway MS, Sharifi R, Wajsman Z, *et al.* Randomized prospective study comparing radical prostatectomy alone versus radical prostatectomy preceded by androgen blockade in clinical stage B2 (T2bNxM0) prostate cancer: the Lupron Depot Neo-Adjuvant Prostate Cancer Study Group. *J Urol* 1995;**154**:424–428.

35 Lange PH, Lightner DJ, Medini E, *et al.* The effect of radiation therapy after radical prostatectomy in patients with elevated PSA levels. *J Urol* 1990;**144**:927–932.

36 Andriole GL. Finasteride induced PSA reduction in patients with early stage prostate cancer. *J Urol* 1994;**151(Suppl)**:450A.

37 Huroszewitz JS, Kawinski E, Murphy GP. Monoclonal antibodies for a new antigenic marker in epithelial prostatic cells and serum of prostate cancer patients. *Anti Cancer Res* 1987;**7**:927–935.

38 deKernion J, Belldegrun A, Naitoh J. Surgical treatment of localized prostate cancer. Indications, technique and results. In. Belldegun A, Kirby RS, Oliver T, eds. *New Perspectives in Prostate Cancer*. Oxford: Isis; 1998:185–203.

39 Dorey F, Franklin J, deKernion JB, Smith RB. Use of multiple PSA values for predicting clinical disease recurrence after radical retropubic prostatectomy? *J Urol* 1996;**155(Suppl)**:487A.

40 Link P, Freiha F, Stamey T. Adjuvant radiation therapy in patients with detectable prostate-specific antigen following radical prostatectomy. *J Urol* 1991;**145**:532–534.

41 Zincke H. Extended experience with surgical treatment of stage D1 adenocarcinoma of prostate. Significant influence of immediate adjuvant hormonal treatment (orchiectomy) on outcome. *Urology* 1993;**33(Suppl)**:27–36.

42 Hanks GE. Radical prostatectomy or radiation therapy for early prostate cancer: Two roads to the same end. *Cancer* 1988;**61**:2153–2160.

43 Amdur RJ, Parsons JT, Fitzgerald LT, Million RR. Adenocarcinoma of the prostate treated with external-beam radiation therapy: 5-year minimum follow-up. *Radiother Oncol* 1990;**18**:235–246.

44 Perez C, Pilepich M, Garcia D, *et al.* Definitive radiation therapy in carcinoma of the prostate localized to the pelvis: experience at the Mallinckrodt Institute of Radiology. NCI *Monogr* 1988;**7**:85–94.

45 Schellhammer PF, El-Mahdi AM. Pelvic complications after definitive treatment of prostate cancer by interstitial or external beam radiation. *Urology* 1983;**21**:451–457.

46 Hanks G. Radiotherapy or surgery for prostate cancer: ten and fifteen year results of external beam therapy. *Acta Oncol* 1991;**30(2)**:231–237.

47 Bagshaw M, Cox R, Ray G. Status of radiation treatment of prostate cancer. NCI *Monogr* 1988;**7**:47–60.

48 Gibbons R, Correa R Jr, Brannen G, *et al.* Total prostatectomy for clinically localized prostatic cancer: Long-term results. *J Urol* 1989;**131**:564–566.

49 Jewett H, Bridge R, Gray G, *et al.* The palpable nodule prostatic cancer: Results 15 years after radical excision. *JAMA* 1968;**203**:403–406.

50 Zagars GK, von Eschenbach AC, Johnson DE, *et al.*

Stage C adenocarcinoma of the prostate: An analysis of 551 patients treated with external beam radiation. *Cancer* 1987;**60**:1489–1499.

51 Epstein BE, Hanks GE. Prostate cancer: evaluation and radiotherapeutic management. *Ca-Cancer J Clin* 1992;**42**:223–240.

52 Soffen EM, Hanks GE, Hwang CC, et al. Conformal static field therapy for low volume low grade prostate cancer with rigid immobilization. *Int J Radiat Oncol Biol Phys* 1991;**20**:141–146.

53 Soffen EM, Hanks GE, Hunt MA, et al. Conformal static field radiation therapy for treatment of early prostate cancer versus non-conformal techniques: a reduction in acute morbidity. *Int J Radiat Oncol Biol Phys* 1992;**24**(3):485–488.

54 Asbell SO, Schlager BA, Baker AS. Revision of treatment planning for carcinoma of the prostate. *Int J Radiat Oncol Biol Phys* 1980;**6**:861–865.

55 Lee DJ, Leibel S, Shiels R, et al. The value of ultrasonic imaging and CT scanning in planning the radiotherapy for prostatic carcinoma. *Cancer* 1980;**45**:724–727.

56 Zagars GK, von Eschenbach AC. PSA: an important marker for prostate cancer treated by external beam therapy. *Cancer* 1993;**72**:538–548.

57 Zietman AL Coen JJ, Shipley WU, et al. Adjuvant irradiation after radical prostatectomy for adenocarcinoma of prostate: analysis of freedom from PSA failure. *Urology* 1993;**42**:292–299.

58 Kaplan ID, Cox RS, Bagshaw MA. Prostate-specific antigen after external beam radiotherapy for prostatic cancer: Follow-up. *J Urol* 1993;**149**:519–522.

59 Schellhammer P, El-Mahdi A, Wright G, et al. Prostate-specific antigen to determine progression-free survival after radiation therapy for localized carcinoma of prostate. *J Urol* 1993;**42**:13–20.

60 Zietman AL, Coen JJ, Shipley WU, et al. Radical radiation therapy in the management of prostatic adenocarcinoma: the initial prostate-specific antigen value as a predictor of treatment outcome. *J Urol* 1994;**151**:640–645.

61 Freiha F, Bagshaw M. Carcinoma of the prostate: Results of post-irradiation biopsy. *Prostate* 1984;**5**(1):19–25.

62 Scardino PT, Frankel JM, Wheeler TM, et al. The prognostic significance of postirradiation biopsy results in patients with prostatic cancer. *J Urol* 1986;**135**(3):510–516.

63 Kabalin J, Hodge K, McNeal J, et al. Identification of residual cancer in the prostate following radiation therapy: Role of transrectal ultrasound guided biopsy and prostate-specific antigen. *J Urol* 1989;**142**:326–331.

64 Kuban DA, el-Mahdi AM, Schellhammer PF, et al. The significance of post-irradiation biopsy with long-term follow-up. *Int J Radiat Oncol Biol Phys* 1992;**24**(3):409–414.

65 Brawer M, Nagle R, Pitts W, et al. Keratin immunoreactivity as an aid to the diagnosis of persistent adenocarcinoma in irradiated human prostates. *Cancer* 1989;**63**(3):454–460.

66 Stamey T, Ferrari, M, Schmid H. Value of serial prostate-specific antigen determinations 5 years after radiotherapy: steeply increasing values characterize 80% of patients. *J Urol* 1993;**150**:1845–1850.

67 Ritter MA, Messing EM, Shanahan TG, et al. Prostate-specific antigen as a predictor of radiotherapy response and patterns of failure in localized prostate cancer. *J Clin Oncol* 1992;**10**:1208–1217.

68 Zagars GK, Pollack A, Kavadi VS, von Escherbach AC. Prostate-specific antigen and RT for clinically localized prostate cancer. *Int J Radiat Oncol Biol Phys* 1995;**32**:293–306.

69 Hart KB, Shamsa F, McLaughlin W, Forman JD, Jeffrey D, Forman MD. Correlation of post-treatment histologic and biochemical results with long-term outcome in prostate cancer patients following radiation therapy. J Urol 2000 (Submitted).

70 Roach M, Pickett B, Holland J, et al. The role of the uretrogram during simulation for localized carcinoma of the prostate. *Int J Radiat Oncol Biol Phys* 1993;**25**:299–307.

71 Corn BW, Hanks GE, Schultheiss TE. Conformal treatment of prostate cancer with improved targeting: superior prostate-specific antigen. *Int J Radiat Oncol Biol Phys* 1995;**32**:325–330.

72 Vijaykumar S, Awan A, Davuson T, et al. Acute toxicity during external beam radiotherapy for localized prostate cancer: comparison of different treatment techniques. *Int J Radiat Oncol Biol Phys* 1993;**25**:359–364.

73 Emami B, Purdy JA, Manolis JM, et al. 3-D static conformal radiotherapy: preliminary results of a prospective clinical trial. *Int J Radiat Oncol Biol Phys* 1991;**21**:197.

74 Dearnaley DP, Nahum A, Lee M, et al. Radiotherapy of prostate cancer. Reducing the treated volume. Conformal therapy, hormone cytoreduction and protons. *Br J Cancer* 1994;**70**(Suppl 22):16.

75 Banker FL. The preservation of potency after treatment of prostate cancer with external beam irradiation. *Int J Radiat Oncol Biol Phys* 1988;**15**:219–221.

76 Hanks GE, Asbell S, Krall JM, et al. Outcome for lymph node dissection negative T16, T2 prostate cancer treated with external beam radiotherapy in RTOG 77-06. *Int J Radiat Oncol Biol Phys* 1993;**27**(Suppl 1):106.

77 Bagshaw MA. External radiation therapy of carcinoma of the prostate. *Cancer* 1980;**45**:1912–1921.

78 Hanks GE, Martz KL, Diamond JJ. The effect of dose on local control of prostate cancer. *Int J Radiat Oncol Biol Phys* 1988;**15**:1299–1305.

79 Leibel SA, Fuks Z, Zelefsky MJ, et al. The effects of local and regional treatment on metastatic outcome in prostate cancer with lymph node involvement. *Int J Radiat Oncol Biol Phys* 1994;**28**:7–16.

80 Laramore GE, Krall JM, Thomas FJ, Griffin TW, Maor MH, Henrickson FT. Fast neutron radiotherapy in the treatment of locally advanced prostate cancer. *Int J Radiat Oncol Biol Phys* 1985;**11**:1621–1627.

81 Russell RJ, Caplan RJ, Laramore GE, *et al.* Photon versus fast neutron external beam radiotherapy in the treatment of locally advanced prostate cancer. *Int J Radiat Oncol Biol Phys* 1993;**28**:47–54.

82 Pilepich MV, Al-Sarraf M, John MJ, McGowan DG, Krall JM. Phase II RTOG study of hormonal cytoreduction with flutamide and goserelin in locally advanced carcinoma of the prostate treated with definitive radiation therapy. *Am J Clin Oncol* 1990;**13**:461–464.

83 Pilepich MV, Sause WT, Shipley WV, *et al.* Androgen deprivation with radiation therapy compared to radiation alone for locally advanced prostatic carcinoma: a randomized comparative trial of the Radiation Therapy Oncology Group. Urology 1995;**45**:616–622.

84 Bolla M, Gonzalez D, Warde P, *et al.* Improved survival in patients with locally advanced prostate cancer treated with radiotherapy and gosserelin. *N Engl J Med* 1997;**337(5)**:295–300.

85 Cohen JK, Rooker GM, Shuman BA, Miller RJJ, Merlotti L. Cryosurgical ablation management alternative for localized prostate cancer. In: Smith AD, ed. *Textbook of Endourology.* St Louis: Quality Medical Publishing; 1996:1217–1233.

86 Cohen JK, Miller RJJ, Rooker GM, Benoit RM, Merlotti L. Four year PSA and biopsy results after cryosurgical ablation of the prostate (CSAP) for localized adenocarcinoma of the prostate. *J Urol* 1997;**157**:419A.

87 Kirby RS. Treatment options for early prostate cancer. *Urology* 1998;**52**:948–962.

88 Weldon VE. Radical perineal prostatectomy. In: Das S, Crawford ED, eds. *Cancer of the Prostate.* New York: Marcel Dekker; 1993:225–266.

89 Van Poppel H, De Ridder D, Elgamal AA, *et al.* Neoadjuvant hormonal therapy before radical prostatectomy decreases the number of positive surgical margin in stage T2 prostate cancer: interim results of a prospective randomized trial. The Belgium Uro-oncological Study Group. *J Urol* 1995;**154**:429–434.

90 Goldenbergy SL, Krotz LH, Srigley J, *et al.* Randomized, prospective, controlled study comparing radical prostatectomy alone and neoadjuvant androgen withdrawal in the treatment of localized prostate cancer. *J Urol* 1996;**165**:873–877.

91 Culp OS. Radical perineal prostatectomy: its past, present, and possible future. *J Urol* 1968;**98**:618–626.

92 Walsh P, Jewett H. Radical surgery for prostatic cancer. *Cancer* 1980;**45**:1906–1911.

93 Tomlinson R, Currie D, Boyce W. Radical prostatectomy: palliation for stage C carcinoma of the prostate. *J Urol* 1977;**117(1)**:85–87.

94 Robey E, Schellhammer P. Local failure after definitive therapy for prostatic cancer. *J Urol* 1987;**137(4)**:613–619.

95 Middleton R, Smith J Jr, Melzer R, *et al.* Patient survival and local recurrence rate following radical prostatectomy for prostatic carcinoma. *J Urol* 1986;**136**:422–424.

96 Catalona W, Miller D, Kavoussi L. Intermediate-term survival results in clinically understaged prostate cancer patients following radical prostatectomy. *J Urol* 1988;**142(3)**:832–833.

97 Zincke H, Utz DC, Taylor WF. Bilateral pelvic lymphadenectomy and radical prostatectomy for clinical stage C prostatic cancer: role of adjuvant treatment for residual cancer and in disease progression. *J Urol* 1986;**135**: 1199–1205.

98 Steinberg G, Epstein J, Piantados S, *et al.* Management of Stage D1 adenocarcinoma of the prostate: the Johns Hopkins experience 1974–1987. *J Urol* 1989;**141**:310A.

99 Rosenberg S, Loening S, Hawtrey C, *et al.* Radical prostatectomy with adjuvant radioactive gold for prostatic cancer: a preliminary report. *J Urol* 1985;**133(2)**:225–227.

100 Bahnson R, Garnett J, Grayhack J. Adjuvant radiation therapy in stages C and D1 prostatic adenocarcinoma: preliminary results. *Urology* 1986;**27(5)**:403–406.

101 Ray G, Bagshaw M, Freiha F. External beam radiation salvage for residual or recurrent local tumor following radical prostatectomy. *J Urol* 1984;**132(5)**:926–930.

102 Jacobson G, Simith J Jr, Stewart J. Postoperative radiation therapy for pathologic stage C prostate cancer. *Int J Radiat Oncol Biol Phys* 1987;**13(7)**:1021–1024.

103 Lange P, Reddy P, Medini E, *et al.* Radiation therapy as adjuvant treatment after radical prostatectomy. NCI *Monogr* 1988;**7**:141–149.

104 Pilepich M, Walz B, Baglan R. Postoperative irradiation in carcinoma of the prostate. *Int J Radiat Oncol Biol Phys* 1984;**10(10)**:1869–1873.

105 Forman J, Wharam M, Lee D, *et al.* Definitive radiotherapy following prostatectomy: Results and complications. *Int J Radiat Oncol Biol Phys* 1986;**12**:185–189.

106 Kuban DA, El-Mahdi AM, Schellhammer PF. Interstitial implantation for prostate cancer. What have we learned 10 years later? *Cancer* 1989;**63**:2415–2420.

107 Kim RY, Bueschen AJ. Interstitial iodine-125 seed implantation in the management of prostate cancer: preliminary report at UAB. *Ala Med* 1986;**55(7)**:27–33.

108 Giles GM, Brady LW. Iodine implantation after lymphadenectomy in early carcinoma of the prostate. *Int J Radiat Oncol Biol Phys* 1986; **12**:2117–2125.

109 Morton JD, Peschel RE. Iodine-125 implants versus external beam therapy for stages A2, B and C prostate cancer. *Int J Radiat Oncol Biol Phys* 1988;**14**:1153–1157.

110 DeLaney TF, Shipley WU, O'Leary MP, *et al.* Preoperative irradiation, lymphadenectomy, and 125 iodine implantation for patients with localized carcinoma of the prostate. *Int J Radiat Oncol Biol Phys* 1986;**12**:1779–1785.

111 Reddy EK, Mebust WK, Weigel JW. Iodine 125 implantation in localized prostatic cancer. *Endocuriether Hyperthern Oncol* 1990;**6**:239–244.

112 Fuks Z, Leibel SA, Wallner KE, *et al.* The effect of local control on metastatic dissemination in carcinoma of the prostate: long-term results in patients treated with 125I implantation. *Int J Radiat Oncol Biol Phys* 1991;**21**:537–547.

113 Schellhammer PF. Radical prostatectomy; patterns of local failure and survival in 67 patients. *Urology* 1988;**31**:191–197.

114 Gibbons R, Correa R Jr, Brannen G, *et al.* Total prostatectomy for localized prostatic cancer. *J Urol* 1984;**131**(1):73–76.

115 Wallner K. Iodine 125 brachytherapy for early stage prostate cancer: new techniques may achieve better results. *Oncology* 1991;**5**:115–122.

116 Dearnaley D. The way ahead for radiotherapy in prostate cancer. In: Belldegrun A, Kirby RS, Oliver T, eds. *New Perspectives in Prostate Cancer*. Oxford: Isis Medical Media; 1998:227–243.

Chapter 10

Alternative strategies for localized prostate cancer

INTRODUCTION

Although the standard management of localized prostate cancer (at least in younger men) has usually been either radical prostatectomy or external beam radiotherapy, a number of publications have highlighted the fact that a policy of 'watchful waiting' and the deferral of therapy until symptoms arise may be appropriate in smaller volume, well-differentiated lesions, especially in patients with a life expectancy of less than 10 years[1–3]. The difficulties with a policy of watchful waiting include, of course, the anxieties shared by both the patient and urologist that the tumour may advance silently to an incurable stage before definitive therapy is initiated. For this reason there has been a move by some towards alternative strategies to deal with localized prostatic cancer that do not involve the small (but significant) morbidity associated with standard therapies discussed in the previous chapter. It has to be pointed out that however attractive these new more conservative treatment strategies may be, there are as yet no long-term outcome data to inform us about their safety and efficacy. Accordingly, all of them, with the exception of watchful waiting, should be regarded as investigational at present.

WATCHFUL WAITING

Although the concept of watchful waiting often seems difficult to countenance in the presence of proven malignant disease, there is now mounting evidence that in certain patients with prostate cancer this may well be the appropriate course of action. In T1a cancers, diagnosed incidentally at transurethral resection of the prostate for obstructive symptoms, for example, the probability of disease progression over 8 years has been reported to be as low as 3%[4] in one series, and 16% in another[5]. Certainly, in patients with a life expectancy of less than 10 years, most clinicians would adopt a 'wait and see' policy with regular prostate-specific antigen (PSA) monitoring, proceeding to therapy only if there were clear evidence of disease progression.

Even in patients with more significant volumes of localized prostate cancer present, long-term follow-up studies have suggested a relatively low metastatic rate[3,6]. Although most patients exhibited local disease progression, the majority died of intercurrent diseases rather than prostatic cancer[3].

In a meta-analysis of conservative treatment of non-metastatic prostate cancer, Chodak *et al.*[2] concluded that histological grading provided the best indicator of the probability of significant disease progression. Those patients with grade 1, well-differentiated lesions had a low metastatic rate and an excellent disease-specific survival of 87% at 10 years. By contrast, only 26% of individuals with grade 3, poorly differentiated tumours were still alive 10 years after diagnosis.

Using a decision-analysis mathematical model, Fleming *et al.*[7] have calculated that conservative therapy may well be the best option for men with well-differentiated, localized prostate cancer, whose life expectancy does not exceed 10 years. However, this study focused on potent men over the age of 60 – those most likely to have side-effects from treatment – and used a rather simplified model of the natural history of prostate cancer. In addition, the data used to predict outcome of treatment did not truly reflect the results attainable with modern methods of detection and treatment.

CRYOABLATION

Cryoablation – that is, the use of freezing techniques to destroy prostatic tissue, was first utilized by Gonder *et al.* in 1964[8]. The original concept was that this form of therapy could permanently eliminate all primary tumour in the prostate, while preserving functional and structural integrity of surrounding structures, including the neurovascular bundles. In addition, it was hoped that cryosurgery might induce some form of protective immune response within the host[9]; however, there has never been any scientific evidence to support this concept.

Current techniques of cryoablation employ newly developed technology. The patient is anaesthetized and placed in the lithotomy position. The perineum is prepared and draped, and a suprapubic catheter inserted percutaneously. Urethral warming is accomplished by circulating heated water (at 44°C) through a urethral catheter. Real-time transrectal ultrasound is then performed to determine the prostatic dimensions. An 18-gauge needle is placed into the prostate and a J-shaped guide wire placed through the needle, deep into the prostatic substance. The track is then dilated and a 7 mm cryoprobe inserted. Three to eight cryoprobes may be inserted in this manner and transrectal ultrasound is employed to monitor correct probe placement (**10.1**). Next, liquid nitrogen is passed into the probes and the freezing process is observed on transrectal ultrasound; as the so-called 'ice balls' develop, their location can be visualized on transrectal ultrasound as they advance through the prostatic tissue to include the prostatic capsule, but they must stop short of the rectal wall. Each of the cryoprobe tips achieves a temperature of between −180°C and −190°C, and produces tissue destruction by inducing

intracellular ice crystals which cause cell membrane rupture and protein denaturation in the frozen zone.

While Gonder[8] originally utilized transurethral cryosurgery, which of course limited his ability to treat the peripheral zone of the prostate, Flocks[10], in 1969, used an open perineal exposure for controlled application of cryotherapy under direct vision. Rather later, Bonney and associates[11] used a similar open transperineal approach with visual monitoring of prostate freezing in 229 patients. At five-year follow-up, they noticed a stage-survival probability equivalent to that of radical prostatectomy, but reported an incidence of urethro-rectal fistula of 1.4%, urethro-cutaneous fistula rate of 10.7%, and erectile dysfunction in 7.4% of patients. In a subsequent publication, Bonney[12] reported that although 66% of patients had elimination of palpable tumour, at least 41% suffered recurrent disease and more than 50% of patients received concomitant endocrine therapy. The addition of this adjuvant therapy, unfortunately, confounds attempts to evaluate the true efficacy of this particular modality. Onik and associates[13] have reported the use of transrectal ultrasound-guided percutaneous transperineal cryosurgery on the prostate of 6 dogs. They reported that with this technique they were able to complete the freezing process successfully and avoid any injury to the rectum and urethra. Following this work, their preliminary results on 55 patients were published. The report was too early to provide reliable information about the efficiency of tumour ablation. However, complications were noted; in particular, four patients suffered freezing of the rectum, leading to urethro-rectal fistula in two and sloughing of prostatic urethral tissue in three. In addition, 65% of patients who were potent pre-therapy were impotent following treatment, indicating probable involvement of the neurovascular bundles in the freezing process. More recent reports have been more favourable[14].

In the final analysis, the safety and efficacy of cryosurgery for prostatic cancer can only be evaluated by careful long-term follow-up of large numbers of patients, ideally in a long-term randomized study comparing it against standard treatment therapies. At the time of writing, no such data are available.

HYPERTHERMIA TREATMENT

Hyperthermia has for many years been recognized as inducing destruction of various tissues, and it

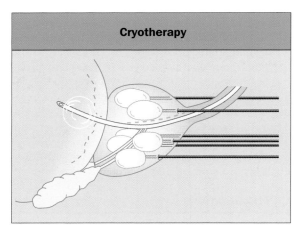

Cryotherapy

10.1 Cryotherapy: under ultrasound control, up to 8 cryoprobes are introduced into the prostate by the transperineal route. Freezing is accomplished by circulation of liquid nitrogen through the needles while the urethra is protected by warming through a catheter.

has been suggested that it has a selective cytotoxic effect on tumour cells both *in vitro* and *in vivo*. Although the explanation for this is not entirely clear, it has been proposed that abnormal tumour vessels are incapable of dilating in the presence of heat (as normal vessels are able to do) and that this may render the tumour more susceptible to heat damage. In addition, neoplastic cells appear in some way intrinsically more sensitive to heat than normal cells. The prostate is easily accessible for hyperthermia via the transrectal route (**10.2**).

Investigations into the clinical effects of hyperthermia on neoplastic prostate tissue have so far been limited. Yerushalmi and co-workers were the first to report the use of microwave hypothermia delivered transrectally for local or locally advanced prostate cancer[15]. In their small series of 15 patients, ten were stage C, one was stage B and four were stage D. All but one had severe local symptoms and each was given at least six treatments, lasting an average of one hour, at temperatures of between 42°C and 43°C. Each patient was treated on an outpatient basis without anaesthesia. Unfortunately, some patients were also given adjunctive post-treatment radiotherapy and some were also treated with either oral oestrogens or orchiectomy prior to hyperthermia treatment. Marked improvements in symptoms were reported in all patients. Minimal complications were described, although follow-up was rather short. The same author followed this report in 1986 with a further report of 32 patients similarly treated, again with sporadic employment of adjunctive radiation or hormonal therapy[16]. In this report, the few patients treated with hyperthermia alone appeared to have objective tumour

regression, but there was usually evidence of relapse after six months. The best results seemed to be obtained in the 20 patients who were treated with both combined radiotherapy and hyperthermia. Montorsi *et al.*[17] reported the results in 46 patients with locally extensive prostatic cancer presenting with urinary retention or perineal pain in spite of total androgen blockade. Hyperthermia was delivered transrectally in ten one-hour sessions delivered over five weeks, with a calculated intra-prostatic temperature of around 43.5°C. This group reported significant improvement of obstructive symptoms and 50% of patients who were in urinary retention were rendered free of their catheter with only minimal complications.

More recently, Servadio and Leib reported a series of 44 patients treated with transrectal hyperthermia in combination with either radiotherapy or hormonal therapy[18]. Twenty-seven of these patients had locally advanced disease, and all had severe local obstruction and irritative symptoms of urinary retention. They noted no complications attributable to hyperthermia, and a significant subjective improvement of symptoms was reported in the majority of patients. Only two of the 27 patients had progression of the disease at four-year follow-up, and nine of the 11 patients who underwent follow-up biopsy were reported to have negative biopsy results. Most recently, Sorensen[19] reported 12 patients undergoing transurethral microwave thermotherapy using the Prostatron™ microwave thermotherapy device (**10.3**). All patients underwent radical prostatectomy 6–9 days after microwave

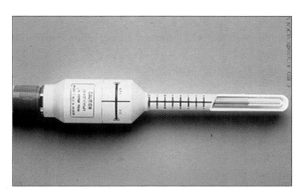

10.2 A transrectal microwave probe for hyperthermia treatment of the prostate.

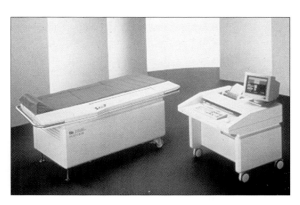

10.3 The Prostatron™ thermotherapy device. This machine delivers microwave energy transurethrally to the prostate while the urethra is cooled by fluid circulated through the urethral catheter.

treatment. The depth of the effective injury was 1–1.5 cm, with a well-demarcated line of thermal damage. Tumours situated posteriorly in the peripheral zone, which constitute the majority of prostate cancers, appeared unaffected by this treatment.

From these data it seems clear that microwave hyperthermia as a treatment for localized prostate cancer is currently only at an early stage of development. Unfortunately, its true efficacy is difficult to judge from those studies that have been performed, either because no clear protocol was followed, or because adjunctive therapies were employed as well as hyperthermia. Nonetheless, the technique does seem to hold some promise, and hopefully more properly controlled longer-term data will be available in the future.

LASER THERAPY

Laser treatment of localized prostate cancer has also been investigated. Lasers transform light energy into heat within the prostatic tissue, resulting in an intraprostatic temperature considerably above 60°C for a few seconds. At this temperature, rapid protein denaturation and cell necrosis result. The depth of penetration of light (and therefore the volume of affected tissue) is primarily dependent upon the wave-length of the applied laser light. The recent advent of right-angled laser fibres has allowed more precise application of the laser energy to the prostate (**10.4**).

Sander and Beisland[20] pioneered the use of the neodymium yag (Nd:YAG) laser for the treatment of localized prostate cancer. Nd:YAG laser radiation seemed to produce a homogeneous coagulation to a depth of 3–4 mm without the necessity to remove tissue. The necrotic zone that was created gradually

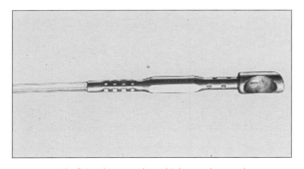

10.4 A side-firing laser probe which may be used to treat the prostate through a cystoscope (Bard Urolase[R]).

converted into fibrotic scar tissue, with only minor shrinkage. Between 1981 and 1986, over 100 patients with localized lesions were treated with either transurethral or suprapubic access to the gland. A suprapubic trocar for cystoscopy was utilized to access all of the capsular areas of the prostate that were not treatable with the laser fibre transurethrally. All patients initially underwent extended transurethral resection of the prostate, exposing capsular fibres throughout the extent of the resection. Three to five weeks later, a thorough lasering of the prostatic capsular bed was performed using 40–50 watts of laser power applied in bursts of 1–4 seconds; a total of 7000–21 000 joules were applied. The transformation of tissue into a grey-white mass (checked by visual inspection) was used as an end point for adequate treatment in a given area of the prostate. At a two-year follow-up, 56 of the original 63 patients were deemed disease free, and only 7 cases were regarded as treatment failures. The failures occurred in patients in whom only the transurethral approach was used.

Samdal and Brevick[21] reported rather similar results in 26 patients with localized prostate cancer: all patients underwent extended transurethral resection (TURP) followed in 6 weeks by Nd:YAG laser treatment at 45 W with a total of 11 000–35 000 J being applied. They reported minimal perioperative complications, but did describe eight late complications: four patients developed bladder neck contracture, two developed stress urinary incontinence, and one developed erectile dysfunction. A further individual developed urethral stenosis and one bilateral hydronephrosis secondary to fibrosis of the ureteric orifices. These authors stressed the importance of careful monitoring of rectal temperature to prevent development of prostato-rectal fistulae. At a rather short follow-up period, 22 of the 26 patients were reported to be disease free. At follow-up, most patients had a reduction in PSA levels, but in no patient did the PSA decrease to undetectable levels.

Lately, interest has been increasing in the use of interstitial laser therapy for prostate cancer, using percutaneous placement of the needles in order to deliver Nd:YAG laser energy (**10.5**). Littrup and associates[22] reported a study in dogs demonstrating focal intraprostatic areas of necrosis and coagulation extending up to 14 mm. Although needles could be placed accurately using ultrasound, the extent of laser treatment was rather imprecise, as the penetration depth of tissue damage was variable.

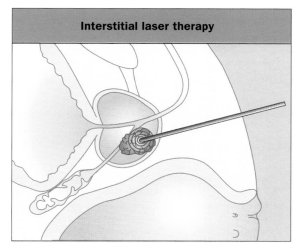

Interstitial laser therapy

10.5 Interstitial laser therapy of the prostate involves the transperineal placement of a laser fibre into the prostate. Laser energy is converted into thermal energy within the gland, resulting in localized tissue destruction.

Other means of delivering laser energy to the prostate are currently being investigated. Liong and colleagues[23] have reported the use of a transurethral balloon 'laserthermia' device that emits circumferential laser energy. Initial studies in dogs revealed extensive coagulation necrosis of the prostatic tissue together with subsequent cavitation formation. Early studies in men with benign prostatic hyperplasia (BPH) have been encouraging, but clearly this device also carries possibilities for the treatment of patients with localized prostate cancer. As yet, however, no data are available concerning its efficacy for this application.

ADJUVANT ANDROGEN DEPRIVATION

The recent publication of so many reports suggesting benefit from combining androgen deprivation with other local therapies directed at the prostate

tumour itself, probably reflects the fact that no currently available therapy for localized prostate cancer is completely effective[24,25]. As described in Chapter 9, neoadjuvant therapy with luteinizing hormone-releasing hormone analogues before either radical prostatectomy[26] or conformed radiotherapy[27] has been reported as improving the results of treatment. It seems likely that in the future anti-androgens such as Casodex™ or flutamide will be used in combination with other local therapies such as cryosurgery[28] or brachytherapy. Such combinations are currently under investigation. The real benefits in terms of freedom from progression and overall survival of such combination therapies will need to be carefully evaluated by long-term randomized studies.

CONCLUSIONS

Watchful waiting with deferred introduction of endocrine ablation when symptoms develop is now a legitimate treatment option for patients with low-volume, well-differentiated prostate cancer and/or limited life expectancy. There has been a recent, rapid development of new, minimally invasive technologies for dealing with bladder-outflow obstruction due to BPH. It seems likely that a similar trend may be seen in prostatic cancer. Of course, this problem is an intrinsically more difficult one in that urologists will wish to be confident that all cancer tissue has been reliably ablated by new competitor therapies to radical prostatectomy and external-beam radiotherapy. To date, there is no conclusive evidence to suggest that any of the new technologies available thus far is capable of producing long-term tumour ablation with reliable serum PSA suppression and minimal side-effects. However, there is little doubt that there is considerable potential for further developments in this area. One of the most promising developments, brachytherapy, is the subject of an entire chapter (see Chapter 11).

REFERENCES

1 Adolfsson J. Deferred treatment of low grade stage T3 prostate cancer without distant metastases. *J Urol* 1993; **149**:326–329.
2 Chodak GW, Thisted RA, Gerber GS, *et al.* Results of conservative management of clinically localized prostate cancer. *New Eng J Med* 1994;**4**:242–248.
3 George NJR. Natural history of localised prostatic

cancer managed by conservative therapy alone. *Lancet* 1988;494–497.
4 Cantrell BB, DeKlerk DP, Eggleston JC, *et al.* Pathological factors that influence prognosis in stage A prostatic cancer: the influence of extent versus grade. *J Urol* 1981;**125**:516–521.
5 Epstein JI, Paull G, Eggleston JC, *et al.* Prognosis of untreated stage A1 prostatic carcinoma: a study of 94 cases with extended follow-up. *J Urol* 1986;**136**:837–839.

6 Johansson JE, Adami HO, Andersson SO, *et al.* High 10-year survival rate in patients with early, untreated prostatic cancer. *JAMA* 1992;**267**:2191–2196.

7 Fleming C, Wasson JH, Albertsen PC, *et al.* A decision analysis of alternate treatment strategies for clinically localized prostate cancer. JAMA 1993;**269**:2650–2658.

8 Gonder MH, Soanes WA, Smith V. Experimental prostate cryosurgery. *Invest Urol* 1964;**1**:610–618.

9 Soanes WA, Ablin RJ, Gonder MJ. Remission of metastatic lesions following cryosurgery in prostate cancer. *J Urol* 1970;**104**:154–159.

10 Flocks TH, Nelson CMK, Boatman CL. Perineal cryosurgery for prostatic carcinoma. *J Urol* 1972;**108**:933–935.

11 Bonney WW, Platz CE, Fallon B, *et al.* Cryosurgery in prostatic cancer: survival. *Urology* 1982;**19**:37–42.

12 Bonney WW, Fallen B, Gerber WL, *et al.* Cryosurgery in prostate cancer: elimination of the local lesion. *Urology* 1983;**22**:8–15.

13 Onik GM, Cohen JK, Reyes GD, *et al.* Transrectal ultrasound-guided percutaneous radical cryosurgical ablation of the prostate. *Cancer* 1993;**72**(4):1291–1299.

14 Cohen JK, Miller RJJ, Rooker GN, Benoit RM, Merlotti L. Four-year PSA and biopsy results after cryosurgical ablation of the prostate (CSAP) for localized adenocarcinoma of the prostate. *J Urol* 1997;**157**:419A.

15 Yerushalmi A, Servadio C, Leib C, *et al.* Local hyperthermia for treatment of carcinoma of the prostate: a preliminary report. *Prostate* 1982;**3**:623–629.

16 Yerushalmi A, Shani A, Fishelovitz Y, *et al.* Local microwave hyperthermia in the treatment of carcinoma of the prostate. *Oncology* 1986;**43**:299–305.

17 Montorsi F, Guazzoni G, Colombo R, *et al.* Transrectal microwave hyperthermia for advanced prostate cancer: long-term clinical results. *J Urol* 1992;**148**:342–345.

18 Servadio C, Leib Z. Local hyperthermia for prostate cancer. *Urology* 1991;**38**:342–345.

19 Sorensen RB, McGarragle MP, Grignon DJ, *et al.* Transurethral microwave thermotherapy (TUMT) using the Prostatron: a histopathological evaluation of the thermal effects on carcinoma of the prostate. *J Urol* 1993;**149**:232A.

20 Sander S, Beisland HO. Laser in the treatment of localized prostatic cancer. *J Urol* 1984;**132**:280–281.

21 Samdal F, Brevik B. Laser combined with TURP in the treatment of localized prostatic cancer. *Scand J Urol Nephrol* 1990;**24**:175–181.

22 Littrup PJ, Lee F, Borlaza GS, *et al.* Percutaneous ablation of canine prostate using transrectal ultrasound guidance absolute ethanol and Nd:YAG laser. *Invest Radiol* 1988;**23**:734–739.

23 Liong ML, Suzuki T, Yamanaka H, *et al.* Prostalase: Basic clinical research and preliminary clinical results with laser thermotherapy for symptomatic benign prostatic hyperplasia. *J Clinic Laser Med & Surg* 1994;**12**(2):85–92.

24 Schulman CC, Sassine AM. Neoadjuvant hormonal deprivation before radical prostatectomy. *Eur Urol* 1993;**24**: 450–455.

25 Gibbons RP, Jonsson E. Adjuvant radiation therapy following radical prostatectomy for pathologic stage C prostate cancer. *Eur Urol* 1995;**27**(Suppl):24–25.

26 Soloway MS, Sharifi R, Wood D, *et al.* Randomized comparison of radical prostatectomy alone or preceded by androgen deprivation for cT2B prostate cancer. *J Urol* 1995; **153**(4):391A.

27 Zelefsky MJ, Leibel SA, Burman CM, *et al.* Neoadjuvant hormonal therapy improves the therapeutic ratio in patients with bulky prostatic cancer treated with three-dimensional conformal radiation therapy. *Int J Rad Oncol Biol Phys* 1994;**29**(4):775–761.

28 Lee F, Bahn DK, McHugh TA, *et al.* US-guided percutaneous cryoablation of prostate cancer. *Radiology* 1994;**192**:769–776.

Chapter 11

Brachytherapy

Perhaps for no other malignancy has the optimal treatment strategy gone through as many pendulum swings as for clinically localized carcinoma of the prostate. Owing to a number of factors, brachytherapy, the interstitial implantation of radioactive sources has been resurrected and is rapidly gaining widespread recognition by clinicians as well as patients in the USA and elsewhere.

This chapter will review the historical events that have led to this resurrection of interest, describe the modern methods, and review the pertinent results from the Northwest Hospital in Seattle, the institution that has the world's longest and largest experience.

Brachytherapy is not new. Indeed, Pasteau and Degrais performed prostate brachytherapy: the insertion of a radium capsule into the prostatic urethra in Paris in 1909[1] (**Table 11.1**). Barringer at the then Memorial Hospital in New York (subsequently known as the Memorial Sloan-Kettering Cancer Center) employed radium needles[2]. However, the term brachytherapy was not used until 1931[3]. The term comes from the Greek *brachy* implying near. In 1952, Flocks *et al.*[4] used interstitial injection of colloidal solutions of radioactive gold into the prostate during open operation.

In the early 1960s iodine-125 radioisotope became available, sealed in minute biocompatible titanium cylinders that could be implanted with needles. Whitmore and colleagues[5] described his retropubic implantation methodology using iodine-125. This pivotal paper was met with a wave of enthusiasm and the technique became an attractive method for the treatment of localized prostate cancer. After open exploration and following a bilateral pelvic lymph node dissection iodine-125 seeds were implanted into the prostate freehand. The depth of needle insertion was facilitated by digital rectal guidance. The goal was to place the needles less than 1 cm apart.

This approach had several theoretical advantages over the commonly utilized external beam (cobalt) irradiation. Most importantly, due to a combination of low radiation, conformal seed placement and the inverse square law, brachytherapy resulted in a higher tumour dose of radiation and decreased injury to surrounding tissues (bladder, rectum). The entire treatment could be performed in one setting rather than using the multiple fractions required for an external beam approach, resulting in considerable time savings for both patients and personnel.

Table 11.1 History of prostate brachytherapy		
1909	Pasteau, DeGrais	Insertion of radium capsule into prostate urethra
1915	Barringer	Radium needle interstitial prostatic brachytherapy
1931	Forssell	Coined term 'brachytherapy'
1951	Flocks	Use of colloidal gold
1972	Whitmore	Iodine-125 prostate brachytherapy (open digitally guided)
1974	Pedersen	Percutaneous ultrasound-guided puncture
1981	Holm	Ultrasound guided iodine-125 prostate cancer brachytherapy
1983	Holm	Transperineal Iodine-125 prostate brachytherapy
1997	Ragde	7–8-year results for prostate brachytherapy
1998	Ragde	10-year results for prostate brachytherapy

Dr Whitmore's approach was widely adapted by numerous authorities and initial results were encouraging[6-13].

However, disadvantages to this approach became apparent and included the need for an open procedure, hospitalization and associated complications. Problems resulted from the relatively crude techniques used, accurate assessment of prostate volume, and most importantly, the difficulty of establishing uniform distribution of the seeds with crude manual palpation of the gland. This often resulted in considerable overdosing in some areas of the gland (hot spots) and underdosing of other areas (cold spots) (**11.1**). With longer follow-up[7,9-12] an unacceptable local failure rate soon lessened the enthusiasm for this method of treating prostate cancer. The fact that these later reports began to emerge when there was concomitant enthusiasm for external beam irradiation and radical prostatectomy[14-17] within time led to radical surgery becoming the treatment of choice.

Technical advances on a number of fronts gradually renewed interest in brachytherapy. Foremost is Dr Holm's publication of transperineal prostate implantation of iodine-125 seeds under transrectal insertion of ultrasound guided seeds[18-21].

Brachytherapy pre-planning using computed tomography (CT)-based dosimetry computers for more accurate dose determination and palladium-103 with a shorter half life than iodine-125 becoming commercially available, together with early promising outcome results from a few select centres, led to greater interest in brachytherapy[22-24].

With the advent of prostate-specific antigen (PSA) testing, it became apparent that external beam radiation was not as effective as earlier thought and surgery gradually became the treatment of choice.

This followed the use of PSA as a screening tool and gradually led to stage and grade migration towards a more favourable patient population.

In 1990, Holm et al.[21] reported on 32 patients who had been treated between 1982 and 1987. This cohort of men had aggressive disease compared with cohorts nowadays: 16 patients had poorly differentiated carcinoma and only 1 had well-differentiated malignancy. The results were not unexpected: 18 men died of metastatic disease. Interestingly, 12 patients showed no progression. Five patients had severe proctitis and six patients had chronic radiation cystitis. Five men required surgical diversion. Among 25 men undergoing post-radiation biopsy performed 12–48 months after the procedure, it was noted that although 80% of the patients who had a positive biopsy died of disease, only 47% who had negative biopsies succumbed. The significant failure rate coupled with the morbidity resulted in the discontinuation of this treatment approach by Dr Holm.

It is fortunate that before Holm's discontinuation of this technique, Haakon Ragde visited his facility and transferred the methodology to the USA with his own improvements. Dr Ragde has headed the brachytherapy programme at Northwest Hospital since the mid 1980s where over 4000 men have been treated to date.

BRACHYTHERAPY TECHNIQUES

The current methodology employed at Northwest Hospital will be described. It is important to note that all brachytherapy procedures are carried out by a team including a urologist, radiation oncologist, medical physicist, specially trained operating room nurses, as well as numerous support individuals. It is only through such a team approach that optimal patient care can be provided.

Although no randomized trials comparing alternative approaches have been completed, overall similar results between brachytherapy, radical prostatectomy and external beam radiation therapy have been realized. Brachytherapy affords the opportunity to deliver a high tumour dose with minimum radiation to surrounding tissue. Ultrasound guidance affords the opportunity to attain accurate seed distribution at the time of implantation (**11.2, 11.3** and **11.4**). Favourable morbidity has been realized and this approach is highly cost-effective because it is performed on an outpatient basis.

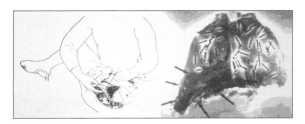

11.1 Digitally guided brachytherapy. Note in the autoradiograph performed on a radical prostatectomy specimen in a man who had previously undergone digitally guided seed implantation the cold spot (arrows) indicating uneven seed distribution.

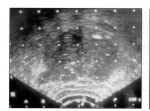 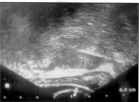

11.2 Ultrasound-guided prostate brachytherapy. Left, transverse; right, sagittal image. Note precise needle placement in the sagittal image affording excellent seed distribution.

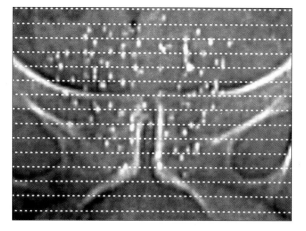

11.3 Post-brachytherapy implant pelvic radiograph. Note uniform seed distribution.

Modern diagnostic approaches and widespread early detection efforts have resulted in a greater proportion of men being diagnosed at a time when their cancer is amenable to this approach.

Modern permanent prostate brachytherapy is performed with iodine-125 or palladium-103 (**Table 11.2**). Iodine-125 has a half-life of 60 days, whereas palladium-103 has a half-life of 17 days, which results in more rapid energy delivery and potentially more tumour kill in higher-grade cancer with higher mitotic rates. Patient selection criteria are similar to those employed for other modalities including radical prostatectomy and external beam therapy. Basically these include patients who have stage T1–T2 disease and are judged on clinical evaluation to have localized disease. Ease of the minimally invasive surgical procedure has resulted in less restriction of eligible patients based on comorbid conditions. However, in our opinion, most men who have less than a 10-year survival probably do not warrant aggressive therapy, including brachytherapy.

One potential important selection criterion is so-called pubic arch interference. In those men who have an exceedingly large gland, the anterior and lateral portions of the prostate may be blocked by the pubic arch rendering accurate perineal insertion of needles difficult. Several technical tricks may be used to guide the needles around the bone. In large glands, neoadjuvant androgen suppression may reduce the gland and allow men who have very large prostates to be treated. Generally this is our major indication for hormonal therapy before planned implant.

Pubic arch interference may be identified during preplanning both by transrectal ultrasound and CT.

Another potential contraindication to brachytherapy is previous transurethral resection of prostate (TURP). If there is a substantial TURP defect it is unlikely that sufficient tissue remains to allow implantation. In men who have had TURP in the distant past the prostate will generally have reconfigured and adequate tissue is available to allow implantation. The TURP defect is evaluated during the pre-brachytherapy volume study.

Table 11.2 Isotopes commonly used for prostate brachytherapy			
Isotope	**Administration**	**Half-life (days)**	**Energy (MEV)**
Iodine-125	Permanent	60	0.027–0.032
Palladium-103	Permanent	17	0.02
Gold-98	Permanent	2.7	0.41
Iridium-192	Temporary	74	0.38

A current issue is whether brachytherapy should be performed in conjunction with external beam radiation therapy. We believe such combination therapy is indicated in high-risk patients – those who have either high-grade large volume lesions or elevated PSA levels. At Northwest Hospital, a neural network programme had been developed to help patient selection for mono and combination brachytherapy. The neural network is based on outcome results from 152 brachytherapy patients followed for 10 years with the combination therapy.

If external beam therapy is performed, 45 Gy in 25 fractions with a fourfield limited pelvic technique is used. Seed implantation follows within 2 weeks of completion of external beam radiation therapy. In combination with external beam radiation therapy, in men who have Gleason scores 6 or less, iodine-125 is used to 108 Gy matched peripheral dose (MPD) and in those who have higher grade carcinoma: palladium-103 is generally used taking the boost to 90 Gy.

In patients treated with brachytherapy alone, iodine-125 is used in patients who have Gleason scores of 6 or less and a maximum prostate dose of 144 Gy is the goal. For those who have higher grade malignancy palladium-103 is generally selected, and the MPD used is 115 Gy.

TREATMENT PLANNING

An initial volume study is carried out using a transrectal ultrasound with a 4.5 MHz transducer. The same 'stepping unit' that will be employed in the operating room is used. This device allows accurate and highly reproducible capture of transverse images of the prostate to be obtained at 5 mm intervals. The patient is placed in the exaggerated dorsal lithotomy position that will be used during the operation to provide reproducible images at the time of peripheral imaging seed implantation. The target volume consists of the prostate plus about 5 mm. These images are then entered into a dosimetry computer to obtain a three-dimensional prostate reconstruction. Computer-based calculations at various individual seed strengths are performed to provide the optimal radiation distribution throughout the target volume. The ideal implant model is then converted to an implant worksheet, which is used during the seed implantation procedure.

PATIENT PREPARATION

Patient preparation includes a careful history and physical examination, chest radiography and serum PSA determination. In those who have a PSA greater than 10 ng/ml, a radionuclide bone scan is performed. Routine preoperative laboratory determination is carried out. Patients are placed on a clear liquid diet 48 hours before the procedure and 'nil by mouth' after midnight. An enema is given the night before and 2 hours before the procedure. Broad-spectrum antimicrobial agents are administered at the time of implant and continued for 1 week.

OPERATIVE PROCEDURE

General or spinal anasthesia is administered and the procedure is carried out in the same exaggerated dorsal lithotomy position used for the pre-implant planning. The bladder is filled with 150 cc of water and the catheter is usually removed. The scrotum is secured to the abdominal wall with an adhesive drape. The ultrasound and stepping unit is then secured to the operating table. The stepping unit is used to move the transducer with transverse producing transverse images from the base to the apex. It is imperative that the ultrasound images generated are identical to those used in the volume study.

Before the procedure, 21 cm 18 gauge needles are preloaded with seeds and Vicryl spacers called for in the preplan. Alternatively, the Mick 200-TP applicator may be used. In this case, empty needles are inserted at the time of the procedure and following insertion of rows of needles the seeds are inserted with the applicator.

A perineal template is secured to the stepping device. This is the same template as used in the volume study and has coordinates set out with numbers and letters, for example, E3. The coordinates correspond to the point in the transverse plane, and the correct needle with the appropriate seeds is inserted in the prostate at this point. The position of the needle within the prostate is established by the ultrasound image that corresponds to the prostate tissue plane at this point. Template coordinates are reproduced on the ultrasound image to facilitate accurate needle placement.

Currently we begin the implantation with the most posterior row, which allows fixation of the prostate. Generally needles are placed 1 cm apart according to the pre-implant plan and inserted to the cephalad extent indicated. Establishment of the cephalad location is readily achieved by examining the ultrasound image and inserting the needle until the tip is identified with a bright echo. After the posterior rows have been inserted, we move to the most anterior row in stepwise fashion and complete each intervening row. After each row of needles has been inserted, the seeds are delivered by withdrawing the needle sheath leaving the obturator fixed in place (**11.4–11.9**). After insertion of all seeds repeat careful ultrasonography is carried out to confirm accurate and uniform seed implantation. Flouroscopy is then used to help identify apparent cold spots and extra seeds may be inserted if any appear. Although routine cystoscopy is not performed if the fluoroscopy identifies seeds in the bladder, these are removed.

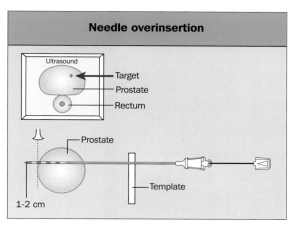

11.6 The needles are over inserted initially just beyond the prostate under ultrasound guidance.

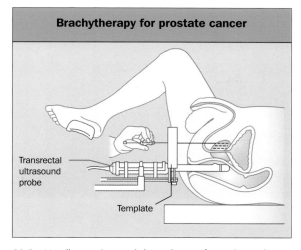

11.4 Needles are inserted through a perforated template under ultrasound control.

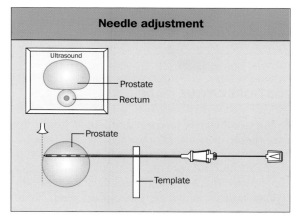

11.7 The needle is then adjusted under ultrasound control by slight withdrawal.

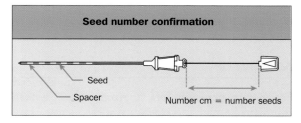

11.5 The distribution of seeds and spaces is tailored to the proportion of the prostate for each individual case. (Copyright 1998 with permission from Elsevier Science.)

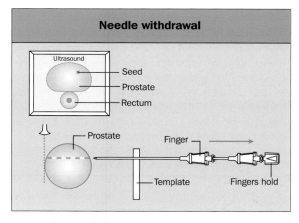

11.8 When seed placement is judged to be appropriate the needle is withdrawn.

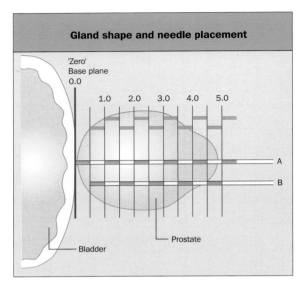

11.9 The shape of the prostate varies. This factor needs to be taken into account when planning seed implantation.

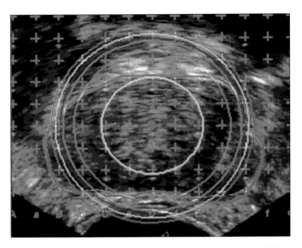

11.10 Computer-generated dosimetry depicting a model in which one seed is implanted. Note fall-off of radiation activity at points distant from the source.

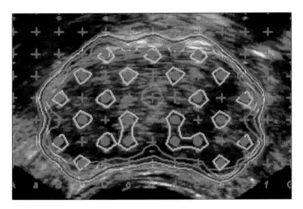

11.11 Post brachytherapy computer-generated dosimetry. Note uniform dosimetry throughout the gland with multiple seed placement.

POST-OPERATIVE CARE

A Foley catheter is inserted and left in until after anaesthesia wears off. The few men who have marked haematuria are discharged with the catheter in place. Virtually all patients are able to be discharged 2–3 hours following the procedure and rapidly resume normal activities. Discomfort tends to be minimal and is usually treated with non-steroidal anti-inflammatory agents; bladder analgesics are rarely prescribed. We routinely also use alpha-adrenergic blocking therapy to minimize bladder outlet obstruction in the first month postoperatively.

The rapid fall-off of radiation with distance from the prostate, low energy of the isotope and low total activity render severe radiation precautions un-necessary. We advise patients to avoid prolonged physical contact with pregnant women or young children for 2 months. Sexual activity may resume after 2 weeks using a condom the first few times to capture any seeds that may escape in the semen.

POST-IMPLANT INVESTIGATION

Computed tomography is performed on the day of the procedure or the next day. Images are obtained with 'bone technique' as well as soft tissue windows, the former to identify the seed accurately,

the latter to distinguish the prostate margins from surrounding tissue. The pre-operative ultrasound volume study and the CT scan images are used to obtain a post-implant dosimetry model (**11.10, 11.11**).

FOLLOW-UP

Patients are generally seen approximately 1 month following implantation and then subsequently every 3 months for the first year. After this, follow-up is bi-annual. At the time of follow-up, physical exam-ination including careful rectal examination and serum PSA are obtained. Routine ultrasound-guided prostate biopsies are obtained 18 months following the implantation.

RESULTS

Having learned the technique of brachytherapy from Holm and associates, Ragde initiated a programme at Northwest Hospital in Seattle. Reports of 7- and 8-year follow-up demonstrated PSA-based disease-free survival comparable to that for external beam radiation and radical prostatectomy studies with less morbidity[25]. Other investigators have reported similar intermediate follow-up[26–30] (**11.12**).

Recently, Ragde and associates reported on 152 consecutive patients followed for 10 years[31]. Between January 1987 and June of 1988 162 patients were treated with brachytherapy at Northwest Hospital in Seattle. For this study patients were excluded as a result of previous hormonal or radiation therapy: 152 men were available for the 10-year evaluation. Of these 98 patients (Group 1) were treated with brachytherapy alone to a target MPD dose of 160 Gy and 54 men (Group 2) received initial 45 Gy external beam radiation followed by 120 Gy MPD with iodine-125. This latter group primarily comprised patients who had higher Gleason scores or clinical stage, although no randomization or uniform selection of therapy was used. The clinical stage pre-operative serum PSA levels and Gleason scores are shown in **Tables 11.3–11.5**. Based on these parameters this series comprises a patient population not dissimilar from the majority of patients presenting today with clinically localized carcinoma of the prostate (**11.13**).

Recurrence was defined as those men that had a positive post-radiation biopsy, radiographic evidence of metastasis or both. Biochemical failure was defined as a PSA greater than 0.5 ng/ml. Biopsies were generally performed at 18 months following the implant. These were classified as negative, positive or indeterminate, the latter category comprising specimens revealing nests of radiation damaged tumour cells.

The median patient age was 70 years (range 53–92) and the medium follow-up was 119 months (range 3–134 months); 82% of men had palpable lesions. Mean pre-treatment PSA for Group 1 was 8.5 ng/ml and 15.6 ng/ml for Group 2. Five men were lost to follow-up. Therefore 147 were evaluated: 67 patients (46%) were alive with no evidence of

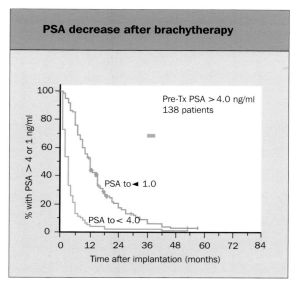

a

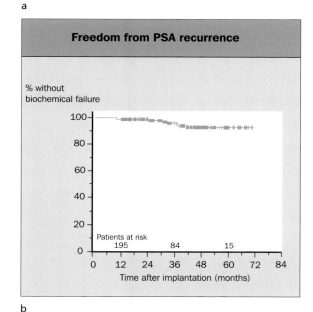

b

11.12 (**a**) PSA decrease after brachytherapy; (**b**) brachytherapy: freedom from PSA recurrence.

disease; 53 patients died during the 10-year period (65% overall survival). Of the 53 men who died, 50 did not have evidence of disease and only three men succumbed to prostate cancer. Therefore the disease-specific survival was 98%. **11.13** demonstrates the overall survival. The disease-specific survival is demonstrated in **11.14**. The observed

Table 11.3 Clinical stages at presentation according to UICC TNM classification (n = 151)

T classification	No. of patients in Group 1	No. of patients in Group 2	Total no. of patients
T1a	4	0	4 (2.6%)
T1b	10	2	12 (7.9%)
T1c	6	4	10 (6.6%)
T2a	56	20	76 (50.3%)
T2b	22	14	36 (23.8%)
T2c	0	10	10 (6.6%)
T3a	0	3	3 (2%)

The difference in clinical stage between Group 1 and Group 2 was significant (p = 0.001), using the Mann–Whitney test. (Data from Ragde et al.[31])

Table 11.4 Preoperative serum PSA levels determined in 147 patients, divided by group

PSA level (ng/ml)	No. of patients in Group 1	No. of patients in Group 2	Total no. of patients
PSA <4	46	10	56 (38.1%)
PSA 4–10	29	20	49 (33.3%)
PSA > 10	20	22	42 (28.6%)

Five patients (three in Group 1 and two in Group 2) had no preoperative PSA level. The difference in PSA levels between Group 1 and Group 2 was significant (p = 0.001) using the Mann–Whitney test. (Data from Ragde et al.[31])

Table 11.5 Preoperative tumour biopsy grade determined by Gleason grade in 150 patients divided by group

Gleason grade	No. of patients in Group 1	No. of patients in Group 2	Total no. of patients
≤ 4	44	2	46 (30.6%)
5–6	52	39	91 (60.7%)
≥7	0	13	13 (8.7%)

Two patients from Group 1 had no tumour grade assigned.
The difference in Gleason grade between Group 1 and Group 2 was significant (p = 0.001) using the Mann–Whitney test. (Data from Ragde et al.[31])

disease-free survival for group 1 was 60% and for group 2, 76%. Although it was observed that after implantation the PSA declined in all patients the rate of decline was slower than expected. A PSA level less than 1.0 ng/ml was reached within 24 months in 68% of successfully treated patients and continued a downward slope to PSA levels less than 0.05 ng/ml.

Post-radiation biopsies were obtained from 123

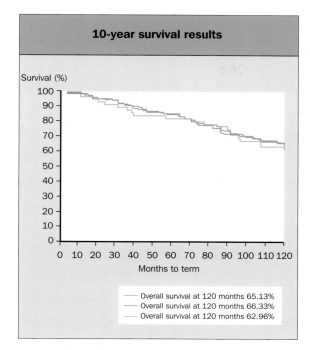

11.13 Observed 10-year overall survival by groups for the study population (n = 152). Group 1 was comprised of 98 patients treated with iodine-125 brachytherapy alone. Group 2 was comprised of 54 patients treated with a combination of 45-Gray external beam irradiation and iodine-125 brachytherapy.

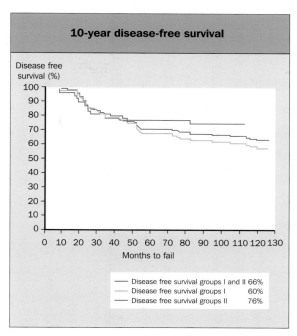

11.14 Observed 10-year disease-free survival by groups (PSA ≤ 0.5 ng/ml). The difference in outcome between Group 1 and Group 2 was not significant (p = 0.09). Positive bone scan, and/or positive biopsy, and/or PSA > 0.5 ng/ml signified treatment failure. Group 1 was comprised of 96 patients treated with iodine-125 brachytherapy alone. Group 2 was comprised of 51 patients who were treated with a combination of 45-Gray external beam irradiation and iodine-125 brachytherapy. Five patients – two in Group 1 and three in Group 2 – were lost to follow-up.

men: 85 were classified as negative, 23 demonstrated persistent cancer and 15 were considered to be indeterminate. On repeat biopsy of this later cohort, 11 reverted to negative and four to positive. Cytokeratin immunohistochemistry may be used to help in this differentiation[32].

Table **11.6** compares Ragde's brachytherapy series with those of contemporary external beam radiation therapy series[31]. As is readily apparent it appears that brachytherapy patients do better, although the limitations of comparative studies must be considered.

Table **11.7** demonstrates a comparative study between Ragde's 10-year brachytherapy follow-up and modern radical prostatectomy series[31]. This table demonstrates the substantially equivalent outcome between brachytherapy and radical prostatectomy.

Recently, Polascik and associates[33] reported on a subset analysis of the Johns Hopkins radical prostatectomy series in which patients were selected in an attempt at matching those reported by Ragde

et al.[31]. This study showed a more favourable biochemical disease-free survival rate for those men treated at Johns Hopkins with radical prostatectomy using in both series a nadir PSA of 0.2 ng/ml (**11.15**). Post hoc analysis in which patients are selected to match a published series is problematic. Although no statistically significant differences were noted in parameters such as serum PSA and Gleason score, it is noteworthy that the radical prostatectomy series involved a greater proportion of men who had a low PSA (< 10.0 ng/ml as shown in **Table 11.8**).

Obviously until prospective randomized trials contrasting these two treatment approaches are reported (an unlikely scenario at best) the methodology is limited to that employed by Polascik and associates. However, the reader is cautioned that selection bias may in part explain these differences. Moreover, the appropriate nadir PSA levels

153

Table 11.6 Disease-free survival for patients undergoing prostate brachytherapy with or without 45-Gray external beam irradiation compared with external beam irradiation alone for clinically localized prostate carcinoma with no evidence of disease at 5-year and 10-year follow-up

References and institutions	No. of cases	Definition of PSA failure or PSA cutoff (ng/ml)	NED (% at 5-year FU)	NED (% at 10-year FU)	Average FU	Treatment radiation	Notes/clinical stage
Hancock et al.[36] Stanford University	110	>4.0	NA	38 (at 12.4-year FU)	12.4 years	XRT XRT	T1–T4 Observed data, at 12.4-year FU
Hanks et al.[37] Fox Chase CC	502	>1.5	44	NA	50 months median FU	Conventional/ conformal	T1–T3 Projected, ↓ to 41% irradiation at 7-year FU
Kuban et al.[33] E. Virginia Medical School	652	<4.0	60	20	14–17 years	XRT XRT	T1–T4 Observed data, long-term FU
Rosenzweig et al.[38] Yale Univ. Medical School	285	>4.0	NA	33	NA	XRT	T1–T2 Projected data, ↓ to 22% in T3
Schellhammer et al.[39] E. Virginia Medical School	434	>4.0 >0.5	NA NA	21.7 13	10-year minimum FU	123 patients I-125/311 XRT	Stage A,B,C (i.e., T1–T4) Different results for PSA cutoffs
Stamey et al.[40] Stanford University	113	≥1.0	20 25.4	NA	6 years	XRT XRT	Stage A,B,C (Jewett staging) (i.e., T1–T4) Projected data, – to 25% in T1–T2

Table 11.6 (contd)

References and institutions	No. of cases	Definition of PSA failure or PSA cutoff (ng/ml)	NED (% at 5-year FU)	NED (% at 10-year FU)	Average FU	Treatment radiation	Notes/clinical stage
Zagars[41] M.D. Anderson CC	269	>1.0	64	NA	33 months	XRT	T1–T2 Projected (actuarial) data
Zietman et al.[42] Massachusetts General Hospital	85	>1.0	41	NA	>2 years	XRT Radical XRT	T1–T2 Projected data, ↓ to 15% in T3–T4
Ragde et al.[22] Northwest Hospital	126	>1.0	87	NA	69 months Median FU	Brachytherapy I–125 solely	T1–T2 Projected data at 7-years FU
Current study Group 1 alone	98	>0.5	71	60	10-years Median FU	Brachytherapy I–125 alone	T1–T2 Observed data, 10-years FU
Current study Groups 1 and 2	152	>0.5	74	66	10-years Median FU	Brachytherapy 125/XRT-45 Gy	T1–T3 Observed data, 10-year FU

PSA: Prostate specific antigen; NED: no evidence of disease; FU: follow-up; CC: cancer centre; NA: not available. I-125: iodine-125; Gy: gray; XRT: external beam irradiation.
Note the difference between projected and objected results, and the varying PSA end-points used. As observed in the current study, the actuarial results previously reported (PSA level ≤ 1.0 ng/ml) were more optimistic than the observed result.
(Data from Ragde et al.[31])

Table 11.7 Disease-free survival for patients undergoing brachytherapy with or without 45-Gray external beam irradiation compared with radical prostatectomy for clinically localized prostate carcinoma – no evidence of disease at 5-year and 10-year follow-up

References and institutions	Average age (years)	Peroperative PSA (ng/ml)	Average FU	No. of cases	Definition of PSA failure or PSA cutoff (ng/FU)	NED (% at 5-year FU)	NED (% at 10-year FU)	Notes/clinical stage
Catalona and Smith[43] Washington University	63.9±7	67% <10.0 33% ≥ 10.0	27 months	925	>0.6	78±	NA	T1–T2 Projected (actuarial) data
Ohori et al.[44] Baylor College	63 range 43–79	68% ≤ 10.0 32% > 10.0	36 months	500	>0.4	76 ±5	73 ±6	T1–T3 Projected (actuarial) data
Partin et al.[45] Johns Hopkins	59 ± 64	78% ≤ 10.0 22% > 10.0	4.1 years	955	>0.2	83	70	T1–T2 Actual (observed) data
Paulson[46] Duke University	65 Median age	NA	13.5 years	613	≥0.5	75	NA	Localized (i.e., T1–T2) Actual data
Trapasso et al.[47] UCLA	NA	Average 11.9 range 0.3–96.0	34 months Median FU	601	≥0.4	69 ±2	47 ±3	T1–T2 Projected (actuarial) data

Table 11.7 (contd)

References and institutions	Average age (years)	Peroperative PSA (ng/ml)	Average FU	No. of cases	Definition of PSA failure or PSA cutoff (ng/FU)	NED (% at 5-year FU)	NED (% at 10-year FU)	Notes/clinical stage
Zincke et al.[48] Mayo Clinic	65.3 ± 6.4	NA	5 year	3170	>0.4	77	54	T1–T2 Actual data, ↓ to 40% at 15-years FU
Current study Groups 1 and 2	70 Range 53–92	Average, 11.0 Range 0.4–138.0	10 years Median FU	152	>0.5	74	66	T1–T3 Observed data, 10 year FU
Current study Group 2 alone	70 Range 53–67	Average, 15.6 Range 0.4–138.0	10 years Median FU	54	>0.5	80	76	T1–T3 Observed data, 10 year FU

PSA: Prostate specific antigen; FU: follow-up; NED: no evidence of disease; UCLA: University of California-Los Angeles; NA: not available.
Group 1 was comprised of 98 patients treated with brachytherapy with iodine-125 alone.
Group 2 was comprised of 54 patients treated with a combination of iodine-125 brachytherapy and 45-Gray external beam irradiation.
(Data from Ragde et al.[31])

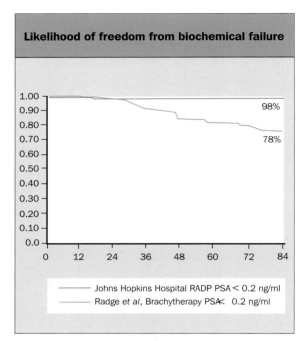

Likelihood of freedom from biochemical failure

98%

78%

— Johns Hopkins Hospital RADP PSA < 0.2 ng/ml
— Radge et al, Brachytherapy PSA< 0.2 ng/ml

11.15 Biochemical failure following brachytherapy versus radical prostatectomy. These data were generated using a case matching between men treated with brachytherapy at Northwest Hospital and radical prostatectomy at the Johns Hopkins Hospital. Although these data support the contention that radical prostatectomy may have a higher cure rate, methodological problems in the absence of a randomized trial preclude definitive statements. (Adapted from Polascik et al.[33] © 1998 with permission from Elsevier Science.)

Table 11.8 Radical prostatectomy versus brachytherapy

Variable	Brachytherapy %	No.	Radical prostatectomy %	No.	p
PSA (ng/ml)					
0–4	44.3	54	54.0	41	NS
4–10	34.4	42	32.9	25	NS
10–20	15.6	19	11.8	9	NS
>20	5.7	7	1.3	1	NS

(Data from Polascik et al.[33])

following brachytherapy or external beam radiation have not yet been determined. Although most experts agree that the lower the nadir and the longer it is held the better, whether 0.2 ng/ml is indeed the appropriate nadir following brachytherapy remains uncertain. Furthermore, the American Society of Therapeutic Radiologists and Oncologists has issued a consensus statement defining external beam radiatic failure as three consecutive PSA rises.

In conclusion, brachytherapy provides an effective method for treatment of men who have clinically localized prostatic carcinoma. Although the 10-year data from Northwest Hospital are encouraging, even longer follow-up is required before the ultimate outcome is known. At a 10-year follow-up the results appear to be similar to those generated by external beam radiation therapy or radical prostatectomy.

REFERENCES

1 Pasteau O, Degrais P. The radium treatment of cancer of the prostate. *Arch Roentgen Ray* 1914; **18**:396–410.
2 Barringer BS. Radium in the treatment of carcinoma of the bladder and prostate: review of one year's work. *J Am Med Assoc* 1917; **68**:1227–1230.
3 Forssell G. La lutte sociale contre le cancer. *J de Radiol et d'Electrol* 1931; **15**:621–634.
4 Flocks RH, Kerr HD, Elkins HB, Culp D. Treatment of carcinoma of the prostate by interstitial radiation with radioactive gold. *J Urol* 1952; **68**:510–522.
5 Whitmore WF Jr, Hilaris B, Grabstald H. Retropubic implantation of iodine-125 in the treatment of prostatic cancer. *J Urol* 1972; **108**:918–920.
6 DeLaney TF, Shipley WU, O'Leary MP, Biggs PJ, Prout GJ. Pre-operative irradiation, lymphadenectomy and 125 iodine implantation for patients with localized carcinoma of the prostate. *Int J Radiat Oncol Biol Phys* 1986; **12**(10):1779–1785.
7 Giles GM, Brady LW. [125]Iodine implantation after lymphadenectomy in early carcinoma of the prostate. *Int J Radiat Oncol Biol Phys* 1986; **12**:2117–2125.
8 Morton JD, Peschel RE. Iodine-125 implants versus external beam therapy for stages A2, B and C prostate cancer. *Int J Radiat Oncol Biol Phys* 1988; **14**:1153–1157.
9 Schellhammer PF, Whitmore RB, Kuban DA, Ladaga LA. Morbidity and mortality of local failure after definitive therapy for prostate cancer. *J Urol* 1989; **141**:567–571.
10 Kuban DA, El-Mahdi AM, Schellhammer PF. I-125 interstitial implantation for prostate cancer: What have we learned 10 years later? *Cancer* 1989;**63**:2415–2420.
11 Fuks Z, Leibel SA, Wallner KE, et al. The effect of local control on metastatic dissemination in carcinoma of the prostate: long-term results in patients treated with [125] implantation. *Int J Radiat Oncol Biol Phys* 1991; **21**:537–547.
12 Koprowski CD, BerKenstock KG, Borofski AM, et al. External beam irradiation versus 125 iodine implant in the definitive treatment of prostate carcinoma. *Int Radiat Oncol Biol Phys* 1991;**21**:955–960. Comment in *Int Radiat Oncol Biol Phy* 1992;**23**:254–255.

13 Critz FA, Tarlton RS, Holladay DA. Prostate-specific antigen-monitored combination radiotherapy for patients with prostate cancer, I-125 implant followed by external-beam radiation. *Cancer* 1995;**75**:2383–2391.

14 Walsh PC, Lepor H, Eggleston JC. Radical prostatectomy with preservation of sexual function: Anatomical and pathological considerations. *Prostate* 1983;**4**:473–485.

15 Walsh PC. Radical retropubic prostatectomy. In: Walsh PC, Gittes RF, Perimutter AD, *et al.*, eds. *Campbell's Textbook of Urology.* 5th edition. Philadelphia: WB Saunders; 1986; 2754–2775.

16 Walsh PC. Radical prostatectomy of sexual function, cancer control: The controversy. *Urol Clin North Am* 1987;**14**:663–673.

17 Walsh PC, Epstein JI, Lowe FC. Potency following radical prostatectomy with wide unilateral excision of the neurovascular bundle. *J Urol* 1987;**138**:823–827.

18 Holm HH, Gammelgaard J. Ultrasonically guided precise needle placement in the prostate and the seminal vesicles. *J Urol* 1981;**125**:385–387.

19 Holm HH, Juul N, Pederson JF, *et al.* Transperineal 125-iodine seed implantation in prostatic cancer guided by transrectal ultrasonography. *J Urol* 1983;**130**:283–286.

20 Iversen P, Bak M, Juul N, *et al.* Ultrasonically guided 125-I seed implantation with external radiation in management of localized prostatic carcinoma. *Urology* 1989;**34**:181–186.

21 Holm HH, Torp-Pedersen S, Myschetzky P. Transperineal seed implantation guided by biplanar transrectal ultrasound. *Urology* 1990;**36**:249–252.

22 Wallner K, Roy J, Zelefsky M, *et al.* Short-term freedom from disease progression after I-125 prostate implantation. *Int J Radiat Oncol Biol Phys* 1994;**30**:405–409.

23 Wallner K, Chie-Tsao ST, Roy J, *et al.* An improved method for computerized tomography-planned transperineal 125 iodine prostate implants. *J Urol* 1991;**146**:90–95.

24 Roy JN, Wallner KE, Harrington PJ, *et al.* A CT-based evaluation method for permanent implants: application to prostate. *Int Radiat Oncol Biop Phys* 1993;**26**:163–169.

25 Ragde H, Blasko JC, Grimm PD, *et al.* Brachytherapy for clinically localized prostate cancer: results at 7- and 8-year follow-up. *Semin Surg Oncol* 1997;**13**:438–443.

26 Stone NN, Forman JD, Sogani PC, *et al.* Transrectal ultrasonography and I-125 implantation in patients with prostate cancer. *J Urol* 1988;**139**:604A.

27 Stock RG, Stone NN, DeWyngaret JK. PSA findings and biopsy results following interactive ultrasound guided transperineal brachytherapy for early stage prostate cancer. Paris: Proceedings of the American Radium Society 78th Annual Meeting; 1995;58.

28 Grado GL, Larson TR. Fluoroscopic and ultrasound guided prostate implant: Technique and experience at Mayo Clinic Scottsdale. Scottsdale; American Brachytherapy Society 18th Annual Meeting: 1995.

29 Dattoli MJ, Wasserman SG, Hoval JM, *et al.* Conformal brachytherapy boost to external beam irradiation for localized high risk prostate cancer. *Int J Radiat Oncol Biol Phys* 1995; **32**:251.

30 Kaye KW, Olson DJ, Payne JT. Detailed preliminary analysis of 125 iodine implantation for localized prostate cancer using percutaneous approach. *J Urol* 1995;**153**:1020–1025.

31 Ragde H, Abdel-Aziz AE, Snow PB, *et al.* Ten-year disease free survival after transperineal sonography-guided iodine-125 brachytherapy with or without 45-Gray external beam irradiation in the treatment of patients with clinically localized, low to high Gleason grade prostate carcinoma. *Cancer* 1998;**83**(5):989–1001.

32 Brawer MK, Nagle RB, Pitts W, Freiha FS, Gamble SL. Keratin immunoreactivity as an aid to the diagnosis of persistent adenocarcinoma in irradiated human prostates. *Cancer* 1989; **63**(3):454–460.

33 Polascik TJ, Pound CR, DeWeese TL, Walsh PC. Comparison of radical prostatectomy and iodine 125 interstitial radiotherapy for the treatment of clinically localized prostate cancer: a 7-year biochemical (PSA) progression analysis. *Urology* 1998;**51**(6):884–889.

34 Hancock SL, Cox RS, Bagshaw MA. Prostate-specific antigen after radiotherapy for prostate cancer: a reevaluation of long-term biochemical control and the kinetics of recurrence in patients treated at Standford University. *J Urol* 1995;**154**:1412–1417.

35 Hanks GE, Lee WR, Schultheiss TE. Clinical and biochemical evidence of control of prostate cancer at 5 years after external beam radiation. *J Urol* 1995;**154**:456–459.

36 Kuban DA, El-Mahdi AM, Schellhammer PF. Prostate-specific antigen for pretreatment prediction and posttreatment evaluation of outcome after definitive irradiation for prostate cancer. *Int J Radiat Oncol Biol Phys* 1995;**32**:307–316.

37 Rosenzweig KE, Morgan WR, Lytton B, Peschel RE. Prostate-specific antigen following radiotherapy for local prostate cancer. *J Urol* 1995;**153**:1561–1564.

38 Schellhammer PF, El-Mahdi AM, Wright GL, Kolm P, Ragle R. Prostate-specific antigen to determine progression-free survival after radiation therapy for localized carcinoma of prostate. *Urology* 1993;**42**:13–20.

39 Stamey TA, Ferrari MK, Schmid HP. The value of serial prostate-specific antigen determinations 5 years after radiotherapy: steeply increasing values characterize 80% of patients. *J Urol* 1993;**150**:1856–1859.

40 Zagars GK. Prostate-specific antigen as an outcome variable for T1 and T2 prostate cancer treated by radiation therapy. *J Urol* 1994;**152**:1786–1791.

41 Zietman AL, Coen JJ, Shipley WU, Willett CG, Efird JT. Radical radiation therapy in the management of prostatic adenocarcinoma: the initial prostate-specific antigen value as a predictor of treatment outcome. *J Urol* 1994;**151**:640–645.

42 Ragde H, Blasko JC, Grimm PD, et al. Interstitial Iodine-125 radiation without adjuvant therapy in the

treatment of clinically localized prostate carcinoma. *Cancer* 1997;**80**:442–453.

43 Catalona WJ, Smith DS. 5-year tumor recurrence rates after anatomical radical retropubic prostatectomy for prostate cancer. *J Urol* 1994;**152**:1837–1842.

44 Ohori M, Goad JR, Wheeler TM, Eastham JA, Thompson TC, Scardino PT. Can radical prostatectomy alter the progression of poorly differentiated prostate cancer? *J Urol* 1994;**152**:1843–1849.

45 Partin AW, Pound CR, Clemens JQ, Epstein JI, Walsh PC. Serum PSA after anatomic radical prostatectomy. *Urol Clin North Am* 1993;**20**:713–725.

46 Paulson DF. Impact of radical prostatectomy in the management of clinically localized disease. *J Urol* 1994;**152**:1826–1830.

47 Trapasso JG, deKernion JB, Smith RB, Dorey F. The incidence and significance of detectable levels of serum prostate-specific antigen after radical prostatectomy. *J Urol* 1994;**152**:1821–1825.

48 Zincke H, Oesterling JE, Blute ML, Bergstralh EJ, Myers RP, Barrett DM. Long-term (15 years) results after radical prostatectomy for clinically localized (stage T2c or lower) prostate cancer. *J Urol* 1994;**152**:1850–1857.

Chapter 12

Treatment options for locally advanced disease

As previously emphasized, there has been a progressive downward migration in stage with which patients with prostate cancer present in many developed countries since the advent of prostate-specific antigen (PSA) testing, which is especially marked in the USA. Worldwide, however, not inconsiderable numbers of men continue to present with, or subsequently develop after treatment, locally advanced malignant prostatic cancer.

The term 'locally advanced prostate cancer' implies a tumour that is no longer gland-confined, but which has metastasized neither to local lymphatics nor to other more distant sites such as bone. It has to be conceded that the inaccuracy of local staging methods, other than pathology after surgery, can result in either overstaging or, more commonly, understaging of this $T_3N_0M_0$ (Stage C) disease. In general, patients with locally advanced prostate cancer have biopsies revealing either moderately well-differentiated, or poorly differentiated, adenocarcinoma, a considerably elevated PSA (>20 ng/ml), a transrectal ultrasound or magnetic resonance imaging suggesting extra-prostatic disease, together with negative pelvic computed tomography and radionuclide bone scans.

Unfortunately, as in so many areas in the treatment of prostate cancer, there have been few properly conducted, randomized, long-term trials to help us advise patients and their families with any certainty of their best therapeutic option in this situation. Indeed, it is in the management of locally advanced disease where medical opinions are often most sharply divergent. In such circumstances *all* treatment options should be carefully and clearly discussed with the patient. Not the least is the unwanted effects of therapy, such as the development of testosterone flare and length of time to recovery of sexual potency with current luteinizing hormone-releasing hormone (LHRH) analogues. It must also be remembered that many men with locally advanced

prostate cancer are elderly (some very elderly) and, as for gland-confined disease in those with a limited life expectancy, observation only by 'so-called' watchful waiting may be a legitimate option.

The currently available treatment options are discussed below.

SURGERY ALONE

Although the results of several series of surgical therapy by radical retropubic prostatectomy for $T_3N_0M_0$ cancers have revealed prolonged survivals[1,2], most patients with extracapsular prostatic cancer will eventually succumb to disseminated disease (unless, of course, they die of something else first). Because of this, the risks of morbidity or mortality following radical extirpative surgery are generally considered unjustified for these patients.

SURGERY AFTER HORMONAL DOWNSTAGING

In an attempt to improve cure rates in patients with $T_3N_0M_0$ prostate cancer, some urologists have employed a period of pre-operative androgen ablation therapy. This has usually taken the form of 3 months of an LHRH analogue, in combination with an antiandrogen such as Casodex™ (bicalutamide), prior to radical retropubic prostatectomy. Several phase 2 studies of this approach have been reported, usually compared against historical 'controls'[3,4]. The results suggested that 'hormonal downstaging' reduces the incidence of positive margins. Subsequent randomized studies[5,6] confirmed this finding, but failed to confirm any reduction in PSA progression, or to date, any improvement in overall survival.

EXTERNAL-BEAM RADIOTHERAPY ALONE

Although, theoretically, it might appear that patients

with locally advanced prostatic cancer without evidence of distant metastases might be ideal candidates for external-beam radiotherapy, in fact it is in these circumstances that the limitations of this modality of treatment are most apparent. Although reasonable survival data have been reported[7], there has been a worryingly high incidence of post-treatment prostatic biopsies showing viable adenocarcinoma cells[8]. Those patients whose biopsies do show residual cancer cells also appear to have a poorer prognosis than biopsy-negative individuals (due to the development of metastatic disease). Of more clinical importance, perhaps, is the failure of radiotherapy to reliably suppress PSA to within the normal range. A persistently elevated or rising PSA after radiotherapy worries both the patient and clinician alike, and usually suggests the need for further adjunctive therapy. The frequent failures of external-beam radiation as monotherapy in such circumstances have provided the impetus for using neoadjuvant endocrine therapy with radiotherapy.

EXTERNAL-BEAM RADIOTHERAPY PLUS HORMONAL THERAPY

The theory that lies behind the combination of hormonal ablation and external-beam radiation maintains that the pre-treatment reduction of tumour burden by endocrine ablation will increase the chances of 100% kill of cancer cells by irradiation. The prospect that the clones of hormonally insensitive cells that eventually result in hormonal relapse could be thus irradicated is certainly appealing. Certainly the significant reduction in prostatic tumour volume should permit the use of smaller boost fields and potentially reduce adverse radiotherapy effects.

Bolla *et al.*[9] evaluated the effectiveness of adjuvant hormonal therapy with goserelin 3.6 mg given at the outset of radiotherapy on local control, disease-free survival and overall survival. There were 415 patients who had locally advanced non-metastatic prostatic cancer and they were randomized to radiotherapy alone or radiotherapy plus LHRH analogue therapy every 4 weeks for 3 years. Overall survival was 79% for the goserelin adjuvant group compared with 62% for the radiation alone group (p=0.0001). Disease-free survival was also significantly increased for patients receiving adjuvant LHRH therapy with the proportion of disease-free patients at 5 years being 85% compared with 48% in the radiation alone group. The 5-year

control rate for the goserelin adjuvant group was 97% compared with 77% for the radiation alone patients.

The Radiation Therapy Oncology group (RTOG) 86–10 trial[10] investigated the use of maximum androgen blockade with the combination of goserelin 3.6 mg depot for 4 months and flutamide 250 mg three times daily in 226 patients who had large palpable T2c, T3 and T4 prostate tumours and unknown nodal status before and during radiotherapy. The outcome of this group was compared with that of 230 patients receiving radiation alone. After 4.5 years of follow-up there were clear benefits for the combined modality therapy. Progression-free survival at 5 years was reported to be 36% in the patients receiving neoadjuvant therapy, versus 15% for patients receiving radiation therapy alone. The difference was statistically significant (p<0.001). The cumulative incidence of local progression at 5 years was 46% in the neoadjuvant group compared with 71% in the radiation therapy group.

ANDROGEN DEPRIVATION THERAPY

Antiandrogen monotherapy alone as therapy for patients who have locally advanced non-metastatic prostate cancer is gaining in popularity. In an ongoing study 480 patients who had non-metastatic disease (M_0) and 805 who had metastatic disease (M_1) were randomized to either castration or bicalutamide 150 mg/day. The end-points are survival, time to progression, time to treatment failure and quality of life.

An analysis of the data was performed after a median follow up of 203 weeks. This analysis demonstrated that the effect of bicalutamide 150 mg may differ for patients who have M_0 disease compared with those who have M_1 disease. At this analysis there were no apparent differences between bicalutamide and castration for patients who had M_0 disease, but there was a small, but significant difference in favour of castration for men who had clear evidence of metastases (the difference in median time to death was 42 days). Consequently this group of patients was withdrawn from the bicalutamide arm of the studies and offered standard treatment for advanced prostate cancer[11]. Subsequent and final analyses have confirmed that there is no significant difference between bicalutamide and castration for patients who have M_0 disease (**12.1**), with the added benefit of preservation of sexual interest (**12.2**) and

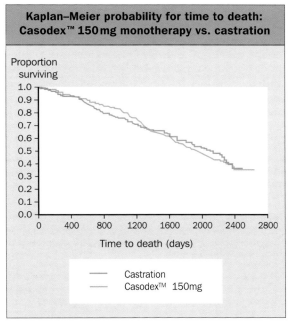

Kaplan–Meier probability for time to death: Casodex™ 150 mg monotherapy vs. castration

12.1 Casodex™ 150 mg is equivalent to castration therapy in men with locally advanced disease. (Reproduced from Iversen *et al.*[13])

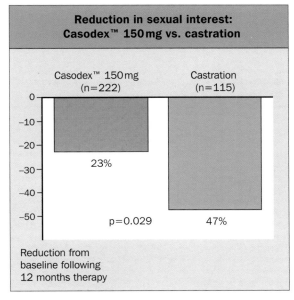

Reduction in sexual interest: Casodex™ 150 mg vs. castration

12.2 Casodex™ causes less loss of sexual interest than castration. (Reproduced from Iversen P. Quality of life issues relating to endocrine treatment options. *Eur Urol* 1999;**36(Suppl 2)**;20–26.)

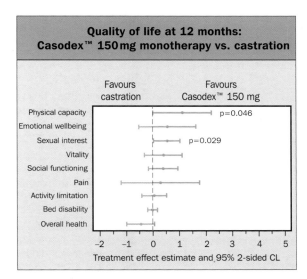

Quality of life at 12 months: Casodex™ 150 mg monotherapy vs. castration

12.3 Most quality of life indices favour Casodex™ over castration. (Reproduced from Iversen *et al.*[13])

physical capacity (**12.3**) in bicalutamide-treated patients[12,13]. Gynaecomastia is common in men treated with antiandrogen monotherapy due to the aromatization of testosterone to oestrogens. However, not all patients find this troublesome.

INTERMITTENT ANDROGEN SUPPRESSION THERAPY FOR LOCALLY ADVANCED PROSTATE CANCER

The ablation of testicular function for the palliative treatment of locally advanced prostate cancer was first attempted in the 1930s with orchidectomy[14]. This proved much less effective than surgical orchidectomy, which was introduced nearly a decade later by Huggins and Hodges[15]. No other treatment exists that equals or surpasses androgen ablation in checking the growth of prostate cancer and reducing its volume in 60–80% of patients. However, for reasons that remain uncertain, the cell-death process induced by androgen ablation fails to eliminate the entire malignant-cell population. Another limitation of conventional androgen ablation is that it may conceivably increase the rate of progression of prostate cancer to an androgen-independent state[16]. In contrast, theoretically progression may be delayed by intermittent androgen suppression, a form of ablative therapy delivered in pulses[17]. For this reason, intermittent androgen suppression therapy is now being evaluated by Bruchovsky and others.

Three Essential Mechanisms of Regulation

Intermittent androgen suppression may work because essential mechanisms that determine the size of the prostate can be activated to check malignant growth[18]. As discussed in Chapter 4, normal control over cell divisions is established by three levels of androgen-mediated regulation: positive effects on initiation of DNA synthesis and cell proliferation, negative or inhibitory effects which limit the number of cells in the prostate, and apoptosis, an androgen-repressed process of programmed cell death which actively eliminates cells from the prostate when androgens are withdrawn.

Androgen Dependence and Independence

Androgen dependence is the clinical manifestation of apoptosis after androgen withdrawal in both normal and malignant tissues. In fact, in the early stages of prostate cancer, only the negative type of regulation is missing[19]. Since the other two mechanisms are still functional, androgen ablation has the double effect of triggering apoptosis and inhibiting DNA synthesis and cell proliferation. Even in malignancy, the ability to undergo apoptosis is acquired as a feature of differentiation under the influence of androgens; thus in the absence of androgens, it is impossible for dividing cells to differentiate and become pre-apoptotic again[17,19]. This may explain why recurrent tumour growth is characterized by androgen independence.

In attempting to avert or delay progression to the androgen-independent state, it has been hypothesized that if malignant cells which survive androgen withdrawal are forced into a normal pathway of differentiation by androgen replacement, then apoptotic potential might be restored – hence setting the stage for a further response to therapeutic androgen withdrawal (**12.4**). Another postulate results from studies that have shown follicle-stimulating hormone (FSH) promotes growth in androgen-independent, metastatic prostate cancer cell lines, PC3[20]. These results have raised the possibility that FSH and its receptor may regulate growth in androgen-refractory prostate cancer.

Experimental Observations

The androgen-dependent Shionogi carcinoma tumour model responds to androgen ablation in a manner strongly reminiscent of prostate cancer. When the parent tumour is transplanted into a male mouse, it grows with a short doubling time, regresses almost completely after castration, and recurs in an androgen-independent state[17]. Intermittent exposure of the parent Shionogi carcinoma to androgens has been carried out experimentally by transplanting the tumour into a succession of male mice, each of which was castrated when the estimated tumour weight was approximately 3 g. After the tumour regressed to 30% of the original weight, it was transplanted into the next non-castrated male. This cycle of transplantation and castration-induced apoptosis was successfully repeated four times before growth

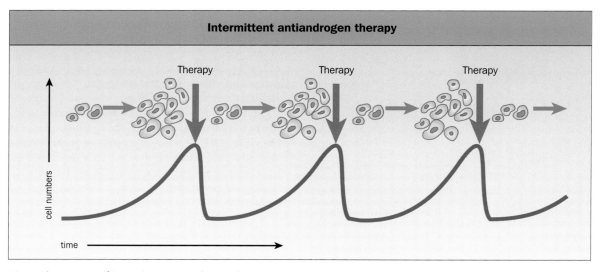

12.4 The concept of intermittent antiandrogen therapy.

became androgen-independent during the fifth cycle[17]. The mean time to androgen independence of 147 days compared to 51 days after one-time castration was in keeping with a retarding effect of cyclical therapy on tumour progression.

Intermittent Androgen Suppression in Clinical Practice

With the advent of antiandrogens (such as bicalutamide and flutamide) and of LHRH agonists (including leuprolide acetate and goserelin acetate), new methods of androgen suppression which mimic the effects of orchidectomy by lowering the intranuclear concentration of dihydrotestosterone by 80% or more have become available. Emphasis has been placed on the combined use of such agents with antiandrogens[21,22] to, among other reasons, reduce the incidence of flare and the 'acute on chronic' phenomenon observed with traditional LHRH analogues; however, little attention has yet been given to their reversibility of action, the significance of which is potentially far-reaching. The possibility of a full recovery from therapy makes it possible to alternate a patient between periods of treatment and no-treatment. When the patient is off-treatment, the function of the testes and the concentration of serum testosterone slowly return to normal, usually over a period of 8–14 weeks. In response to this incremental androgenic stimulus, atrophic cells may be recruited into a normal pathway of differentiation where the risk of progression is small. With the associated movement through the division cycle, the cells become pre-apoptotic again, making it possible to repeat androgen deprivation therapy (**12.4**).

When to Interrupt Therapy?

A decrease of serum PSA to a stable nadir in a normal range, or a decreasing level, is an important aspect of the response to therapy[23,24]. If the serum PSA remains above 4 ng/ml between 24–32 weeks of treatment, it has been found that the median survival time is only 18 months[24]. On the other hand, if the serum PSA is below 4 ng/ml between 24–32 weeks of therapy, the median survival time is much greater at 40 months[25]. Only those patients whose serum PSA has reached a stable or decreasing value in a normal range at 24 and 32 weeks should be considered eligible for studies of intermittent androgen suppression with interruption of the therapy at around 36 weeks.

When to Resume Therapy?

In patients with advanced prostate cancer, the serum PSA at the time of diagnosis may range in value from the upper limit of the normal range to a level of several thousand ng/ml. In those patients with a pre-treatment serum PSA below 20 ng/ml, the second cycle of treatment may be started when the serum PSA increases to the pre-treatment level again. If the serum PSA at presentation is greater than 20 ng/ml, the second cycle of therapy is started when the serum PSA increases to approximately 20 ng/ml. Following these guidelines, up to 5 cycles of therapy have been administered before there has been evidence of developing androgen-independence[26].

Applications of Intermittent Androgen Suppression

In theory, intermittent androgen suppression should be suitable for the long-term management of not only locally advanced prostate cancer, but also incompletely excised or locally recurrent prostate malignancy. Quality of life for the patient may potentially be improved with reduced toxicity from medication, recovery of sexual function and normal sense of well-being as well as a decreased incidence of osteoporosis. The new gonadotropin-releasing hormone (GnRH) antagonists may have a role in this context.

Whether intermittent androgen suppression and its effects on tumour progression alter survival in a beneficial or adverse way is unknown; however, both time to progression and survival in a small number of patients with metastatic prostate cancer so far are similar to the expected results with continuous androgen ablation[25]. More information will become available from randomized trials of intermittent androgen suppression which are currently in progress.

MANAGEMENT OF COMPLICATIONS FROM LOCALLY ADVANCED DISEASE

Patients with locally advanced prostate cancer are prone to either present with, or subsequently develop, local complications that severely affect the quality of life. The most common of these are bladder outflow obstruction with eventual acute or chronic urinary retention. Haematuria from tumour infiltration of the prostatic urethra or bladder base may also be troublesome. Although transurethral resection (TURP) of the obstructing and/or bleeding tissue is usually feasible, caution should be exercised in these circumstances because there is a higher incidence of urinary incontinence after TURP for malignant as opposed to benign prostatic obstruction. This phenomenon is conventionally ascribed to infiltration of the distal urinary sphincter by malignant tissue, but, in fact, may be the result of technical difficulties caused by the loss of anatomical landmarks.

An alternative approach to the management of urinary retention due to prostate cancer is to employ androgen ablation therapy (usually with an LHRH analogue, or GnRH antagonist, or bilateral orchidectomy) during an extended period of catheterization. At the initiation of therapy, the patient must be monitored carefully for complaints of pain since this indicates the onset of spinal cord compression from a flare reaction. On removal of the catheter after three months has elapsed, the majority of patients are able to void, although many probably remain obstructed[27]. A recent study randomized patients presenting with malignant prostatic obstruction to either TURP or hormonal therapy and catheterization, and found similar outcomes in both groups, but a lower incidence of incontinence in the conservatively managed cohort[28].

Many patients, however, are understandably reluctant to endure a three-month period of catheterization while the reduction of prostate volume is taking place. In such circumstances, the placement of a temporary intraurethral stent – such as a Porges 'Urospiral'™ (**12.5**, see also **12.6**) – to permit restoration of normal voiding over this time can be considered. However, problems with stent migration, urethral discomfort and lower urinary tract infection occur not uncommonly, and careful follow-up is mandatory.

Management of Malignant Obstruction of the Ureters due to Prostate Cancer

Locally advanced prostate cancer may also produce either unilateral or bilateral ureteric obstruction (**12.7**). This may be due either to direct malignant infiltration of the ureters at the bladder base, or to compression by enlarged lymph nodes within the pelvis.

The former scenario may make management by retrograde insertion of double-pigtail ureteric stents (**12.8**) technically impossible, because of difficulties visualizing the ureteric orifices when infiltrated by

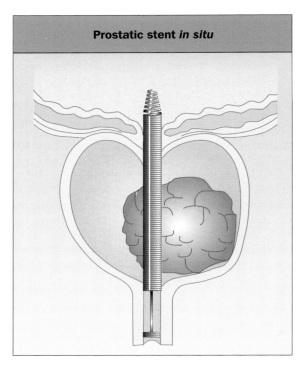

Prostatic stent *in situ*

12.5 Porges Urospiral™ *in situ* relieving obstruction due to locally advanced prostatic tumour.

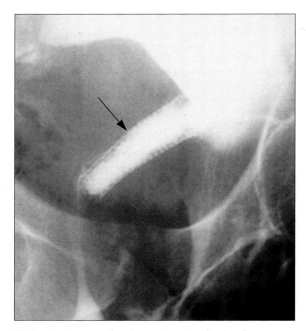

12.6 A cystogram showing a patient with a locally extensive prostate cancer voiding through a Urolume™ intraprostatic stent (arrowed).

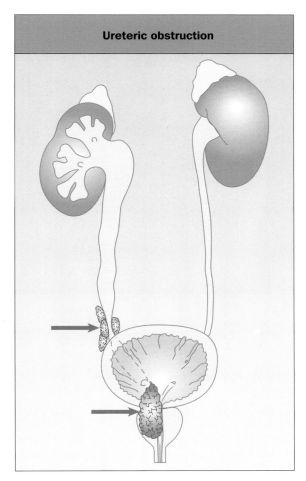

Ureteric obstruction

12.7 Ureteric obstruction in prostate cancer may occur at the level of the vesico–ureteric junction or at the pelvic brim due to lymph-node enlargement (arrowed).

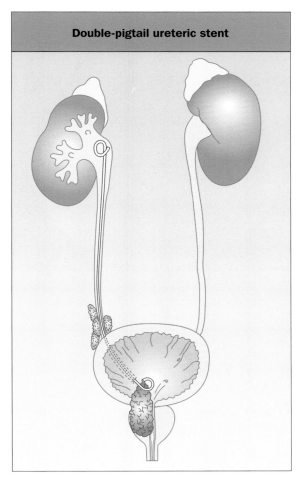

Double-pigtail ureteric stent

12.8 A double-pigtail ureteric stent may be inserted retrogradely.

malignant tissue. A way around this problem is to enlist the help of the radiologists in antegrade stent insertion (**12.9**); often a guide wire can be negotiated through the obstruction under radiographic control. Another option is to place a percutaneous nephrostomy or bilateral nephrostomies, to preserve renal function, while a response to either hormonal manipulation and/or external-beam radiotherapy is awaited (**12.10**). Those elderly patients, however, who develop malignant bilateral ureteric obstruction after, or in spite of, hormonal manipulation, are sometimes best managed palliatively without percutaneous nephrostomies, since the quality of the short period of life prolongation achievable by these means is usually poor. Informed discussion

with the patient and his family in these situations is paramount.

Other Problems Associated with Locally Advanced Prostatic Malignancy

In certain circumstances a bulky, locally advanced prostatic cancer may impinge posteriorly on the rectum (**12.11**). This development may result in the patient complaining of tenesmus and a sensation of incomplete rectal emptying. As the tumour continues to advance, severe constipation may develop, with eventual large-bowel obstruction. If all conservative measures fail, it is occasionally necessary to create a defunctioning colostomy to relieve symptoms in these unfortunate individuals.

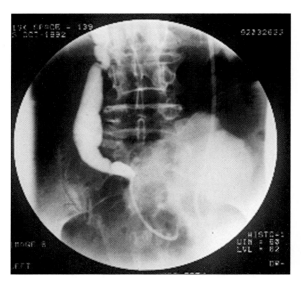

12.9 Antegrade passage of a guide wire to allow placement of a double-pigtail stent. (Courtesy of Dr David Rickards.)

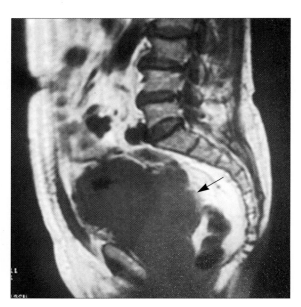

12.11 An MRI scan showing a locally extensive prostate cancer (arrowed) compressing the rectum posteriorly.

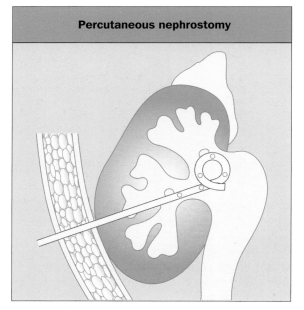

Percutaneous nephrostomy

12.10 Percutaneous nephrostomy to relieve ureteric obstruction.

CONCLUSIONS

Locally advanced prostate cancer often produces debilitating local symptoms that can markedly diminish the individual's quality of life. Correct management for the patient depends upon a combination of staging that is as accurate as possible, and an informed discussion with the individual and his family about the safety and efficacy of available treatment options. Until the results of randomized studies comparing various treatment options are available, the choice of therapy will continue to depend greatly on the personal experience of the urologist handling the case and the individual preferences of the patient and his close family.

REFERENCES

1 Catalona WJ, Bigg SW. Nerve-sparing radical prostatectomy: Evaluation of results after 250 patients. *J Urol* 1990;**143**:538–544.

2 deKernion JB, Neuwirth H, Stein A, *et al.* Prognosis of patients with stage D1 prostate carcinoma following radical prostatectomy with and without early endocrine therapy. *J Urol* 1990;**144**:700–703.

3 Flamm J, Fisher M, Holil W, *et al.* Complete androgen

deprivation prior to radical prostatectomy in patients with stage T3 cancer of the prostate. *Eur Urol* 1991;**19**:192–195.

4 Labrie F, Dupont A, Gomez JL, *et al*. Beneficial effect of combination therapy administered prior to radical prostatectomy. *J Urol* 1993;**149**(**Abstract**):348A.

5 Witjes WPJ, Schulman CC, DeBruyne FMJ, *et al*. Results of a European randomised study comparing radical prostatectomy and radical prostatectomy plus neoadjuvant hormonal combination therapy in stage $T_{2-3}N_0M_0$ prostate carcinoma. *Mol Urol* 1998;**2**:181–185.

6 Soloway MS, Shatiri R, Wajsman Z, *et al* Randomized prospective study comparing radical prostatectomy alone versus radical prostatectomy preceded by androgen blockade in clinical stage B2 (T2bNxM0) prostate cancer. *J Urol* 1995;**154**:424–428.

7 Bagshaw MA. Radiation therapy for cancer of the prostate. In: Skinner DG, Lieskovsky G (eds.) *Diagnosis and Treatment of Genito-urinary Cancer*. Philadelphia: W B Saunders, 1988; 425–445.

8 Freiha FS, Bagshaw MA. Carcinoma of the prostate: results of post-irradiation biopsy. *Prostate* 1984;**5**:19–23.

9 Bolla M, Gonzalez D, Warde P, *et al*. Improved survival in patients with locally advanced prostate cancer treated with radiotherapy and goserelin. *N Engl J Med* 1997;**337**:295–300.

10 Pilepich MV, Krall JM, Al-Sarraff M, *et al*. Androgen deprivation with radiation therapy compared with radiation therapy alone for locally advanced prostate carcinoma: a randomised trial of the Radiation Therapy Oncology Group. *Urology* 1995;**45**:616–623.

11 Tyrrell CJ, Kaisary AV, Iversen P, *et al*. A randomised comparison of Casodex (bicalutamide) 150 mg monotherapy versus castration in the treatment of metastatic and locally advanced prostate cancer. *Eur Urol* 1998;**33**:447–456.

12 Iversen P, Tyrrell CJ, Kaisary AV, *et al*. Casodex (bicalutamide) 150 mg monotherapy compared with castration in patients with previously untreated non-metastatic prostate cancer: results from two multicentre randomised trials at a median follow up of 4 years. *Urology* 1998;**51**:389–396.

13 Iversen P, Tyrrell CJ, Kasiary AV, *et al*. Bicalutamide (Casodex) 150 mg monotherapy compared with castration in patients with non-metastatic locally advanced prostate cancer: 6.3 years follow up. *J Urol* 2000 (in press).

14 Sharifi R, Kiefer J. History of endocrine manipulation in the treatment of carcinoma of the prostate – who was first? *J Endocrinol Invest* 1987;**10**(**Suppl 2**):91.

15 Huggins C, Hodges CV. Studies of prostatic cancer: I Effect of castration, oestrogen and androgen injections on serum phosphates in metastatic carcinoma of the prostate. *Canc Res* 1941;**1**:293–297.

16 Bruchovsky N, Lesser B, Van Doorn E, *et al*. Hormonal effects on cell proliferation in rat prostate. *Vitamin Horm* 1975;**33**:61–102.

17 Akakura K, Bruchovsky N, Goldenberg SL, *et al*. Effects of intermittent androgen suppression on androgen-dependent tumours: apoptosis and serum prostate-specific antigen. *Cancer* 1993;**71**:2782–2790.

18 Bruchovsky N. Androgens and antiandrogens. In: Holland JF, Frei III E, Bast RC, *et al*. (eds.) *Cancer Medicine*. Philadelphia: Lea & Febiger, 1993;884–896.

19 Bruchovsky N, Brown EM, Coppin CM, *et al*. The endocrinology and treatment of prostate tumour progression. In: Coffey DS, Bruchovsky N, Gardner WA Jr, *et al*. (eds.) *Current concepts and approaches to the study of prostate cancer. Progress in clinical and biological research*. New York: Alan R. Liss Inc., 1987;348–387.

20 Ben-Josef E, Yang SY, Ji TH, *et al*. Hormone refractory prostate cancer cells express functional follicle-stimulating hormone receptor (FSHR). *J Urol* 1999;**161**:970–976.

21 Crawford ED, Eisenberger MA, McLeod DG, *et al*. A controlled trial of leuprolide with and without flutamide in prostatic cancer. *N Engl J Med* 1989;**321**:419–424.

22 Denis L, Murphy GP. Overview of phase III trials on combined androgen treatment in patients with metastatic prostate cancer. *Cancer* 1993;**72**(**Suppl**):3888–3895.

23 Miller JI, Ahmann FR, Drach GW, *et al*. The clinical usefulness of serum prostate-specific antigen after hormonal therapy of metastatic prostate cancer. *J Urol* 1992;**147**:956–961.

24 Bruchovsky N, Goldenburg SL, Akakura K, *et al*. Luteinizing hormone-releasing hormone agonists in prostate cancer: Elimination of flare reaction by pretreatment with cyproterone acetate and low-dose diethylstilboestrol. *Cancer* 1993;**72**:1685–1691.

25 Goldenberg SL, Bruchovsky N, Gleave ME, *et al*. Intermittent androgen suppression in the treatment of prostate cancer. *J Urol* 1994;**151**:240A.

26 Goldenberg SL, Bruchovsky N, Gleave ME, *et al*. Intermittent androgen suppression in the treatment of prostate cancer: a preliminary report. *Urology* 1995;**45**(5):839–845.

27 Hampson SJ, Davies JH, Charig CR, *et al*. LHRH analogues as primary treatment for urinary retention in patients with prostatic carcinoma. *Br J Urol* 1993;**71**:583–586.

28 Thomas DJ, Babaji VJ, Coptcoat MJ, *et al*. Acute urinary retention secondary to carcinoma of the prostate. Is initial channel TURP beneficial? *Proc Roy Soc Med* 1992;**85**:318–319.

Chapter 13

Management of metastatic disease

Unfortunately, despite the trend to earlier diagnosis already referred to, many patients with prostate cancer still present with either bony and/or soft tissue metastases. Others develop disseminated disease in spite of the best curative endeavours employed at a stage when the disease was still localized.

The mainstay of therapy for metastatic prostate cancer generally involves androgen deprivation, to which an initially favourable response will be seen in more than 80–90% of patients. Almost inevitably, however, disease progression ('hormone escape') occurs eventually, due to the clonal selection of hormone-independent cancer cells. In this respect, there is some evidence that, at least a proportion of patients, the addition of an antiandrogen at an early stage to achieve so-called maximal androgen blockade (MAB) may delay clinical disease progression and also prolong overall survival. When progression does eventually occur, and this is now usually heralded by a rise in serum prostate-specific antigen (PSA) values, there is an understandable desire to implement effective second-line therapy. Unhappily, such manoeuvres do not always meet with success, although a number of new approaches are currently under evaluation and seem promising. Contrary to popular belief, metastatic prostate cancer is often a lethal condition – 70% or so of patients dying *from*, rather than *with*, the disease, usually within 5 years of diagnosis.

METHODS OF ANDROGEN DEPRIVATION

Bilateral Orchidectomy

The most cost-effective way of inducing permanent androgen deprivation is to undertake either bilateral orchidectomy or bilateral subcapsular orchidectomy (**13.1**). The procedure can be accomplished easily as a day case under a light general or regional anaesthetic, or even under local anaesthesia. The morbidity is low, and there are no concerns about either

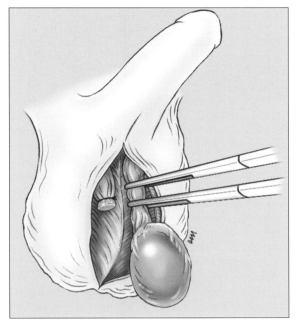

13.1 Bilateral orchidectomy is accomplished through a midline scrotal incision.

tumour flare or subsequent patient compliance. However, many patients find the concept of surgical castration worrisome, and when offered the choice of either this or a luteinizing hormone-releasing hormone (LHRH) analogue, or gonadotropin-releasing hormone (GnRH) antagonist, the majority (78% in one study) will now elect for the medical rather than surgical option[1]. The main side-effects of bilateral orchidectomy are minor local complications, such as haematoma formation and wound infection, as well as loss of libido and erectile impotence, and hot flushes. The psychological and cosmetic stigmata of castration can probably be reduced by performing the subcapsular excision of only the functional part of the organs, leaving a nubbin of residual testicular tissue on each side. A clinical response, usually manifested by a relief of bone pain, and rapid decline in serum PSA values, is seen in more than 75% of patients treated by this means. The procedure is, of course, irreversible.

Administration of LHRH Analogues

Soon after the decapeptide structure of LHRH was elucidated, work began to develop LHRH analogues. These were synthesized by substitution or modification of one or more of the ten constituent amino acids. The result has been to produce super-active agonists which possess a prolonged duration of action. The administration of these agents causes an initial stimulation of luteinizing hormone (LH) and follicle-stimulating hormone (FSH) production with a resultant rise in serum testosterone to 140–170% of basal levels. Within 21 days, however, LHRH analogues cause an inhibition of LH and FSH release, and a subsequent suppression of testosterone secretion similar to that seen after surgical castration (**13.2**). Chronic administration of LHRH analogues makes the pituitary resistant to further stimulation by endogenous LHRH, and the production of testicular androgens is therefore prevented. However, adrenal secretion of the 5% or so of residual androgens is regulated by adrenocorticotropic hormone (ACTH), and is therefore unaffected by the administration of LHRH analogues.

The most commonly used LHRH analogues are goserelin acetate (**13.3**), buserelin and leuprolide acetate. Goserelin acetate 3.6 mg and leuprolide acetate 3.75 mg are available as monthly copolymer and depot suspension formulations respectively. Goserelin is administered by subcutaneous injection, usually into the abdominal wall through a wide bore needle (**13.4**), leuprolide is given intramuscularly through a conventional needle. A new long-acting 10.8 mg depot formulation of goserelin has now been developed and is effective when administered on a three-monthly basis[2,3].

Discomfort at the injection site can be minimized by the prior administration of local anaesthetic. The principal side-effect is the potential 'tumour flare' that can accompany the initial rise in plasma testosterone. This may manifest itself as an increase in either bone pain or obstructive voiding symptoms; occasionally, catastrophic spinal-cord compression, due presumably to transient androgen stimulation of tumour cells, may develop. Because of this, it is advisable that LHRH analogues be administered

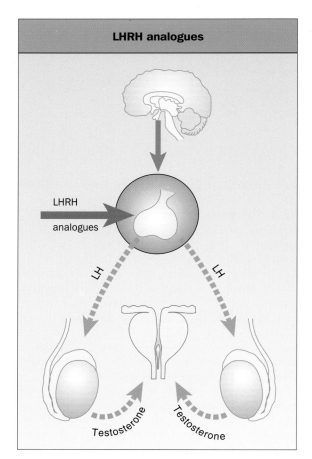

LHRH analogues

13.2   Mechanism of action of LHRH analogues.

Structure of naturally-occurring LHRH and goserelin

Glp-His-Trp-Ser-Tyr-Gly-Leu-Arg-Pro-Gly-NH$_2$

LHRH

Glp-His-Trp-Ser-Tyr-D-Ser(Bu)-Leu-Arg-Pro-Azgly-NH$_2$

goserelin

13.3   Structure of goserelin and LHRH.

concomitantly with an antiandrogen for the first 4 weeks of therapy to prevent this potentially devastating adverse effect. Other side-effects of LHRH analogues are those generally of androgen deprivation, namely, loss of libido, erectile impotence,

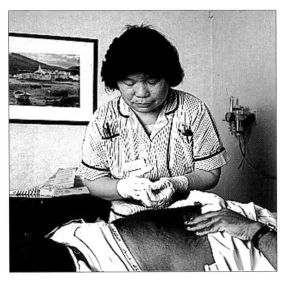

13.4 Depot preparations of LHRH analogues (such as goserelin acetate) are injected into the subcutaneous tissues of the abdomen; leuprolide acetate depot suspension is given intramuscularly.

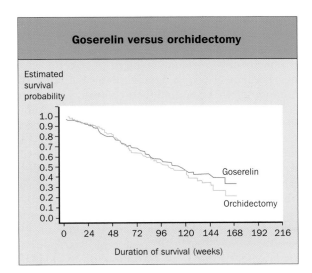

Goserelin versus orchidectomy

Estimated survival probability

Goserelin

Orchidectomy

Duration of survival (weeks)

13.5 Overall survival as a result of treatment with goserelin versus orchidectomy.

reduction of body hair, similar to that seen after surgical castration, as well as hot flushes.

Several large studies have demonstrated the equivalence of leuprolide, goserelin and orchidectomy in terms of both time to progression and overall survival[4–6] (**13.5**).

Monotherapy with LHRH Analogues versus Maximal Androgen Blockade (MAB)

Although numerous studies have confirmed that an initial response may be obtained in 70–80% of patients with metastatic prostate cancer, this remission following alteration of the hormonal milieu is unfortunately not usually maintained in the longer term. The average time to subsequent tumour progression is less than 18 months, with a mean overall survival time of around 18–28 months. Huggins and Scott[7] were the first to recognize the ephemeral nature of the response to testicular androgen ablation, and, as early as 1945, attempted to treat relapsing patients surgically by bilateral adrenalectomy. Unfortunately, adrenal replacement therapy was less than adequate in these early days and no patient survived longer than 4 months. Nonetheless, with their classic studies, these Nobel-prize winning researchers not only laid the framework for most future clinical studies of prostatic cancer, but also first raised the important question of the role of adrenal androgens in sustaining tumour growth once testicular androgens have been withdrawn.

While most urologists have been content to manage their patients with advanced prostatic cancer by testicular androgen ablation (using either bilateral orchidectomy or depot preparations of LHRH analogues such as leuprolide or goserelin acetate), for more than a decade Labrie and co-workers have been urging the therapeutic addition of an antiandrogen to suppress a postulated stimulatory effect by residual androgens of adrenal origin. This manoeuvre, they have argued, enhances initial response rates, delays the development of subsequent androgen independence, and improves both time to progression and overall survival. However, this approach of 'total androgen blockade' has important implications in terms of additional drug toxicity and in adding considerably to the health economic burden of the disease. Therefore, the evidence for and against this contention – both in the laboratory and more importantly from clinical trials – needs to be carefully weighed before clinicians in general are encouraged to adopt this approach.

Evidence from Animal Models for a Contribution by Adrenal Androgens

The mechanisms by which prostatic cancer cells develop the ability to grow despite androgen depletion are still incompletely understood, but may involve a series of events including mutations of androgen receptors, the over-expression of onco-genes (which encode various mitogenic growth factors), and the deletion of tumour-suppressor genes. Critical from the viewpoint of the efficacy, or otherwise, of total androgen blockade are the androgen requirements of the developing tumour.

In the Shionogi mammary-tumour cell line, which is very sensitive to dihydrotestosterone (DHT), Labrie and Veilleux[8] have, by plating single cells, identified clones of cells that are extremely sensitive to the growth stimulating effects of low concentrations of androgens. Stimulation of cell division of different clones of Shionogi cells by DHT were seen *in vitro* at very low concentrations, ranging from 10^{-8} to 10^{-11} molar. The same group of workers have also demonstrated stimulatory effects of adrenal androgen precursors on ventral prostate weight, as well as androgen-dependent gene expression in the castrated rat model. Importantly, these effects were observed at plasma concentrations of dehydroepiandrosterone (DHEA) and androstenedione comparable to those found in the sera of adult castrated men[9].

By contrast, other workers using alternative androgen-sensitive cell lines have not been able to identify clones exhibiting sensitivity to such low levels of androgens or androgen precursors. They have also argued that the development of androgen insensitivity *in vitro* and *in vivo* is more likely to be the result of the natural selection of cell lines which can flourish independently of any need for androgen stimulation. In such circumstances, more complete suppression of androgen levels by total androgen blockade might be anticipated to be of little or no beneficial use.

Ellis and Issacs[10] performed a series of experiments and compared the effects of partial versus complete androgen ablation in the treatment of rats with the Dunning 3327H (well-differentiated) and 3327R (poorly differentiated) tumour. Using control groups, tumour-bearing rats were treated with either orchidectomy alone or with orchidectomy and cyproterone acetate, a progestational antiandrogen. There was no significant difference in either tumour growth or overall survival between the two groups, but cyproterone is not the most effective antiandrogen.

CLINICAL STUDIES OF MAXIMAL ANDROGEN BLOCKADE

For a number of reasons, prostatic cancer is an inherently difficult tumour to study. As previously discussed, histological foci of prostate cancer have been demonstrated to be present in up to 30% of men over the age of 50, yet clinical cancer only develops in 7–9% of individuals; unequal inclusion of cases of low-volume, well-differentiated carcinomas in single-arm studies or in trials of competing therapies may therefore lead to misleading information concerning their efficacy. The doubling time of prostate cancer is often slow (6 months to 4 years, or even longer) compared with other tumours, which means a long observation period is necessary before the results of clinical studies can be correctly evaluated. Finally, the behaviour of individual prostatic tumours – even when extensive metastases are present – is rather unpredictable; some respond for prolonged periods to androgen withdrawal while others progress relentlessly in spite of all therapy. Large numbers of patients of similar disease status must therefore enter each arm of any study, as unequal stratification of patients will certainly result in significant bias. Many of the reports relating to efficacy of total androgen withdrawal can be criticized for the inadequate numbers of patients studied, the unequal stratification of comparison groups and, especially, the lack of maturity of data in terms of period of patient observation at the time of reporting. Another may be that testosterone is not the only hormone involved. A role for FSH has been described and may cause a rethink of humoral mechanisms and their control.

The main protagonists of total androgen blockade have been Labrie and co-workers from Quebec, Canada, who have produced a series of publications on the subject[11-13]. Unfortunately, much of their data were based on phase II observational studies which have employed rather weak criteria by which objective response to therapy is defined. Protocols have not always been strictly followed; for example, in one prospective multicentre study of 94 patients with histologically proven prostatic adeno-carcinoma[14] treated by castration or by LHRH agonist plus an antiandrogen, the castration arm was discontinued when 4 of 7 patients entering this arm of the study died after 11, 16, 17 and 29 months respectively. The remaining group of 87 patients who received combined treatment were reported to have an initial response of 100% and a probability of a continuing positive response at 2 years of 81%. Of the 8 (11.9%) patients in this arm who relapsed, only 1 perished from prostate cancer and 3 from other causes. These results compare extremely favourably with standard therapy in which only testicular androgens are ablated – where progression may be anticipated in roughly one third of patients within one year – and were initially greeted with considerable scepticism by the urological community. However, further impetus towards a more rigorous evaluation of the clinical effect of maximal androgen blockade came from the demonstration that as much as 10–15% of intraprostatic DHT remains after medical or surgical castration[15]. Moreover, Harper *et al.* confirmed that, in fact, adrenal androgens may be responsible for as much as 15–20% of total intraprostatic DHT[16].

In response to the claims of Labrie and co-workers, a prospective, randomized placebo-controlled trial was established with the assistance of the National Cancer Institute (NCI) in 1984 in the USA. The protocol was simple in its design, comparing leuprolide 1 mg subcutaneously per day with placebo, against leuprolide 1 mg subcutaneously per day plus flutamide 250 mg tds in patients with metastatic cancer of the prostate confirmed on radioisotope bone scan. Crossover from placebo to flutamide was allowed at the first signs of tumour progression. Six hundred and three patients from 93 contributing institutions were recruited within 18 months[17] and results stratified according to the severity of the disease and patient performance status at the time of presentation. Overall median, progression-free survival favoured the group receiving flutamide (16.5 months versus 13.9 months), as did overall survival (35.6 months for the flutamide arm versus 28.3 months for the placebo arm) (**13.6**).

In the subset analysis, patients with good performance status and minimal disease on bone scan (defined as absence of disease in ribs, long bones, skull, or soft tissues other than lymph nodes), who were treated with total androgen blockade at diagnosis (41 patients in each arm), experienced a longer time to objective progression (48 months for the flutamide arm, 19 months for the placebo arm) and prolonged overall survival (median 61 months versus 42 months) (**13.7**). The majority of patients fell into the category of good performance status, but with severe disease (241 patients in each arm). In this group, median time to progression was prolonged by 3 months through the addition of flutamide (16 months versus 13 months) and overall survival was enhanced by 6 months in the combination therapy group. Diarrhoea was the main side-

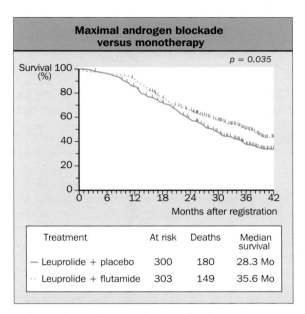

13.6   Kaplan–Meier survival curves of patients with metastatic prostate cancer treated with leuprolide alone versus leuprolide + flutamide 250 mg tds (i.e. maximal androgen blockade)[17].

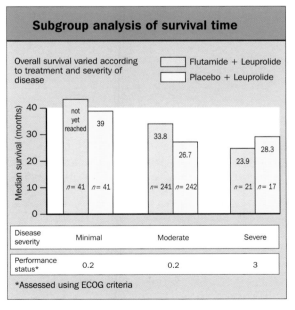

13.7   Differences in survival in patients with metastatic prostate cancer treated with LHRH analogue alone versus maximum androgen blockade[17].

effect reported, more frequently by the flutamide group (13.6% of subjects)[18,19].

Not all studies of various alternative regimes of maximal androgen blockade compared with monotherapy have confirmed such unequivocal advantage. Denis[20], however, has reported an update of European Organization for Research and Treatment of Cancer (EORTC) data showing improved cancer-specific survival in an EORTC study comparing goserelin acetate implants (Zoladex™) plus flutamide against orchidectomy, amounting to some 7 months' advantage for the combination therapy (13.8). Keuppens et al.[21] had previously reported a benefit in the flutamide group in delaying the time to first progression (p = 0.004) but, at that stage, survival advantage had not been seen, perhaps because of the lack of maturity of the study.

In a Canadian study in which a different non-steroidal antiandrogen, nilutamide (Anandron™), was compared with an identical placebo plus bilateral orchidectomy[22], it was found that although there was a delay in progression, no clear demonstration of improved survival was apparent. A similar double-blind placebo-controlled study involving 457 patients with metastatic disease has been reported by Janknegt[23]. Statistically significant differences were found in favour of orchidectomy plus nilutamide in complete or partial response (p < 0.001),

and in cancer-related survival (p = 0.046), compared with patients treated by orchidectomy alone.

By contrast, several other studies have failed to demonstrate any definite benefit of maximal androgen blockade over monotherapy with either LHRH analogues or orchidectomy. A large prospective, randomized trial comparing goserelin acetate (3.6 mg sc/month) and flutamide to orchidectomy alone did not confirm any significant difference in subjective response rate, time to disease progression or overall survival in 571 evaluable subjects after a mean follow-up of two years[24]. Another study combining the EORTC data mentioned above[21] with a similar Danish study allowing an evaluation of altogether 591 patients treated by either goserelin acetate plus flutamide or orchidectomy also failed to demonstrate any significant difference in overall survival, although time to progression and the specific death rate from prostate cancer were delayed by the introduction of combination therapy[25].

In an attempt to resolve the controversy surrounding the efficacy of maximum androgen blockade a number of meta-analyses have been performed. The most statistically powerful of these is that of the Prostate Cancer Trialists Collaborative Group (PCTCG), which examined 22 published and unpublished randomized trials and over 3200 clinical events[26]. Smaller meta-analyses using only published data have been performed by Caubet et al. and Klotz et al. in which 13 and 20 clinical trials were examined, respectively[27,28]. The main points to note are that all analyses identified that for non-steroidal anti-androgens, when used in combination, the hazard ratios (relative risks) were in favour of maximum androgen blockade compared with castration alone. The estimated risk of death over a given period of time was between 6 and 22% lower with maximum androgen blockade compared with castration alone. The PCTCG analysis showed a trend, although not statistically significant, in favour of all anti-androgens compared with castration alone. In addition, the recently published South West Oncology Group (SWOG) study identified a 9% non-significant benefit for the estimated risk of death in favour of maximum androgen blockade compared with orchidectomy[29].

Since the advent of serum PSA determination in patients with prostate cancer, a powerful additional tool has been acquired by which the efficacy of various treatment options can be compared. To date, only a few studies have reported the

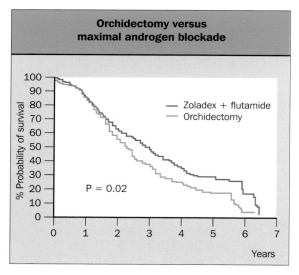

Orchidectomy versus maximal androgen blockade

— Zoladex + flutamide
— Orchidectomy

P = 0.02

% Probability of survival

Years

13.8 Duration of survival following either orchidectomy or maximal androgen blockade[20]. The patients treated with MAB fared best.

comparative extent of PSA decline with maximal androgen blockade compared with that seen with orchidectomy or LHRH analogues. However, Smith and colleagues[30] reported that 98% of 411 prospectively treated patients with metastatic prostate cancer had a decrease in PSA levels with a median reduction of 97.7% 3 months after randomization to leuprolide plus nilutamide or leuprolide plus placebo. A greater proportion (76%) of those on maximal androgen blockade had normalization of their PSA value within three months than those treated with leuprolide alone (52%). The difference was statistically significant (p < 0.0001).

One possible explanation for the delay in tumour progression and survival advantage seen in at least some reports of maximal androgen blockade is that LHRH analogues, when employed without a concomitant antiandrogen, produce a transient surge of luteinizing hormone (LH) release and a consequent rise in testosterone levels. This may result in a 'tumour flare'[31], which usually manifests itself as acute exacerbation of bone pain, though occasionally devastating spinal cord compression may occur. This may be prevented by commencing with LHRH analogues and antiandrogens simultaneously. However, such a tumour flare does not occur when the method of ablation of testicular androgens is bilateral orchidectomy. As mentioned above, the addition of an antiandrogen to bilateral orchidectomy also seems to improve results in some studies[22,23].

OTHER METHODS OF ACHIEVING MAXIMAL ANDROGEN BLOCKADE

Although the majority of data reviewed above suggest that the combination of either leuprolide or goserelin acetate (or alternatively bilateral orchidectomy) with either flutamide or nilutamide, and more recently the once/day antiandrogen Casodex™, may provide some additional benefit to monotherapy (which ablates only testicular androgens) in at least a subgroup of patients, there are several other pharmacological agents available that seem potentially capable of achieving similar effects, although data on these are less complete. Several alternative therapeutic options are discussed below.

Diethylstilboestrol (DES), which has the advantage of being very cheap, has unfortunate and well-documented cardiovascular toxicity at either 5 mg/day or 3 mg/day dosage. At 1 mg/day, however, this does not appear to be too great a problem,

although at this dosage serum testosterone levels are not reliably suppressed into the castrate range[32]. However, the EORTC Protocol 30805, in which patients were randomized to either 1 mg DES/day or bilateral orchidectomy +/– cyproterone acetate, showed no differences in either survival or cardiovascular thromboembolic events[33]. These data suggest that randomized studies of an antiandrogen plus low-dose DES versus the more expensive option of an LHRH analogue plus an antiandrogen may be worthwhile, although the side-effects of DES induced gynaecomastia are still liable to be troublesome, even at 1 mg/day (**13.9**). Gynaecomastia may be prevented by single-dose radiotherapy to the pectoral area. The most intriguing property of DES is that, discounting the cardiotoxicity, it remains probably the most effective agent for prostate cancer. It is also a very potent inhibitor of FSH synthesis which, in turn, results in sustained FSH suppression[34]. Interestingly, the GnRH antagonist abarelix also causes an immediate suppression of FSH, in contrast to LHRH agonists (**13.10**). The addition of one

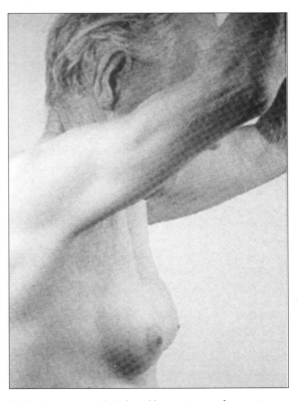

13.9 Gynaecomastia induced by treatment of prostate cancer with diethylstilboestrol.

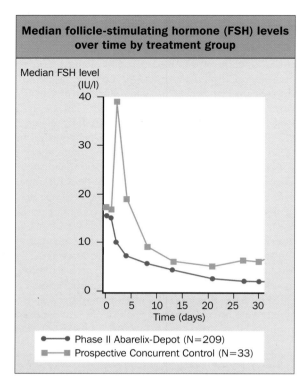

Median follicle-stimulating hormone (FSH) levels over time by treatment group

Median FSH level (IU/l)

Time (days)

● Phase II Abarelix-Depot (N=209)
■ Prospective Concurrent Control (N=33)

13.10 Median follicle-stimulating hormone (FSH) levels over time by treatment group. (Adapted with permission from Garnick MB, Campion M, the Abarelix Depot Study Group. Abarelix depot, a GnRH antagonist V. LHRH superagonists in prostate cancer: differential effects on follicle-stimulating hormone. *Mol Urol* 2000:**4**;275.)

aspirin/day to reduce cardiovascular side effects has been advocated, but there are currently no data to confirm the safety and efficacy of such a manoeuvre.

Cyproterone acetate and *megestrol acetate* are steroidal antiandrogens (**13.11**), both of which have marked progestational activity which inhibits LH release from the pituitary and produces castrate levels of testosterone; they also compete with testosterone and DHT for androgen receptor sites. However, if used as monotherapy, there tends to be a gradual increase in testosterone values with chronic usage (as a result of escape of pituitary inhibition), and they are probably not as effective as DES or orchidectomy. In one three-arm study of cyproterone acetate versus goserelin acetate versus a combination of the two, cyproterone was found to be inferior to goserelin. Combination therapy with this antiandrogen was found to offer no benefit over monotherapy with the LHRH analogue[35]. Side-effects of

cyproterone include an increased risk of thrombosis with cardiovascular consequences as well as an increased tendency towards diabetes. Disturbances of liver function have been reported, including four recent cases of hepatocellular carcinoma among long-term cyproterone users[36,37].

Flutamide, a non-steroidal antiandrogen (**13.12**), has been used by some clinicians as monotherapy for metastatic prostate cancer. However, it has not yet been approved by any regulatory authority for this indication, and most experts have contended that flutamide should usually be used only in conjunction with medical or surgical castration. Calculations based on known affinities of DHT and flutamide for the androgen receptor suggest that when flutamide is used as monotherapy, it leaves at least 40% of androgen receptor sites available for binding by DHT; when combined with castration, however, only 5% of DHT is available to the androgen receptor. Unlike most other agents that are active against prostate cancer, flutamide when used alone does not appear always, or even usually, to affect libido and potency adversely. Diarrhoea, however, is not uncommon, and gynaecomastia and breast tenderness also occur, presumably because of an increased aromatization of testosterone to oestradiol. These latter effects are not seen when flutamide is combined with an LHRH analogue. In a recent study, Boccon-Gibot[38] compared flutamide 250 mg administered 3 times/day to bilateral orchidectomy in 104 patients with newly diagnosed metastatic prostate cancer. In those patients whose PSA was less than 120 ng/ml at inclusion the two arms produced similar responses, not only in terms of PSA suppression, but also for progression-free survival.

Nilutamide (Anandron™) is a non-steroidal, pure antiandrogen which is similar in structure to flutamide. In contrast to cyproterone acetate, it is devoid of progestational and antigonadotrophic properties. It competes with testosterone and DHT at the androgen receptor, not only at the level of the prostate, but also at the hypothalamo–pituitary complex (where androgens exert their negative feedback effect); as a result, LH secretion is enhanced and, in the presence of intact testes, testosterone biosynthesis is increased. However, because of the presence of the antiandrogen, the effects of the rising testosterone at the receptor level are blunted. Its main value seems to be in combination with an LHRH analogue, as has already been discussed[22,23]. Side-effects of nilutamide include gastrointestinal

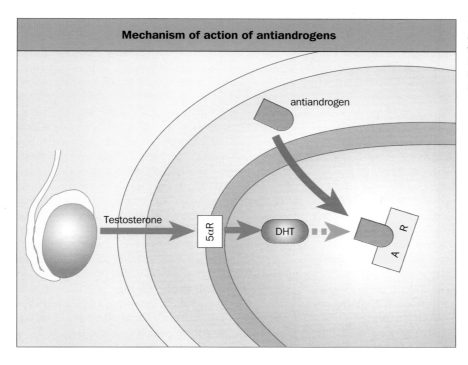

Mechanism of action of antiandrogens

13.11 Mechanism of action of antiandrogens which interfere with DHT interaction with androgen receptors. 5αR, 5 alpha-reductase.

symptoms, anaemia, disturbances of light/dark adaptation and alcohol intolerance.

Casodex™ (bicalutamide) is a non-steroidal anti-androgen that binds to the androgen receptor on the rat prostate with about 2% of the affinity of DHT, but roughly four times the affinity of hydroxy-flutamide (**13.13**). Unlike flutamide, Casodex™ does not cause a marked elevation in serum LH and testosterone in rats or dogs, and has a much longer half-life[39]. A steady state is reached after about a month of therapy. Phase II clinical trials confirmed the efficacy of Casodex™ when used as mono-therapy in patients with metastatic prostate cancer,

Chemical structure of flutamide and its metabolite

Flutamide

Hydroxyflutamide

13.12 Structure of flutamide and its major metabolite.

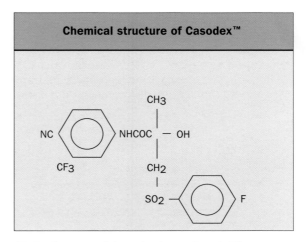

Chemical structure of Casodex™

13.13 Structure of the antiandrogen Casodex™ (bicalutamide).

as judged by both acid phosphatase and PSA level decline. The most frequent side-effects were breast tenderness, gynaecomastia and hot flushes, but the incidence of hot flushes was lower in those receiving Casodex™ monotherapy (9%) than those treated by orchidectomy (41%) or combination with LHRH analogue (49%). In man, in contrast to the pre-clinical studies in other animals, Casodex™, like flutamide, appears to elevate serum testosterone levels somewhat, due to central antagonism of testosterone receptors in the hypothalamo–pituitary complex – there is a consequent increase of LH secretion[40]. However, Casodex™'s long half-life of about one week enables maintenance of high serum concentrations and allows once daily dosing; moreover, serum testosterone concentrations in patients treated with Casodex™ rarely exceed the normal range that the drug must antagonize.

Phase III studies of Casodex™ at both 50 mg and 150 mg per day dosages have been undertaken in North America and Europe[41]. Casodex™ 50 mg monotherapy dose revealed somewhat inferior efficacy results in comparison with castration (**13.14**). Large Phase III randomized trials comparing Casodex™ 150 mg monotherapy with either the LHRH analogue, Zoladex™, or orchidectomy are in progress in patients with non-metastatic disease.

In the context of combination therapy, a multicentre, randomized, double-blind study of Casodex™ 50 mg + LHRH analogue and flutamide 750 mg + LHRH analogue has recently been completed in North America. A total of 813 patients were recruited for a minimum follow-up of 6 months. Casodex™–LHRH analogue therapy was associated with a significant improvement in time to treatment failure than the flutamide–LHRH analogue combination (p = 0.005) (**13.15**). In all, 88 patients withdrew from treatment because of an adverse event: 32 from the Casodex™–LHRH analogue arm and 56 in the flutamide–LHRH analogue arm. Diarrhoea was more frequently reported in patients treated with flutamide–LHRH analogue than Casodex™–LHRH analogue (24% vs 10%, p<0.001) and was the most frequent adverse event leading to withdrawal (25 for flutamide–LHRH analogue and 2 for Casodex™–LHRH analogue. Abnormal liver-enzyme test results were reported in both groups (25 for Casodex™–LHRH analogue, 41 for flutamide–LHRH analogue) and the number of patients who had study therapy withdrawn was similar in both treatment groups (6 for Casodex™–LHRH analogue and 8 for flutamide–LHRH analogue)[42]. Assessment of quality of life questionnaires did not reveal any significant difference between the two treatment groups, but patients in both arms experienced a reduction in pain, improved physical capacity, better emotional well-being and more vitality.

Aminoglutethimide blocks the conversion of cholesterol into pregnenolone, thus inhibiting the production not only of testicular and adrenal androgens, but also of aldosterone, cortisol and

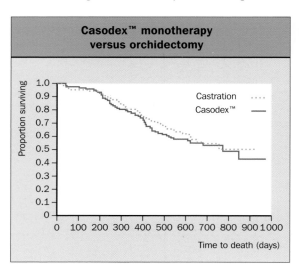

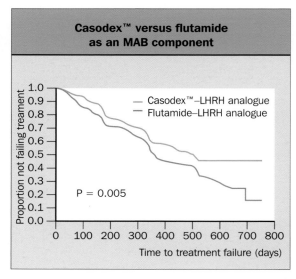

13.14 Phase III studies of Casodex™ 50 mg versus orchidectomy.

13.15 Kaplan–Meier probability of treatment failure in two alternative forms of maximal androgen blockade (MAB)[38].

oestrogens; it also inhibits peripheral aromatase activity. This blocking effect is accomplished by binding to the cytochrome P450 moiety of enzyme complexes. Replacement glucocorticoids must therefore be given with aminoglutethimide to avoid cortisol insufficiency, and to prevent the reflex rise of ACTH which would otherwise act to overcome the effects of chemical blockade. There are no current data available on the use of aminoglutethimide as first-line therapy in metastatic prostate cancer, either used singly or in combination with an LHRH analogue. What data there are have mainly been accrued from patients with relapsed prostate cancer after primary treatment with ablation of testicular androgens. After the initial studies of Robinson *et al.* in 1974[43], a few other reports, mainly with subjective response rates, followed. At most, one third of patients obtained some benefit for only limited periods of time from medical adrenalectomy by aminoglutethimide–cortisol combination therapy. Side-effects were troublesome and included lethargy, rash and drowsiness in a substantial number of patients. Two Australian studies reported around 20% subjective response rates in patients with prostate cancer in relapse, in 126 and 34 patients respectively, for reasonably prolonged periods[44,45]; however, the exact role of the additional cortisone

supplements in achieving these results is unknown, since it has been shown that corticosteroids alone can produce some improvement in patients with advanced prostate cancer[46].

Ketoconazole, a synthetic imidazole dioxalane, is active against a number of fungi by virtue of its inhibitory effect on cytochrome P450. At higher doses than are necessary for fungicidal action, the same effect inhibits the C17-20 lyase biosynthesis in the adrenals, thereby reducing the production of adrenal androgens. In general, plasma glucocorticoids and mineralocorticoids are not affected, although there have been reports of adrenal insufficiency in debilitated patients treated with this medication. In patients with relapsed prostatic cancer treated with ketoconazole, around 50% subjective improve-ment but little objective improvement has been reported[47]. Side-effects at this high dosage, however, are common with this drug, particularly gastrointestinal toxicity, and, more rarely but alarmingly, severe hepatotoxicity; for this reason it is now rarely used.

Finasteride is a 4-aza steroid competitor of 5 alpha-reductase – the enzyme that converts testosterone to DHT within the prostate (**13.16**). Several studies have confirmed that finasteride reduces serum DHT by 75% while maintaining testosterone

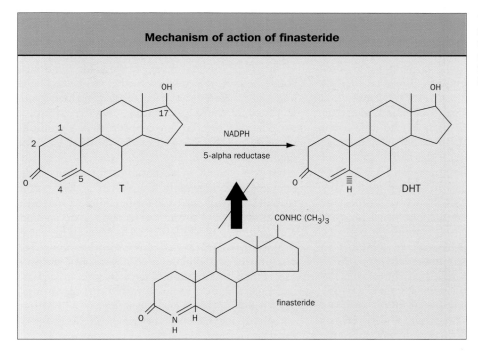

Mechanism of action of finasteride

13.16 Finasteride, a 5 alpha-reductase inhibitor, competitively inhibits the conversion of testosterone to dihydrotestosterone (DHT).

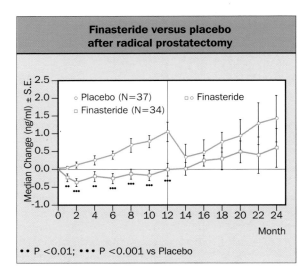

Finasteride versus placebo after radical prostatectomy

○ Placebo (N=37)
□ Finasteride (N=34)
□ ○ Finasteride

•• P <0.01; ••• P <0.001 vs Placebo

13.17 Effect of finasteride on serum PSA of patients who are found to be margin positive on histology after radical prostatectomy[48].

levels, and results in significant regression of the benignly enlarged gland[48,49]. Geller *et al.*[50] have shown that finasteride results in a marked decline of intraprostatic DHT, but a rise in intraprostatic testosterone levels. Animal studies suggested that finasteride would have activity in prostatic cancer[51], and a pilot study in 28 patients with metastatic prostate cancer showed some declines in PSA, but less than seen after orchidectomy or treatment with an LHRH analogue[52]. However, in a randomized study of patients who had positive margins after radical prostatectomy, finasteride delayed the rise in PSA by around 18 months[53] (**13.17**). Finasteride is a competitive inhibitor of 5 alpha-reductase; in contrast, other inhibitors, such as the new agent SK&F 105657, are thought to be uncompetitive inhibitors. A recent report of the use of this agent in androgen-responsive cell lines and in R-3327 tumour-bearing rats suggested some potentially useful anti-tumour activity[54]. However, at the time of writing, there have been no published phase II reports of the effect of this compound in patients. The appeal of a 5 alpha-reductase inhibitor in this context is the very favourable toxicity profile compared with the agents discussed above; virtually the only side-effect seen with finasteride is a 3–5% incidence of impotence and loss of libido, which is reversible on discontinuing the drug. The hypothesis that a combination of a 5 alpha-reductase inhibitor

with an antiandrogen may be of some value has been evaluated in a randomised phase II study. With respect to PSA suppression, finasteride plus flutamide performed as well as either goserelin and flutamide or goserelin and finasteride[55].

TIMING OF ENDOCRINE ABLATION THERAPY FOR METASTATIC PROSTATE CANCER

Traditionally, urologists have often favoured deferred administration of hormonal manipulation in patients with advanced prostate cancer, often waiting until symptoms appear before acting medically or surgically to ablate testicular androgens. The rationale for this decision to defer therapy was to some extent based on the findings from Study I of the Veterans Administration Cooperative Urological Research Group (VACURG). In this study, when patients were randomized between immediate hormonal therapy and placebo therapy, with later hormonal therapy when they became symptomatic, there was no difference in average survival rates between the two groups[56]. Sarosdy[57] however, has reanalysed the VACURG Study I data in detail, withdrawing the deaths due to cardiovascular events in the oestrogen-treated group and calculating cancer-specific death rates. These recalculations show that those who were treated initially with oestrogen therapy in fact fared better than those treated with placebo (3% cancer deaths in the oestrogen group versus 8.4% in the placebo group; p = 0.008).

The studies of total androgen blockade mentioned above have now produced further evidence of the potentially deleterious effects of allowing metastases of prostatic cancer to progress unfettered until a considerable tumour burden eventually produces symptoms. The enhanced results (both in terms of time to progression and overall survival in a subgroup of patients with good performance status and minimal metastatic disease) in at least some studies[17,20,23] now provide further support for those advocating more prompt intervention in patients who present with M1 disease. The Medical Research Council (MRC) Prostate Study Group has completed recruitment of 934 patients with metastatic prostate cancer and has randomized them into immediate androgen ablation versus deferred therapy groups. The results favour early treatment, with more patients dying from or suffering complications of prostate cancer in the deferred therapy arm[58].

CONCLUSIONS

The current gold standard – first-line therapy for metastatic prostate cancer – is androgen ablation by either bilateral orchidectomy or the use of LHRH analogues. However, Labrie's original hypothesis that androgen precursors secreted by the adrenal glands may play a role in maintaining prostate cancer growth and the escape of tumour cells from hormone control after ablation of testicular androgens has gained some scientific credence. The burden of evidence from a number of randomized, multicentre studies is that a subgroup of patients with good performance status and a reasonably restricted volume of metastatic disease may in fact remain in remission longer and have a prolonged survival if treated by maximal androgen blockade rather than conventionally with LHRH analogues or orchidectomy alone. More work is needed to confirm these results, and much of the data needs more time to mature before final evaluation, as the economic implications for already overstretched healthcare budgets are not inconsiderable. However, the current position is that if we wish to offer the very best therapy to our patients, then maximal androgen blockade with an antiandrogen plus either an LHRH analogue or bilateral orchidectomy is now the recommended treatment in the fitter younger individuals who do not present with an unduly heavy burden of prostate cancer, and in whom eventual death from prostate cancer, rather than a comorbid condition, seems likely[59].

For the future, it may well be possible to pre-identify (for example, by biochemical or morphometric means) the subgroup of patients in whom total androgen blockade, rather than orchidectomy or LHRH analogues alone, may produce a definite survival advantage. Moreover, there seems to be the promise of equally effective monotherapy by orally administered antiandrogens, which may obviate the need for either injections or surgery and also preserve sexual interest and potency and thereby quality of life. Current data suggests that early deployment of androgen withdrawal yields better results than deferred therapy[58]. The challenge of confirming these suggestions may be added to the many others that face us as we strive to reduce the morbidity and mortality of this most prevalent disease of men beyond middle age.

REFERENCES

1 Cassileth BR. Patients' choice of treatment in stage D prostate cancer. *Urology* 1989;**33**(Suppl 5):57–59.

2 Dijkman GA, Debruyne FMJ, Fernandez de Moral P, *et al*. A Phase III randomized trial comparing the efficacy and safety of the 3-monthly 10.8 mg depot of Zoladex™ with 3.6 mg depot in patients with advanced prostate cancer. *Eur Urol* 1994;**26**(1):1–2.

3 Debruyne FMJ. Zoladex™ 10.8 mg depot for prostate cancer. *J Urol* 1995;**153**:448A.

4 Peeling WB. Phase III studies to compare goserelin (Zoladex™) with orchidectomy and diethylstilbestrol in treatment of prostatic carcinoma. *Urology* 1989;**33**:45–52.

5 Leuprolide Study Group. Leuprolide versus diethylstilbestrol for metastatic prostate cancer. *N Eng J Med* 1984;**311**:1281–1286.

6 Debruyne FMJ. Long-term therapy with a depot luteinizing hormone-releasing hormone analogue (Zoladex™) in patients with advanced prostatic carcinoma. *J Urology* 1988;**140**:775–777.

7 Huggins C, Scott WW. Bilateral adrenalectomy in prostate cancer. *Ann Surg* 1945;1031–1041.

8 Labrie F, Veilleux R. A wide range of sensitivities to androgens develops in cloned Shionogi mouse mammary tumour cells. *Prostate* 1986;**8**:293–300.

9 Labrie C, Simand J, Begin D. Conversion of precursor adrenal steroids into potent androgens in peripheral tissues. In: Labrie F, Lee F, Dupont A (eds.) *Early stage prostate cancer: diagnosis and choice of therapy*. Amsterdam: Elsevier Science Publishers BV, 1989;1–21.

10 Ellis WJ, Issacs JT. Effectiveness of complete versus partial androgen withdrawal therapy for the treatment of prostate cancer as studies in the Dunning R-3327 system of rat prostatic adenocarcinomas. *Canc Res* 1985;**45**:6041–6045.

11 Labrie F, Dupont A, Belanger A. New approach in the treatment of prostate cancer: complete instead of partial withdrawal of androgens. *Prostate* 1983;**4**:579–594.

12 Labrie F, Dupont A, Belanger A. Combination therapy with flutamide and castration (LHRH agonist or orchidectomy) in advanced prostate cancer: a marked improvement in response and survival. *J Steroid Biochem* 1986;**23**:833–841.

13 Labrie F. Benefits of combination therapy with flutamide in patients relapsing after castration. *Br J Urol* 1988;**61**:341.

14 Labrie F, Dupont A, Belanger A, *et al*. Combination therapy with flutamide and castration (LHRH agonist or orchiectomy) in advanced prostate cancer: a marked improvement in response and survival. *J Steroid Biochem* 1985;**23**:833–841.

15 Geller J, De La Vega DJ, Albert JD. Tissue dihydrotestosterone levels and clinical response to hormone therapy in patients with prostate cancer. *J Clin Endocrinol Metab* 1984;**58**:36–40.

16 Harper ME, Pike A, Peeling WB, *et al*. Steroids of adrenal origin metabolized by human prostate tissue both *in vivo* and *in vitro*. *J Endocrinol* 1984;**60**:117.

17 Crawford ED, Eisenberger MA, McLeod DG, *et al.* A controlled trial of leuprolide with and without flutamide in prostatic cancer. *N Engl J Med* 1989;**321**:419–424.

18 Crawford ED, Nabors WL. Total androgen blockade: American experience. *Urol Clin North Am* 1991;**18**:55–63.

19 Mayer FJ, Crawford ED. Optimal therapy for metastatic prostate cancer. In: Hendry WF, Kirby RS, eds. *Recent advances in urology/andrology*. Churchill Livingstone, 1993;159–176.

20 Denis LD, Carneiro de Moura JL, *et al.* Goserelin acetate and flutamide versus bilateral orchiectomy: a phase III EORTC trial (30853). *Urology* 1993;**42**(2):119–129.

21 Keuppens F, Denis L, Smith P. Zoladex™ and flutamide versus bilateral orchidectomy. A randomized phase III EORTC 30853 study. *Cancer* 1990;**66**:1045–1057.

22 Canadian Anandron Study Group. Total androgen blockade in the treatment of metastatic prostate cancer. *Semin Urol* 1990;**8**:159–162.

23 Janknegt RA. International Anandron Study Group: Efficacy and tolerance of a total androgen blockade with Anandron and orchidectomy. A double-blind, placebo controlled multicentre study. *J Urol* 1991;**145**:425A.

24 Lunglmayr A. The international prostate cancer study group. A multicentre trial comparing the LHRH analogue Zoladex™, with Zoladex™ plus flutamide in the treatment of advanced prostate cancer. *Eur Urol* 1990;**18**(Suppl3):28–29.

25 Iversen P, Sucini S, Sylvester R. Zoladex™ and flutamide versus orchidectomy in the treatment of advanced prostate cancer. A combined analysis of two European studies EORTC and DAPROCA 86. *Cancer* 1990;**66**:1067–1073.

26 Prostate Cancer Trialists Collaborative Group. Maximum androgen blockade in advanced prostate cancer: an overview of 22 randomised trials with 3283 deaths in 5710 patients. *Lancet* 1995;**346**:265–269.

27 Caubet JF, *et al.* Maximum androgen blockade in advanced prostate cancer: a meta-analysis of published randomised trials using non-steroidal antiandrogens. *Urology* 1997;**49**:71–78.

28 Klotz LH, Newman T. Does maximum androgen blockade (MAB) improve survival? A critical appraisal of the evidence. Can J Urol 1996;3:246–250.

29 Eisenberger MA, Blumenstein BA, Crawford ED, *et al.* Bilateral orchidectomy with or without flutamide for metastatic prostate cancer. *N Engl J Med* 1998;**339**:1036–1042.

30 Smith JA, Crawford ED, Lange PH. PSA correlation with response and survival in advanced carcinoma of the prostate. *J Urol* 1991;**145**:384A.

31 Kahan A, Delriu M, Amor B. Disease flare induced by D-Trp-6-LHRH analogue in patients with metastatic prostate cancer. *Lancet* 1984;971–972.

32 Shearer RJ, Hendry WF, Sommerville IF. Plasma testosterone, an accurate monitor of hormone treatment in prostate cancer. *Br J Urol* 1973;**45**:668–671.

33 Robinson MRB. Complete androgen blockade: the EORTC experience comparing orchidectomy versus orchidectomy plus cyproterone acetate versus low dose stilboestrol in the treatment of metastatic carcinoma of the prostate: Proceedings of the Second International Symposium on Prostate Cancer. *Prostate Cancer Part A, Research, Endocrine Treatment and Histopathology* New York, Alan Liss, Inc 1987;383–390.(Abstract)

34 Kitahara S, Yoshida K, Ishizaka K, *et al.* Stronger suppression of serum testosterone and FSH levels by a synthetic oestrogen than by castration or an LHRH agonist. *Endocrine Journal* 1997;**44**:527–532.

35 Thorpe SC, Azmatullah S, Fellows GJ, *et al.* A prospective randomized study to compare goserelin acetate (Zoladex™) vs Cyprostat (cyproterone acetate) vs a combination of the two in the treatment of metastatic prostate cancer. *Eur Urol* 1996;**29**(1):47–54.

36 Watanabe S, Yamasaki S, Tanae A, *et al.* Three cases of hepatocellular carcinoma among cyproterone users. *Lancet* 1994;**344**:1567–1568.

37 Ohri SK, Caer JAR, Keane PF. Hepatocellular carcinoma and treatment with cyproterone acetate. *Br J Urol* 1991;**67**: 213–221.

38 Boccon-Gibot L, Fournier G, Bottet P, *et al.* Flutamide versus orchidectomy in patients with metastatic prostate cancer. *XI Congress of the EAU* 1994;**Abstracts Book**:13.

39 Furr BJA, Valcaccia B, Curry B. ICI 176334. A novel non-steroidal peripherally selective antiandrogen. *J Endocrinol* 1987;**113**:R7–R9.

40 Kennealey GT, Furr BJA. Use of the non-steroidal antiandrogen Casodex in advanced prostatic cancer. *Urol Clin North America* 1991;**18**:99–110.

41 Kaisary V. Current clinical studies with a new steroidal antiandrogen, Casodex. *Prostate* 1994;**5S**:27–33.

42 Schelhammer P, Sharifi R, Block N, *et al.* A controlled trial of bicalutamide (Casodex) versus flutamide each in combination with LHRH analogue therapy in patients with D$_2$ prostatic carcinoma. *Urology* 1997;**50**:330–336.

43 Robinson MRG, Shearer RJ, Fergusson JD. Adrenal suppression in the treatment of carcinoma of the prostate. *Br J Urol* 1974;**46**:555–559.

44 Murray R, Pitt P. Aminoglutethimide in the treatment of advanced prostate cancer. In: Murphy G, Khoury S, Kuss R, *et al.* eds. *Prostate Cancer*. New York: A.R. Liss, 1987;275–282.

45 Harnett DR, Raghavan D, Caterson I. Aminoglutethimide in advanced prostate carcinoma. *Br J Urol* 1987;**59**:323–327.

46 Plowman PN, Perry LA, Chard T. Androgen suppression by hydrocortisone without aminoglutethimide in orchidectomized men with prostate cancer. *Br J Urol* 1987;**59**:255–257.

47 Pont A. Long-term experience with high dose ketoconazole therapy in patients with D2 prostate carcinoma. *J Urol* 1987;**137**:902–904.

48 Gormley GJ, Stoner E, Bruskewitz RC, *et al.* The effect of finasteride in men with benign prostatic hyperplasia. *N Engl J Med* 1992;**327**:1185–1191.

49 Kirby RS, Vale J, Bryan J, *et al*. Long-term urodynamic effects of finasteride in benign prostatic hyperplasia: a pilot study. *Eur Urol* 1993;**24**:20–26.

50 Geller J. Effect of finasteride, a 5-alpha reductase inhibitor on prostate tissue androgens and prostate-specific antigen. *J Clin Endocrinol Metab* 1990;**71**:1552–1555.

51 Brooks JR, Berman C, Nguyen H, *et al*. Effect of castration, DES, Flutamide, and the 5-alpha reductase inhibitor MK906, on the growth of the Dunning rat prostatic carcinoma, R-3327. *Prostate* 1991;**18**:215–217.

52 Presti JC, Fair WR, Andriole G, *et al*. Multicentre, randomised, double-blind, placebo-controlled study to investigate the effect of finasteride (MK-906) on stage D prostatic cancer. *J Urol* 1992;**148**:1201–1204.

53 Andriole GL. Finasteride induced PSA reductions in patients with early stage prostate cancer. *J Urol Abstract* 1994;**151**:450A.

54 Lamb JC, Levy MA, Johnson RK, *et al*. Response of rat and human prostatic tumours to the novel 5-alpha reductase inhibitor, SK&F 105657. *Prostate* 1992;**21**:15–34.

55 Kirby RS, Robertson C, Turkes A, *et al*. Finasteride in association with either flutamide or goserelin as combination hormonal therapy in patients with stage M1 carcinoma of the prostate. *Prostate* 1999;**40**:105–114.

56 Veterans Administration Cooperative Urological Research Group. Carcinoma of the prostate: treatment comparisons. *J Urol* 1967;**98**:516–519.

57 Sarosy MF. Do we have a national treatment plan for stage D1 carcinoma of the prostate. *World J Urol* 1990;**8**:27–31.

58 Medical Research Council Prostate Council Working Party Investigators Group. Immediate versus deferred treatment for advanced prostatic cancer: initial results of the Medical Research Council trial. *Br J Urol* 1997;**79**:235–246.

59 Kirby RS. Is total androgen blockade now mandatory? *Rev Endocrine-Related Cancer* 1994;**42**:31–43.

Chapter 14

Management of hormone-refractory prostate cancer

Unfortunately, as already described, unless some comorbid condition intervenes, virtually every advanced prostate cancer treated by androgen ablation will eventually 'escape' from the growth-restraining effects of low circulating androgen levels, and will show signs of disease progression. The mechanism for this hormone escape is almost certainly the clonal selection of androgen-independent cell lines (**14.1**). A follicle-stimulating hormone (FSH) receptor has been identified in androgen-independent, metastatic prostatic cell lines as well as in human malignant prostate tissues. Furthermore, these tissues can be stimulated by exposure to FSH. This has caused speculation that the FSH receptor and its ligand may play a role in the regulation of growth of androgen-refractory prostate cancer[1]. Now that serial prostate- specific antigen (PSA) determination is readily available and commonly utilized for follow-up, 'PSA relapse' is frequently seen as an inevitable harbinger of clinical disease progression. This leaves the urologist and his or her patient in the position of knowing the worst and therefore wishing to employ second-line therapy before symptoms inexorably develop. Although the prognosis in these circumstances is generally still poor, there are now some manoeuvres that it may be helpful to make.

VARIATIONS ON THE THEME OF ANDROGEN ABLATION

For those patients who have been managed initially by monotherapy (by either orchidectomy or luteinizing hormone-releasing hormone (LHRH) analogues), the addition of an antiandrogen to neutralize the 5% or so of circulating adrenal androgens would seem logical. However, by the time hormone escape has

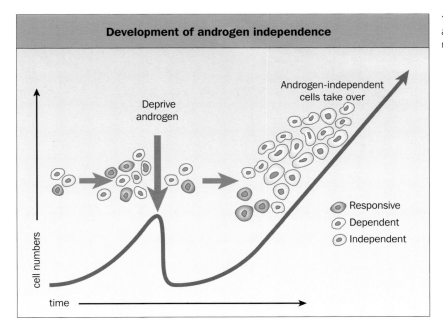

14.1 Clonal selection of androgen-independent cells resulting in hormonal escape.

occurred, this may have disappointingly little beneficial effect. Recently, the observation has been made that certain patients who have been managed from the outset with maximal androgen blockade may benefit from cessation of the antiandrogen[2]. In such circumstances, the rising serum PSA may be temporarily halted or reversed by flutamide withdrawal. Although this phenomenon is presently unexplained, it could be the result of an agonist effect of the antiandrogen on mutated androgen receptors in tumour cells[3]. This would be akin to the mild oestrogenic effect of the antioestrogen tamoxifen, which is sometimes seen in breast cancer, and which is probably due to structural mutation of oestrogen receptors in breast cancer cells. Antiandrogen withdrawal is such a simple and cost-effective measure that it should now always be considered in situations of prostate cancer relapse in spite of maximum androgen blockade. Moreover, it must be borne in mind that if some new form of therapy is initiated at the same time as bicalutamide or flutamide withdrawal, then any clinical or biochemical improvement seen may conceivably be incorrectly ascribed to the new drug rather than to the withdrawal of the original therapy.

Diethylstilboestrol

Another treatment strategy for relapsed prostate cancer is to introduce an oestrogen such as diethylstilboestrol (DES) at this stage. Although the major action of oestrogens in prostate cancer is at the hypothalamo–pituitary level, there is also evidence of a direct cytotoxic effect on prostate cancer cells, conceivably by direct inhibition of DNA polymerase. Evidence for the efficacy of DES in this context, however, is virtually all anecdotal, since randomized studies have seldom proven practical in the situation of disease relapse.

A recent study in experimental animals has suggested that hormonal escape itself might be delayed by the introduction of oestrogens[4]. The side-effects of oestrogens, including gynaecomastia, deep vein thrombosis (4%), and other cardiovascular complications, usually preclude the use of DES as first-line therapy. In situations of hormonal relapse, however, where life expectancy is so limited, a therapeutic trial may be indicated, and it has been suggested, but not yet proven, that the cardiovascular side-effects can be minimized by additional dosing with 75 mg of aspirin per day.

Estramustine Phosphate

Another drug with oestrogenic effects that is currently making something of a comeback is estramustine phosphate (EMP). This agent is a combination of nitrogen mustard linked to a phosphorylated estradiol (**14.2**). EMP is rapidly dephosphorylated in the body to its main metabolites, estramustine and estromustine[5]. Only 10% or so of these metabolites are hydrolysed to estradiol and estrone, which act secondarily to depress testosterone levels (**14.3**). These oestrogenic steroid metabolites are present in considerably lower concentrations than those achieved with the standard doses of oestrogen used in the treatment of metastatic prostate cancer, and are not the primary mode of anti-cancer action of the drug. EMP cytotoxicity is mainly due to its ability to bind to microtubule-associated proteins (MAPs).

As discussed in Chapter 4, MAPs are essential to microtubule stability and microtubules are intimately involved in the cell cycle. Estramustine causes microtubules to disassemble, as well as preventing their *de novo* formation (**14.4**), thereby resulting in mitotic arrest during metaphase and cell death[6].

Estramustine appears to accumulate preferentially in the prostate; in one study, prostate biopsies showed concentrations of estramustine six times higher than those achieved in the plasma. In the relatively hormone-resistant human prostate cancer cell line DU 145, estramustine has been shown to inhibit cell growth[7,8]. Moreover, in a number of phase 2 and phase 3 trials of estramustine as second-line therapy, the drug has been shown to produce an overall subjective response rate of around 60%, and an objective response rate in 30–35% of patients (**Tables 14.1** and **14.2**). Toxicity can be a problem though, especially in the typically frail and elderly

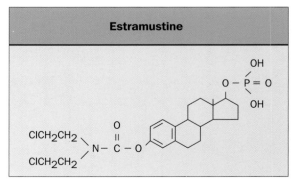

Estramustine

14.2 Chemical structure of estramustine.

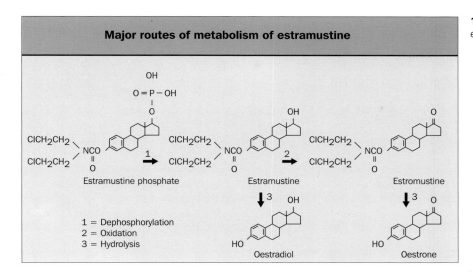

14.3 Metabolism of estramustine.

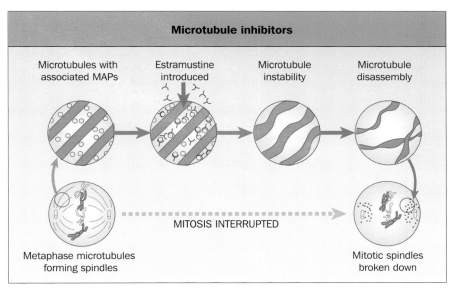

14.4 The action of estramustine in disassembling microtubules and thereby preventing cell division.

patient with hormone-relapsed cancer. Nausea, anaemia and granulocytopenia can all occur, any of which may necessitate the cessation of therapy.

USE OF CYTOTOXIC AGENTS

Cytotoxic agents have often been tried in metastatic prostate cancer, either alone or in combination, both as primary therapy and in situations of hormonal relapse. Unfortunately, although partial responses may be obtained in some cases, in neither circumstance has the objective response rate been of sufficient magnitude to counterbalance the toxicity often seen, which is often especially severe in this group of elderly men who have frequently received prior radiotherapy, and who also often have pre-existing bone marrow suppression due to bone metastases. The original problem of the lack of bidimensionally measurable disease in assessing the response to therapy has to some extent been overcome by the advent of quantitative PSA determination. However, as yet, not many reports of chemotherapeutic agents have included PSA data. The issue is further clouded by the fact that, not

Table 14.1 Summary of selected phase II studies of estramustine in hormone-refractory prostate cancer

Reference	No. of patients	Objective response (%)
Benson and Gill[34]	51	69
Chisholm, O'Donoghue and Kennedy[35]	30	27
Fosså and Miller[36]	17	35
Jönsson, Högberg and Nilsson[37]	91	31
Küss et al.[38]	15	20
Leistenschneider and Nagel[39]	23	35
Lindberg[40]	22	27
Mittelman, Shukla and Murphy[41]	44	18
Veronesi et al.[27]	27	74

Table 14.2 Phase III clinical trials of estramustine in hormone-refractory prostate cancer patients

Reference	Protocol	Treatment (no. of patients)	Objective response (%)
Murphy et al.[42]	NPCP Protocol 200	Estracyt (46)	30
		Streptozotocin (38)	31
		Standard therapy (21)	19
Soloway et al.[43]	NPCP Protocol 800	Estracyt (27)	26
		Estracyt + vincristine (19)	24
		Vincristine (34)	15
Soloway et al.[44]	NPCP Protocol 1200	Estracyt (40)	18
		Estracyt + cisplatinum (42)	33
		Cisplatinum (42)	21

NPCP, National Prostatic Cancer Project

uncommonly, patients exhibit a 'mixed response'; for example, improvement in soft-tissue disease sites, but advancement in other areas, most commonly in bone metastases.

For several years, the National Prostatic Cancer Project (NPCP) has utilized criteria for response that were developed by their group which includes a category for 'stable disease' (SD) as evidence of a response to therapy[9]. By their definition, SD represents no evidence of disease progression during the initial 12 weeks of therapy. Survival analysis of patients with SD appeared to be comparable to those who had evidence of partial response (PR); both groups survived significantly longer than those who did not respond. For these reasons, patients with SD are often considered in the category of 'responders', together with those exhibiting evidence of partial response. Since the tumour-doubling time of many prostatic cancers is notoriously slow, even in advanced disease, it may well be that the apparent disease stabilization observed over 12 weeks was not in fact due to the treatment itself. Inclusion of patients with SD in responder groups may therefore falsely inflate apparent treatment response rates.

Experience with Single Agents and Multidrug Combinations in Single Arm Studies

The experience with single-agent chemotherapeutic regimes in prostate cancer has not been especially encouraging. The methodological problems already alluded to make it difficult to estimate the exact level of antitumour activity of most drugs. The marked variability of reported response rates probably reflects different methodologies as well as widely varying patient selection criteria.

Because of the disappointing response rates to single-agent chemotherapy, a number of investigators have employed multidrug regimens in patients with metastatic prostate cancer. Unfortunately, the number of complete or even partial responses has generally remained low; moreover, the toxicity associated with multidrug therapy is usually greater than that of single-agent treatment. Further studies are ongoing.

Prospective Randomized Studies of Chemotherapy in Endocrine-Resistant Prostate Cancer

For obvious reasons, randomized studies of chemotherapy are easier to interpret than single-arm studies. They also usually serve to evaluate more clinically relevant end-points, such as time to treatment failure and overall survival. Some of the more important randomized studies are summarized in **Table 14.3**. In virtually all of them, the differences between the chemotherapy arm and standard therapy, which usually consisted of various palliative measures including treatment with corticosteroids, analgesics, and palliative radiation to painful metastases, were negligible. In several large NPCP studies of multidrug regimes, the Kaplan–Meier survival curves constructed for both arms were virtually identical (**14.5**).

Table 14.3 National Prostatic Cancer Project (NPCP): randomized trials in prostate cancer				
Treatment	No. evaluable/ entered	Complete and partial response	Stable disease	Median survival (weeks)
NPCP study 100[44,45]				
Cyclophosphamide	41	4	4	47
5-Fluorouracil	33	4	4	44
Standard therapy	36	0	0	38
NPCP study 200[46,47]				
Estramustine	46/54	3	3	26
Streptozotocin	38/46	0	0	25
Standard therapy	21/25	0	0	24
NPCP study 300[48]				
Cyclophosphamide	35/39	0	9	27
DTIC	55/68	2	13	40
Procarbazine	39/58	0	5	31
NPCP study 700[49]				
Cyclophosphamide	43/47	3	12	41
MeCCNU	27/38	1	7	22
Hydroxyurea	28/40	2	2	19
NPCP study 800[50]				
Estramustine	27/38	1	6	26
Vincristine	29/42	1	4	22
Estramustine + Vincristine	34/41	0	7	32
NPCP study 1200[51]				
Estramustine	40/50	0	7	38
Cisplatinum	42/51	0	9	28
Estramustine + Cisplatin	42/48	0	14	40

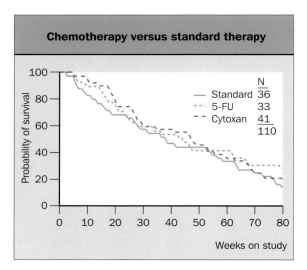

14.5 Kaplan–Meier survival curves of chemotherapy versus palliative measures only in patients with hormone-escaped metastatic prostate cancer. 5-FU, 5-fluorouracil. (Reproduced from Eisenberger[52].)

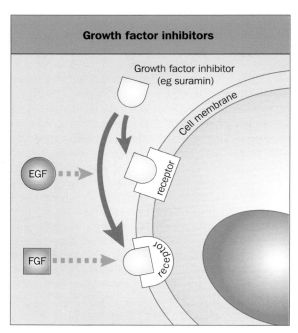

14.6 Mechanism of action of growth factor inhibitors such as suramin.

THE USE OF GROWTH FACTOR INHIBITORS

The accumulating evidence suggesting that growth factors, including epidermal growth factor (EGF), insulin-like growth factor (IGF), platelet-derived growth factor (PdGF), as well as fibroblast growth factor (FGF), may be involved in the development and progression of prostate cancer has stimulated researchers to evaluate the effect of the growth factor inhibitors, such as suramin, in patients with metastatic prostate cancer (**14.6**). Suramin is a polysulphonated naphthylurea analogue of tryptan blue, with several important biological activities including growth factor inhibition[10].

As discussed in Chapter 4, growth factors are involved in the pathogenesis of many cancers because malignant cells become the endogenous producers of polypeptide growth stimulators. Therapeutic interruption of this so-called autocrine loop has been most extensively investigated in systems dependent on PdGF. Human PdGF is a 30 000 molecular weight protein that is a mitogen to connective tissue-derived cells. The B chain of PdGF is virtually identical to part of the transforming protein v-*sis* of simian sarcoma virus (SSV), which suggests that a PdGF-like factor mediates cell transformation. When added to SSV-transformed human fibroblasts, suramin causes a reversible and dose-dependent

reversion to the normal phenotype. Suramin can also interfere with the binding of insulin-like growth factor (IGF) to its receptors[11,12]. Unlike members of the EGF and FGF families, which are for the most part produced and act locally in tissues, IGF-I and IGF-II are produced both locally and systemically. IGF-I is released from the liver under the stimulation of growth hormone, and is the key mediator of growth-hormone effects. Prostatic cancer cells in tissue culture respond to insulin and its related peptides, and the blocking effect of suramin on IGF receptors may therefore account for some of its activity in metastatic prostate cancer.

Clinical trials to evaluate the effects of suramin in hormone-refractory prostate cancer began in 1988[13]. The drug was administered to patients as a continuous infusion to a target plasma level of 300 µg/ml. Of the 38 patients that entered this trial, 17 had measurable soft-tissue disease and the rest bone metastases alone. Thirty-three percent of the patients with soft-tissue metastases demonstrated shrinkage of deposits but more than 50% of those with bone secondaries did so. Seventy per cent had significant relief of bone pain and more than half had a greater than 50% decline in their serum PSA. The magnitude of the pre-treatment PSA was an important predictor of outcome: of those patients whose pre-treatment PSA was <100 ng/ml 70% had a greater than 75% decline in PSA in response to suramin. By contrast, only a quarter of patients with pre-treatment PSA values >100 showed similar responses. From this, it was concluded that the effectiveness of suramin was limited dramatically by the extent of the tumour burden.

Other preliminary reports from the USA of the use of suramin in prostate cancer have also been encouraging[14]. However, although some remissions have been documented, in general the side-effect profile of this agent is insufficiently clean for it to gain general acceptance for the treatment of this condition; skin rashes, prolonged bleeding time, keratopathy and neuromuscular toxicity have all been encountered. Many patients report paraesthesiae involving the lower extremities and a syndrome of fever and chills, and more severe neurotoxicity with progressive peripheral neuropathy may also occur. Adrenal insufficiency and increased susceptibility to infections are also significant clinical problems with this agent. Growth factor inhibitors that are more specific to the prostate are eagerly awaited for deployment in patients with relapsing prostate cancer. Tyrosine kinase inhibitors which prevent the cell proliferation signals from growth factors also appear a promising avenue of therapy.

Taxol™

The diterpine Taxol™ (paclitaxel, Mead Johnson, Princeton, NJ), which is a natural product of the plant *Taxus brevifolia*, seems to hold the promise of some useful activity in hormone-refractory prostate cancer[15] (**14.7**). This compound has a unique mechanism of action, with high-affinity binding to polymerized microtubules at a site distinct from those identified for colchicine, vinblastine or estramustine (**14.4**). Recently, Taxol™ has been demonstrated to possess an ability to inhibit the invasiveness of an *in vitro* human prostate cancer cell line, and to inhibit the growth and metastatic potential of human prostate cancer xenografts[16].

A phase II study looking at paclitaxel in advanced, hormone-refractory carcinoma of the prostate was conducted by Roth *et al.*[17] Twenty-three patients (with bidimensionally measurable disease) were treated with paclitaxel 135–170 mg/m² by 24-hour intravenous infusion, every 21 days for a maximum of 6 cycles. In 21 evaluable patients, there was 1 partial response (4.3%) lasting 9 months. Four

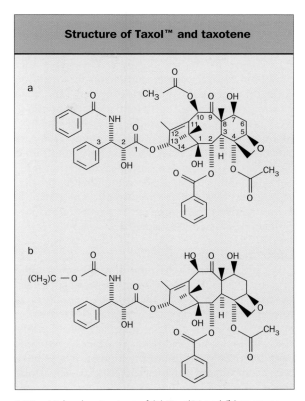

Structure of Taxol™ and taxotene

14.7 Molecular structure of (**a**) Taxol™ and (**b**) taxotene.

other patients with radiographically stable disease had minor reductions in the serum PSA of 16–24%. Eleven patients (47.8%) had stable disease, and progressive disease developed in 9 patients (39.1%) during therapy. The median survival was 9 months.

Leukopenia was generally the dose-limiting toxicity, with 13% of patients having Grade 3 and 61% having Grade 4 toxicity. Granulocytopenic fever developed in 26% of patients. The study concluded that in the setting of hormone-refractory prostate cancer and bidimensionally measurable disease, paclitaxel at this dosage has limited clinical activity.

Hudes *et al.*[18] conducted a phase 1 pharmacological study of a 96-hour infusion of paclitaxel combined with estramustine (600 mg/m² D_1–D_2) every 3 weeks in 18 patients with refractory tumours. Patients had received a median of 2 prior chemotherapy regimens. Paclitaxel was administered at a dose of 80–140 mg/m².

Objective responses occurred in 2 out of 2 patients with measurable hormone-refractory prostate cancer, and the authors concluded that such activity merits further investigation.

Retinoids and Prostate Cancer

Another interesting group of compounds with regard to the treatment of hormone-refractory prostate cancer are the retinoid derivatives of vitamin A. Within the nucleus retinoids act as transcription regulators, generally inhibiting growth and promoting epithelial-cell differentiation. Fenretinide (N-4-hydroxyphenylretinamide) has been shown to be cytotoxic to both rat and human prostate cancer cells *in vitro*. Using various angiogenesis inhibition assays, it was demonstrated that fenretinide not only inhibited angiogenesis but also endothelial cell motility and tubule formation[19]. The potential for retinoids as chemopreventive agents in prostate cancer is discussed in Chapter 11.

Liarozole

Liarozole acts mainly by inhibiting the breakdown of retinoic acid, thus increasing retinoic acid levels. Retinoic acid is one of the principal endogenous compounds that control growth and differentiation of epithelial cells. Besides their anti-proliferative and differentiation-inducing potencies, retinoids have important antitumoral activities. These have been demonstrated in acute promyelocytic leukaemia, as well as in solid tumours such as lung cancers and squamous cell carcinomas of both the head and neck and the skin.

Normally, retinoic acid is metabolized by means of a cytochrome P450-mediated hydroxylase enzyme system; this system is inhibited by liarozole (**14.8**). A further biological activity of liarozole is as an aromatase inhibitor, preventing the peripheral conversion of testosterone to oestrogen. The biosynthesis of testosterone is also cytochrome P450-dependent. Liarozole causes a dose-dependent lowering of testosterone, and a rise in the precursors 17 alpha-hydroxyprogesterone and progesterone for at least 24 hours after a single dose of 300 mg. Unlike ketoconazole, however, liarozole does not significantly effect adrenal androgen levels.

In experimental animals, liarozole has shown antitumoral effects in both androgen-dependent and androgen-independent prostate cancers[20]. The compound is now being evaluated in patients suffering clinical relapse after previous androgen-depletion therapy for prostate cancer. Early data suggested tolerance was acceptable overall, with most adverse events being mild to moderate, and mostly retinoid related (i.e. akin to hypervitaminosis A), such as dry mouth, itchy peeling skin, nausea, asthenia and

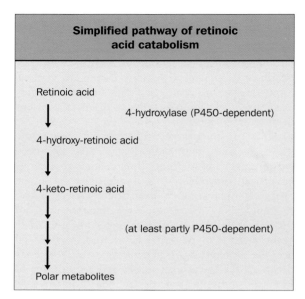

14.8 Retinoic metabolism is inhibited by liarozole.

fatigue. Unfortunately efficacy is less than originally anticipated and approval from the regulatory authorities has not been obtained.

ROLE OF NEWER COMBINATION THERAPIES

As in the 1970s with testicular cancer, we are currently awaiting a major breakthrough in the therapy for hormone-relapsed metastatic prostate cancer. Now that some agents such as Taxol™, suramin and mitoxantrone are beginning to emerge with signs of useful activity, the possibility of improving efficacy with various combination therapies exists – e.g. growth factor inhibitors plus cytotoxic agents or retinoids; there seems to be plenty of scope for advancement in this area.

For example, the combination of estramustine with vinblastine has a logic, because both agents have distinctive and potentially synergistic effects as microtubule inhibitors. *In vitro* studies in the DU 145 human prostate cancer cell line demonstrated additive antimitotic effects. In recent clinical trials involving 82 patients, a PSA decline of more than 50% was achieved in 35 (43%) individuals. Moreover, 6 of 19 (32%) patients with bidimensionally measurable disease achieved a partial response. Vinblastine was usually given as a weekly, intravenous bolus of 4 mg/m² in combination with oral estramustine 10–15 mg/kg/day on days 1–42. There-after, treatment was repeated after a 2-week break if toxicity was acceptable and there was no disease progression. Toxicity was predominantly attributable to the estramustine, which causes cardiovascular side-effects such as venous and arterial thrombosis in up to 10% of cases; mild nausea and haematological disturbances were also reported in up to 50% of patients. Using a 50% PSA decrease as a clinical endpoint, Seidman et al.[21] also showed a promising response rate to this combination of between 30 and 50%.

Another interesting combination therapy is that of etoposide and estramustine. Etoposide is a topoisomerase II inhibitor that inhibits DNA replication directly at the level of the nuclear matrix. The results of etoposide used alone in prostate cancer have been disappointing[22]. However, in vitro etoposide combined with estramustine has been shown to inhibit growth in the human metastatic PC-3 cell line as well as the MAT-LyLu (MLL) rat prostate cancer cell line[23]. In a phase 2 clinical trial, 20 patients with hormone-refractory prostate cancer were treated with estramustine 15 mg/kg/day and etoposide 50 mg/m²/day, both taken orally for 21 out of 28 day cycles. Fifteen patients were available at the time of the first report, 9 of whom had measurable disease. A partial response was seen in 6 patients; the remaining 3 achieved stable disease. Toxicity consisted of nausea, granulocytopenia and anaemia. All patients noted alopecia[24].

Other Forms of Palliation

In some circumstances, a short course of corticosteroids may be worth considering. It has been noted that this intervention may improve anaemia and weight loss and psychological well-being, but there are little scientific data to corroborate this contention.

Bone Pain

One of the most intractable and distressing problems encountered in hormone-escaped prostate cancer is bone pain associated with skeletal metastases. The usual analgesic agents are often of little efficacy in this situation. Doses high enough to provide some relief are associated with unacceptable side-effects of sedation and confusion. The mechanisms for the often especially severe pain are incompletely understood. There may be an increase in intramedullary pressure and local invasion of endosteal, periosteal and marrow nerve endings.

Obviously, pathologic fractures through tumour-affected bone should be excluded by local radiographs.

There is now some evidence that some patients with painful bony metastases may benefit from treatment with diphosphonates. Diphosphonates are pyrophosphate analogues that suppress bone resorption and mineralization by a direct influence on the activity of osteoclasts, and have been used in the treatment of Paget's disease, multiple myeloma and metastatic breast cancer. Clodronate (dichloro-methylene-diphosphonate) has been shown to be effective in palliation of bone pain in prostate cancer when given intravenously in 16 of 17 patients in one study[25], and in 29 of 41 (71%) in another[26]. The only side-effects noted were slight gastrointestinal discomfort when the patients were continued on oral therapy.

Local Radiotherapy

External-beam radiotherapy has been employed for many years as a form of palliation for painful skeletal metastases due to prostate cancer. The probability of effective pain relief is around 70–80% when radiotherapy is given either as a single dose (8 Gy), or as a short two-week (20 Gy) or three-week (30 Gy) course. When, as is often the case, there are multiple sites of bone pain, local therapy is less effective.

Wide-Field Radiotherapy

Wide-field radiation treatment may sometimes be an option for some patients with intractable pain from widespread metastases. In one collaborative study, hemibody irradiation (6 Gy to upper body and 8 Gy to lower body) resulted in pain-free status being achieved in 30% of patients, partial response in 50%, and no change in 20%. Eighty percent of responses had occurred within 1 week, and the mean duration of pain relief was 3 months. Nausea, vomiting and diarrhoea occurred to mild or moderate extent in 35% of patients. In 15%, however, this was classified as severe or life-threatening. Haematological effects were also classified as severe or life-threatening in 9% of cases[27].

Strontium-89 chloride (Metastron)

The use of the beta-emitting isotope Strontium-89 chloride (Metastron) constitutes a useful therapeutic advance for the pain control of patients with prostate cancer. Strontium-89 follows the biological pathways of calcium within the body and decays with a half-life of 50.5 days. Although it is washed out of healthy bone, it localizes preferentially at the sites of increased mineral turnover which characterize osteoblastic metastases. The turnover of Strontium-89 within normal trabecular bone has a half-life of around 14 days, whereas metastatic deposits appear to retain the isotope almost indefinitely.

A number of published trials indicate that Strontium-89 is safe and provides pain relief in up to 78% of patients[28]. For example, in a prospective, randomized study of 32 patients with metastatic cancer using a crossover design against placebo, complete pain relief was only seen after Strontium-89 administration[29]. One recent study showed that it produced a 50% reduction in analgesic requirements in 55% of patients. In the UK Metastron trial 284 patients with painful bone metastases were stratified into two groups according to suitability for local radiotherapy or hemibody (wide-field) irradiation and then randomized within each group to receive either 200 MBq (5.4 mCi) Strontium-89 or the assigned form of external radiotherapy. Pain response at the site of presenting pain was similar in patients treated with either Strontium-89 or external beam radiotherapy, but patients treated with Strontium-89 were less likely to experience new sites of pain. Porter and McEwan[31] have also shown that the isotope delays disease progression and is cost effective by virtue of reduced analgesic and hospitalization costs[32].

Side-effects from Strontium-89 consist mainly of mild haematological toxicity, usually thrombocytopenia. When this is seen, platelet count decreases range from 24–70% and only occasionally meet the criteria for toxicity used to assess cytotoxic chemotherapy. Platelet nadir is dose related and is usually reached 5–7 weeks post-treatment. The leukocyte nadir also occurs around this time, and the effect persists for up to 3 months[33]. As approximately 90% of Strontium-89 is excreted through the kidneys (the remainder undergoing biliary excretion), care

should be taken with patients with renal insufficiency. Patients receiving Strontium-89 should also be instructed to dispose of their urine by double flushing since the urine radioactivity, though slight, is measureable.

Patients receiving Strontium-89 should fulfil the following criteria:

- More than one site of skeletal metastasis and diffuse painful sites.
- WBC count >3000/cubic mm and platelet count >60 000/cubic mm.
- Life expectancy >3 months.
- No change in hormonal treatment or chemotherapy within 30 days.

The standard dose is 148 MBq (4 mCi), administered by a slow intravenous injection into a fast running IV line, avoiding extravasation. Pain relief typically occurs in 1–2 weeks and rarely takes 4 weeks or more. If the first injection is not beneficial, the second will probably be no more effective. In the 80% or so of patients who are responsive, the effects of Strontium-89 should last 3 months or longer, after which a further dose may be required.

PALLIATIVE CARE

Eventually, in spite of all therapeutic efforts, more than 80% of patients with metastatic prostate cancer will deteriorate and die from their disease, the remainder dying from comorbid conditions. The terminal stages of this illness may be distressing for all concerned because of severe pain from metastatic deposits, and are usually best handled by a team effort involving the relatives, an experienced palliative-care team and the family practitioner. The urologist should be readily available for consultation concerning modifications of therapy and the advisability of eventually transferring the patient to either hospital or preferably a unit specialized in the care of the terminally ill[53].

REFERENCES

1 Ben-Josef E, Yang SY, Ji TH, et al. Hormone refractory prostate cancer cells express functional follicle-stimulating hormone receptor (FSHR). *J Urol* 1999;**161**:970–976.

2 Scher HI, Kelly WK. Flutamide withdrawal syndrome: its impact on clinical trials in hormone-refractory prostatic cancer. *J Clin Oncol* 1993;**11**:1566–1572.

3 Kelly WK. Endocrine withdrawal syndrome and its

relevance to the management of hormone refractory prostate cancer. *Eur Urol* 1998;**34**:18–23.

4 Landstrom M, Damber JE, Bergh A. Estrogen treatment postpones the castration-induced dedifferentiation of Dunning R3327-PAP prostatic adenocarcinoma. *Prostate* 1994;**25**(1):10–18.

5 Andersson SB, Gunnarsson PO, Nilsson T, et al. Metabolism of estramustine phosphate (Estracyt) in patients with prostatic carcinoma. *Eur J Drug Metab Pharmacokinet* 1981;**6**:149–154.

6 Stearns ME, Tew KD. Antimicrotubule effects of estramustine, an antiprostatic tumor drug. *Canc Res* 1985;**45**:3891–3897.

7 Hansenson M, Lundh B, Hartley-Asp B, *et al.* Growth-inhibiting effect of estramustine on two prostatic carcinoma cell lines, LNCaP and LNCaP-r. *Urol Res* 1988;**16**:357–361.

8 Hartley-Asp B. Estramustine induced mitotic arrest in two human prostatic cell lines DU 145 and PC-3. *Prostate* 1984;**5**:93–100.

9 Murphy GP, Slack NH. Response criteria for the prostate of the USA National Prostatic Cancer Project. *Prostate* 1980;**1**:375–382.

10 Olivier S, Formento P, Fischel JL, *et al.* Epidermal growth factor expression and Suramin cytotoxicity *in vitro. Eur J Cancer* 1990;**29A**:245–247.

11 Pollak M, Richard M. Suramin blockade of insulin-like growth factor I-stimulated proliferation of osteosarcoma cells. *J Natl Cancer Inst* 1990;**82**:1349–1352.

12 Pollak M, Polychronakos C, Richard M. Suramin interferes with the binding of insulin-like growth factor I (IGF-I) to IGF-I receptors. *Proc Am Assoc Cancer Res* 1990;**31**:47–51.

13 Myers C, Cooper M, Stein C, *et al.* Suramin: a novel growth factor antagonist with activity in hormone-refractory prostate cancer. *J Clin Oncol* 1992;**10**:881–889.

14 Eisenberger MA, Reyno LM, Jodrell DI. Suramin, an active drug for prostate cancer; interim observations in a phase I trial. *J Natl Cancer Inst* 1993;**85**:611–621.

15 Rowinsky EK, Onetto N, Canetta RM, *et al.* Taxol: the first of the taxanes, an important new class of antitumor agents. *Sem Urol* 1992;**19**:646–662.

16 Stearns ME, Wang M. Taxol blocks processes essential for prostate tumor cell (PC-3 ML) invasion and metastases. *Cancer Res* 1994;**52**:3776–3778.

17 Roth BJ, Yeap BY, Wilding G, *et al.* Taxol in advanced, hormone-refractory carcinoma of the prostate. *Cancer* 1993;**72**(8):2457–2460.

18 Hudes G, Obasaju C, McAleer C, *et al.* Phase I pharmacologic study of 96-HR infusional Taxol combined with estramustine. *Proc ASCO* 1994;**13**:188-Abst 465.

19 Pienta KJ, Nguyen NM, Lehr JE. Treatment of prostate cancer in the rat with the synthetic retinoid fenretinide. *Canc Res* 1993;**53**:224–226.

20 Dijkman GA, Van Moorselaar RJA, Van Ginckel R, *et al.* Antitumoral effects of liarozole in androgen-dependent and independent R3327-Dunning prostate adenocarcinomas. *J Urol* 1994;**151**:217–222.

21 Seidman AD, Scher HI, Petrylak D, *et al.* Estramustine and vinblastine: use of prostate-specific antigen as a clinical trial end point for hormone refractory prostatic cancer. *J Urol* 1992;**147**:931–934.

22 Scher HI, Sternberg C, Heston WDW. Etoposide in prostate cancer: experimental studies and phase II trial in patients with bidimensionally measurable disease. *Cancer Chemother Pharmacol* 1986;**18**:24–26.

23 Pienta KJ, Lehr JE. Inhibition of prostate cancer growth by estramustine and etoposide: evidence for interactions at the nuclear matrix. *J Urol* 1993;**149**:1622–1625.

24 Pienta KJ, Redman BG, Hussain M, *et al.* A combination of estramustine and etoposide orally may be an effective regimen in the treatment of hormone refractory prostate cancer. *Proc Am Soc Clin Oncol* 1993;**12**:246–251.

25 Adami S, Salvagno G, Guarrera G, *et al.* Dichloromethylene-diphosphonate in patients with prostatic carcinoma metastatic to the skeleton. *J Urol* 1985;**134**:1152–1154.

26 Vorreuther R. Biphosphonates as an adjunct to palliative therapy of bone metastases from prostatic carcinoma. A pilot study on clodronate. *Br J Urol* 1993;**72**:792–795.

27 Veronesi A, Zattoni F, Frutaci S, *et al.* Estramustine (Estracyt) treatment of T3–T4 prostatic carcinoma. *Prostate* 1982;**3**:159–164.

28 Crawford ED, Balmer C, Kozlowski JM, *et al.* The use of Strontium-89 for palliation of pain from bone metastases associated with hormone-refractory prostate cancer. *Urology* 1994;**44**:481–485.

29 Lewington V, McEwan AJ, Ackery DM, *et al.* A prospective, randomized double-blind crossover study to examine the efficacy of Strontium-89 in pain palliation in patients with advanced prostate cancer metastatic to bone. *Eur J Cancer* 1991;**27**(8):954–958.

30 Bolger JJ, Dearnoley DP, Kirk D, *et al.* Strontium-89 (Metastron) versus external beam radiotherapy in patients with painful bone metastases from prostate cancer: preliminary report of a multicentre trial. *Semin Oncol* 1993;**20**(**Suppl 2**):32–33.

31 Porter AT, McEwan AJB. Strontium-89 as an adjuvant to external beam irradiation improves pain relief and delays disease progression in advanced prostate cancer: results of a randomized, controlled trial. *Semin Oncol* 1993;**20**(**Suppl 2**):38–43.

32 McEwan AJB, Amyotte GA, McGowan DG. A retrospective analysis of the cost-effectiveness of treatment with Metastron (Strontium-89) in patients with prostate cancer metastatic to bone. *Nuc Med Comm* 1994;**15**:499–504.

33 Robinson RG. Strontium-89-precursor targeted therapy for pain relief of blastic metastatic disease. *Cancer* 1993;**72**:3433–3435.

34 Benson RC, Gill GM. Estramustine phosphate compared with diethylstilbestrol. A randomized, double-blind, crossover trial for stage D cancer. *Am J Clinic Oncol* 1986;**9**:341–351.

35 Chisholm GD, O'Donoghue EPN, Kennedy CL. The treatment of oestrogen-escaped carcinoma of the prostate with estramustine phosphate. *Br J Urol* 1977;**49**:717–720.

36 Fosså SD, Miller A. Treatment of advanced carcinoma of the prostate with estramustine phosphate. *J Urol* 1976;**115**: 406–408.

37 Jönsson G, Högberg B, Nilsson T. Treatment of advanced prostatic carcinoma with estramustine phosphate. *Scan J Urol Nephrol* 1977;**11**:231–238.

38 Küss R, Khoury S, Richard F, *et al.* Estramustine

phosphate in the treatment of advanced prostatic cancer. *Br J Urol* 1980;**52**:29–33.

39 Leistenschneider W, Nagel R. Estracyt therapy of advanced prostatic cancer with special reference to control of therapy with cytology and DNA cytophotometry. *Eur Urol* 1980;**6**:111–115.

40 Lindberg B. Treatment of rapidly progressing prostatic carcinoma with Estracyt. *J Urol* 1972;**108**:303–306.

41 Mittelman A, Shukla SK, Murphy GP. Extended therapy of stage D carcinoma of the prostate with oral Estracyt. *J Urol* 1976;**115**:409–412.

42 Murphy GP, Gibbons RP, Johanson DE, *et al.* A comparison of estramustine phosphate and streptozotocin in patients with advanced prostatic carcinoma who have had extensive radiation. *J Urol* 1977;**118**:288–291.

43 Soloway MS, de Kernion JB, Gibbons RP, *et al.* Comparison of estramustine phosphate and vincristine alone or in combination for patients with advanced hormone refractory previously irradiated carcinoma of the prostate. *J Urol* 1981;**125**:664–667.

44 Soloway MS, Beckley S, Brady MF, *et al.* A comparison of estramustine phosphate versus cisplatinum alone versus estramustine phosphate plus cisplatinum in patients with advanced hormone refractory cancer who have had extensive irradiation to the pelvis or lumbosacral area. *J Urol* 1983;**129**:56–61.

45 Eisenberger M, Simon R, O'Dwyer P, *et al.* A re-evaluation of non-hormonal cytotoxic chemotherapy in the treatment of prostatic carcinoma. *J Clin Oncol* 1985;**3**:827–841.

46 Scott WW, Gibbons RP, Johnson DE, *et al.* The continued evaluation of the effects of chemotherapy in patients with advanced carcinoma of the prostate. *J Urol* 1976;**116**:211–213.

47 Murphy GP, Gibbons RP, Johnson DE, *et al.* A comparison of estramustine phosphate and streptozotocin in patients with prostatic carcinoma who had extensive irradiation. *J Urol* 1977;**118**:288–291.

48 Schmidt JD, Scott WW, Gibbons RP, *et al.* Comparison of procarbazine, imidazole-carbamide and cyclophosphamide in relapsing patients with advanced carcinoma of the prostate. *J Urol* 1979;**121**:185–189.

49 Loening SA, Scott WW, de Kernion JB, *et al.* A comparison of hydroxyurea, methyl-chlorohexyl-nitrosourea and cyclophosphamide in patients with advanced prostate cancer. *J Urol* 1981;**125**:812–816.

50 Soloway MS, de Kernion JB, Gibbons RP, *et al.* Comparison of estramustine phosphate and vincristine alone or in combination for patients with advanced hormone refractory previously irradiated carcinoma of the prostate. *J Urol* 1981;**125**:664–667.

51 Soloway M, Beckley S, Brady MF, *et al.* A comparison of estramustine phosphate, versus cis-platinum alone versus estramustine phosphate plus cis-platinum in patients with advanced hormone refractory prostate cancer who had extensive irradiation to the pelvis or lumbosacral area. *J Urol* 1983;**129**:56–61.

52 Eisenberger MA. Chemotherapy and palliation in prostate cancer. In: Prostate Cancer. Das S, Crawford ED (eds) Marcel Dekker; New York, 1993:380.

53 Crawford ED. The role of the urologist in chemotherapy of hormone refractory prostate cancer. *Urology* 1999;**54**:51–52.

Chapter 15

Sexual function

INTRODUCTION

Enormous advances have been made in the treatment of malignant diseases to the extent that surgery, chemotherapy, radiotherapy or a combination of these therapies can cure many. As a consequence patients' expectations for cure are rising. However, in many cases the radical nature of the therapies means that appreciable side-effects are inevitable. In all cases informed consent outlining the potential risks is crucial before commencing treatment. Some patients may consider the potential side-effects to be unacceptable and opt for less aggressive, but suboptimal alternatives that have fewer complications. Quality of life issues are becoming a more prominent consideration. In men who have prostate cancer the potential for sexual dysfunction is of considerable concern. The male population has an increasing life expectancy and improved health to the extent that many are now fit and active enough to engage in sexual activity well into their eighth decade and indeed expect this! Prostatic diseases and their treatments have a major impact on satisfactory sexual intercourse in the elderly male. Awareness of these problems is increasing and newer therapies are now available to minimize risks. Rapid recovery of sexual performance is still a problem with current neo-adjuvant therapies and is a concern for many patients. Agents in development allow a more rapid rise in testosterone after therapy cessation. This may translate to a more rapid return to sexual activity[1]. Sexual dysfunction can entail disturbance of libido, erectile function or ejaculation and fertility or a combination of these. These perturbations can have a major impact on the quality of life, not only of the patient but also of his partner.

ERECTILE DYSFUNCTION

Anatomy and Physiology of Normal Erection

Normal erectile function is dependent upon an unimpaired nerve supply, intact vascular supply to the corpora cavernosa (both arterial and venous), a normal libido and psychological factors. Penile erection results from coordinated neural and vascular processes, which culminate in an increased inflow of blood to the corpora cavernosa, dilatation of venous sinusoids within the penis and a reduction in corporal venous outflow.

Nerve plexuses play a central role in relaying the neurogenic stimuli for erection. Before 1982 the exact location of the branches of the pelvic plexus supplying the corpora cavernosa had not been traced in detail. Most of the branches are small and are difficult to dissect in the adult cadaver because they are encased in fibro-fatty tissue. Walsh and Donker traced their course by dissections in male fetuses and stillborn infants[2]. Their findings were later confirmed in adult cadavers[3].

The pelvic plexus is formed by parasympathetic visceral efferent preganglionic fibres (the nervi erigentes) arising from sacral segments S2, 3 and 4 and postganglionic sympathetic fibres arising from the thoracolumbar region (T11–L2) and travelling to the plexus via the hypogastric nerve. The parasympathetic fibres control erectile function while the sympathetic fibres play an important role in ejaculation. The plexus is a fenestrated rectangular structure situated in the sagittal plane that lies retroperitoneally on the lateral wall of the rectum 5–11 cm from the anal verge with its midpoint related to the tip of the seminal vesicle. Branches from the pelvic plexus innervate the rectum, bladder, prostate, seminal vesicles, urethra and corpora cavernosa. The bulk of the plexus is located lateral and posterior to the seminal vesicles. The cavernous branches travel from the plexus towards the posterolateral aspect of the base of the prostate, gradually coalescing from a group of fibres approximately 12 mm wide to a more organized bundle approximately 6 mm wide at the level of the prostate. At

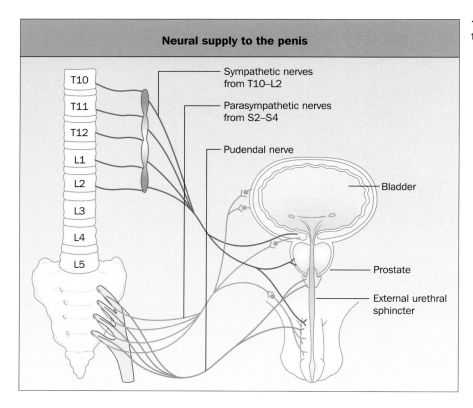

15.1 The innervation of the penis.

Neural supply to the penis

- Sympathetic nerves from T10–L2
- Parasympathetic nerves from S2–S4
- Pudendal nerve
- Bladder
- Prostate
- External urethral sphincter

T10, T11, T12, L1, L2, L3, L4, L5

this point, the cavernous nerves are travelling in association with the capsular arteries and veins of the prostate in the lateral pelvic fascia outside the prostatic capsule and outside Denonvillier's fascia. The association of nerve fibres with the capsular vessels of the prostate to constitute the neurovascular bundle therefore provides a macroscopic landmark for these microscopic nerves. From this position, the nerves ascend at the level of the apex of the prostate posterolateral to the urethra where they penetrate the urogenital diaphragm. The fibres then pass behind the dorsal penile artery and nerve before entering the corpora cavernosa[2–4] (**15.1**).

The arterial supply to the penis derives from the internal iliac arteries via the internal pudendal arteries. The two internal pudendal arteries terminate as the penile arteries, which divide to form the dorsal arteries, the cavernosal arteries (or deep arteries of the penis) and the bulbo-urethral arteries that supply the corpus spongiosum. The cavernosal arteries give off numerous branches called helical arteries that carry blood to the sinusoids of the erectile tissue. Although the corpora cavernosa receive their blood supply primarily from the internal pudendal artery,

supplementary blood supply can also arise from the obturator and inferior and superior vesical arteries[5] (**15.2**).

The venous drainage from the corpora cavernosa initially passes into emissary veins, which penetrate the tunica albuginea and join to form the deep dorsal

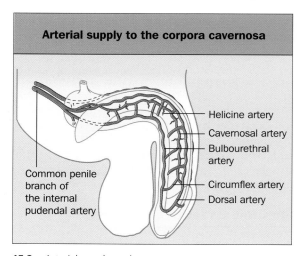

Arterial supply to the corpora cavernosa

- Helicine artery
- Cavernosal artery
- Bulbourethral artery
- Circumflex artery
- Dorsal artery

Common penile branch of the internal pudendal artery

15.2 Arterial supply to the corpora cavernosa.

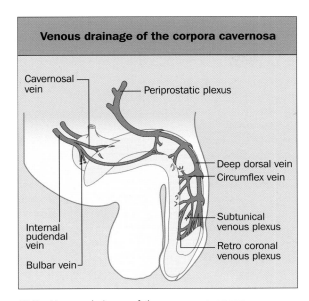

Venous drainage of the corpora cavernosa

Cavernosal vein

Periprostatic plexus

Deep dorsal vein

Circumflex vein

Internal pudendal vein

Subtunical venous plexus

Retro coronal venous plexus

Bulbar vein

15.3 Venous drainage of the corpora cavernosa.

vein. This vein penetrates the suspensory ligament before passing into the periprostatic venous plexus (**15.3**).

Prostate Cancer Treatments and Erectile Dysfunction

Normal erectile function may be disturbed in prostate cancer patients by a number of factors. The erectile nerves may be damaged during surgery, following external beam radiotherapy or late after brachytherapy and the resultant erectile dysfunction may be irreversible. Division of accessory arteries during surgery may impair the vascular supply to the penis and external beam radiotherapy may lead to endarteritis, both of which may lead to erectile dysfunction. Hormonal manipulation therapy for prostate cancer with luteinizing hormone-releasing hormone (LHRH) analogues suppresses sexual interest and commonly reduces libido and in the long term leads to shrinkage of the external genitalia, making sexual intercourse difficult. In addition, the patient's anxiety about his prostate cancer diagnosis can lead to psychogenic impotence[6]. The specific details of each of these causes of erectile dysfunction are outlined below.

Radical prostatectomy

Before 1982 radical prostatectomy was performed without any attempt at preservation of the neurovascular bundles. The erectile nerves were in-advertently damaged during apical dissection, during transection of the urethra, separation of the prostate from the rectum or division of the lateral pedicle[2,4,7,8]. In 1982, Walsh and Donker demonstrated that impotence, which frequently complicated radical prostatectomy, was secondary to injury to the branches of the pelvic plexus that innervate the corpora cavernosa[2]. They undertook detailed studies of the pelvic plexus and used the principles they derived to modify standard methods of radical prostatectomy. Walsh's nerve-sparing technique was designed to minimize the risk of such inadvertent damage. Anatomical knowledge is used to accurately identify the neurovascular bundles intra-operatively. The success of this manoeuvre relies upon the control of blood loss from the dorsal venous complex and Santorini's plexus allowing more precise visualization of the nerves. The anatomy of this vasculature was clarified in 1979 leading to changes in technique that minimized blood loss and improved surgical exposure[9]. The dorsal complex and Santorini's plexus are ligated as a primary manoeuvre. The urethra is then transected and the prostate is separated from the rectum in the midline. In contrast to the conventional approach, the neurovascular bundles are identified at this point, allowing the surgeon to determine whether the extent of the tumour mandates excision of the bundle or whether it can be preserved. If unilateral neurovascular bundle excision is necessary, it may be possible to preserve the contralateral bundle. When this technique is used, all structures can be visualized and a decision made as to whether they can be preserved or must be sacrificed for disease control[4]. One concern with nerve-sparing operations is that they might compromise cancer excision. Walsh's group have examined their surgical specimens since adopting the nerve-sparing approach and compared the findings on whole mount specimens with specimens removed by standard blunt dissection radical retropubic prostatectomy and perineal prostatectomy[7]. They concluded that less periprostatic tissue and skeletal muscle was removed with the perineal approach than either of the other techniques, but that none of the techniques appeared to compromise adequate removal of confined prostatic cancer. A subsequent examination of 100 nerve-sparing radical prostatectomies revealed that capsular penetration was present in 41%, but that only seven patients had positive surgical margins, all of whom had extensive extraprostatic disease[10].

In no case was the margin positive only at the site of the nerve-sparing modification. Further studies have also indicated that patients who have positive surgical margins tend to have extensive disease, often with seminal vesicle or lymph node involvement[11,12]. It is unlikely that surgery of any type will result in complete eradication of these tumours[8,11]. In one series, three patients had positive margins only at the site of the nerve-sparing modification that would probably have been avoided by excision of the neurovascular bundle[13]. It is not clear, however, what effect these positive margins have on long-term survival and recurrence rates. It is widely agreed that the nerve-sparing technique rarely compromises cancer control. It has been claimed that precise identification of the neurovascular bundle with wide excision when necessary may allow more extensive resection than blunt dissection[4].

Potency is generally defined as the ability to achieve an erection sufficient for vaginal penetration and orgasm. The best results for potency after radical prostatectomy have been reported by Walsh and associates with overall potency rates of 68% among men potent pre-operatively[14]. Other groups such as Geary and colleagues report potency rates of only 13.3% for unilateral nerve-sparing procedures and 31.9% for bilateral nerve sparing[13]. Results of other series are shown in **Table 15.1**. Therefore, although rates of recovery of erectile function are better than with non-nerve-sparing techniques, the morbidity in terms of sexual function is not inconsiderable.

A number of other factors affect the risk of impotence following radical prostatectomy. The most important factor in determining preservation of potency is the number of neurovascular bundles injured. Potency rates are reported as 31.9–76% for bilateral nerve-sparing procedures, 13.3–60% for unilateral nerve-sparing procedures and 0–1.1% for non-nerve-sparing procedures[13,14].

The tumour stage is also related to post-operative potency[13-16]. In one series, patients who were potent post-operatively were much more likely to have tumour volumes less than 3 cc and no potent patient had positive lymph nodes or involved seminal vesicles[13]. However, because stage determines the extent of surgery required for tumour excision, it is not an independent predictor of outcome. For example, in one series, only 9% of patients in whom it was possible to spare both neurovascular bundles presented with clinical stage B2 or C disease compared with 51% of those for whom unilateral excision of the neurovascular bundle was required[14].

It is generally agreed that younger patients fare considerably better in terms of post-operative potency than their older counterparts[13-16]. It has been reported that men less than 50 years of age tolerate unilateral neurovascular bundle excision with similar potency rates to those with bilateral nerve-sparing procedures (90% potency). In older men, however, excision of one neurovascular bundle significantly reduces the percentage of patients having erections sufficient for intercourse[14]. It may be relevant that patients in Walsh's series are on average 5 years younger than those from other

Table 15.1 Risk factors for erectile dysfunction after radical prostatectomy

Series	Catalona & Basler[15]	Drago et al.[16]	Geary et al.[13]	Quinlan et al.[14]
Mean age (years)	64	64	64	59
No. of patients evaluated for potency (total no.)	295 (522)	151 (528)	459 (481)	503 (600)
Post-operative potency with nerve sparing (%)	Bilateral 63 Unilateral 41	66	Bilateral 32 Unilateral 13 None 1	Bilateral 76 Unilateral 60 None 0
Factors influencing potency	Age Stage	Age Tumour volume Frequency of intercourse pre-operatively	Age Stage Number of nerves spared	Age Stage Number of nerves spared

centres and this may be one factor in the high potency rates achieved by this group[14]. Patients in whom potency recovers post-operatively are more often sexually active pre-operatively, even when the higher prevalence of sexual activity in younger men is accounted for[13].

There are aspects of erectile dysfunction following radical prostatectomy that are not completely explained by nerve damage. Some patients do not respond to intracavernosal papaverine injection post-operatively[17], suggesting that there may be a vasculogenic component. It has been suggested that division of accessory arteries during radical prostatectomy may compromise arterial supply to the corpora, particularly in older patients who are more likely to have atherosclerotic disease of the internal pudendal vessels. One study has examined the influence of preservation of accessory pudendal arteries on return of sexual function[18]. Accessory arteries amenable to preservation were present in only 4% of patients undergoing radical prostatectomy, but preservation had no effect on potency rates. It is more likely that vasculogenic impotence following radical prostatectomy is due to division of arterial branches running beneath the anterior capsule of the prostate, which are visible following division of the dorsal complex. These vessels are not amenable to preservation and may represent a collateral arterial supply to the penis[18]. The authors have encountered a small number of patients in whom the quality of erections has improved following radical retropubic prostatectomy (unpublished data). These patients probably had a degree of venous leakage pre-operatively that was improved by ligation of penile veins during the procedure.

Most patients who regain potency after radical prostatectomy recover within 6–12 months[13], although improvement can continue for up to 2 years postoperatively. Patients who have undergone excision of one neurovascular bundle lag behind those who have a bilateral nerve-sparing operation[14]. Although patients may retain erections sufficient for vaginal penetration they many notice a definite change in the quality of their erections after surgery which can be associated with reduced sexual satisfaction[13,15]. Geary and associates found that less than half of their patients defined as potent on the basis of erections sufficient for vaginal penetration were satisfied with their erections or achieved intercourse at least once a month[13]. In general, when patients are asked in person about their sexual function, satisfaction rates are lower than those reported in physician-based studies[13,19]. It is therefore probably misleading to offer the average prostate cancer patient undergoing radical prostatectomy a greater than 50% chance of retaining normal potency, even with the use of the Cavermap™ intra-operative nerve stimulation device.

Transurethral prostatectomy

Erectile dysfunction occurs in up to 16% of men undergoing transurethral resection of the prostate (TURP)[20]. The aetiology of post-TURP impotence is not absolutely clear. It is, however, likely that the cavernous nerves and arteries are damaged by perforation of the prostatic capsule, extravasation of irrigant solution or injudicious electrocautery of the capsule, particularly at the apices. Men who have previously undergone radiotherapy or cryotherapy to the prostate for localized prostate cancer have an even greater risk of erectile dysfunction after TURP. Other causes of erectile dysfunction are of course common among the elderly men who constitute the majority of TURP patients.

Radiation therapy

Irradiation of the prostate for cancer by external beam radiotherapy, conformal radiotherapy or interstitial seeds (brachytherapy) can all lead to erectile dysfunction. The aetiology in these men has been shown on pharmacocavernosometry to be a result of arterial insufficiency, which is presumed to be due to endarteritis obliterans, although damage to the erectile nerves is also a factor. There is an increased risk of erectile dysfunction in older men, smokers, hypertensives and diabetics[21]. A prospective study of 289 men undergoing external beam radiotherapy for prostate cancer has shown that 62% of those who were potent before treatment remained potent at 12 months. At 24 months this figure reduced further to 41%[22]. In general conformal radiotherapy appears to have a better side-effect profile than traditional external beam radiotherapy. However, only 62% of men have been shown to have a return of normal erectile function after this treatment[23].

There has been a recent resurgence of interest in interstitial radioisotope seed radiotherapy (or brachytherapy) and the technology for insertion of the seeds is rapidly improving (see Chapter 11). A series of 92 men who had clinical stage T1–T2 disease and transperineal insertion of iodine-125 seeds have undergone follow-up for up to 3 years.

Of the 56 men who were potent before treatment 85% retained satisfactory potency at 3 years[24]. There has also been some recent interest in high-dose combination radiotherapy, which entails insertion of radioisotope seeds followed by a course of external beam radiotherapy. Out of a series of 212 men who had clinical stage T1–T3 prostate cancer who underwent combination therapy using external beam radiotherapy at a dose of 45 Gy, 100 were potent before treatment and of these 62% retained potency[25]. Of all the treatment modalities available for localized prostate cancer brachytherapy appears to carry the lowest risk of treatment-induced erectile dysfunction.

Cryotherapy

In some centres there has been an interest in the use of cryotherapy for localized prostate cancer. Erectile dysfunction following cryotherapy was initially thought to be a consequence of nerve and vascular injury. In an early series 65% of men developed impotence after a course of cryotherapy[26]. In a study of 15 sexually active men who underwent cryotherapy for clinically localized prostate cancer nine (60%) had erectile dysfunction 6 months after treatment, and colour Doppler studies suggested that vascular injury was the major aetiological factor[27]. Another study of 90 non-radiated men treated by cryosurgery for prostate cancer revealed erectile dysfunction at 18 months in 88% of the 74 men who had normal erections before treatment. It appears that the vascular injury caused by cryotherapy leads to a high risk of impotence, above that experienced with other therapies for localized prostate cancer.

Hormonal Therapies

The aim of endocrine therapy for prostate cancer is to suppress the production of androgens, particularly testosterone, and therefore this therapy almost inevitably leads to sexual dysfunction. Castration, historically the original therapy for advanced prostate cancer, leads to a reduction in libido, lethargy, gynaecomastia and depression in many cases. However, some castrated men are still able to have erections and their sexual function may be maintained by the effect of androgens derived from the adrenal glands. Castration is no longer often employed as a treatment for prostate cancer and has been largely superseded by drug therapies in the form of depot injections or oral medication. The LHRH agonists

leuprolide acetate and goserelin acetate are administered as depot injections lasting 1 month or 3 months according to strength. These agents reduce the testosterone to castrate levels and in doing so induce a loss of interest in sex and impotence in the majority of men.

In addition, maximal androgen blockade – a combination of an LHRH agonist (or castration) and an oral anti-androgen – leads to a complete loss of interest in sex and impotence by suppressing androgenic stimulation from both the testes and adrenals. Combined therapy with goserelin acetate and cyproterone acetate has been reported to lead to a loss of libido and impotence in 86% of men[28]. Preservation of normal sexual function features high on the list of quality of life issues for men. In a quality of life study of 230 patients a significant number were prepared to trade a 14% survival advantage for normal sexual function[29]. It would therefore be distinctly advantageous to have a treatment option for men who have advanced prostate cancer that preserves sexual function. Monotherapy with bicalutamide 150 mg/day has been shown to produce a loss of sexual interest in 23% of men compared with 47% of men treated by castration without resulting in a significant difference in long-term survival (in press). Therefore bicalutamide may prove to be a preferable treatment option for men who have advanced prostate cancer who wish to preserve their libido and sexual function providing that they do not have demonstrable bone metastases.

Treatment of Erectile Dysfunction

Most patients who have erectile dysfunction following prostate surgery usually respond well to standard treatments, especially if the impotence is primarily neurogenic. Intracavernosal injections, intraurethral prostaglandin pellet insertion, oral sildenafil citrate and vacuum devices are the most popular modalities. The insertion of penile prostheses is an option for selected patients who have failed to respond to more conservative treatments.

A variety of agents can be used for intracavernosal injection therapy. They can be broadly divided into phosphodiesterase inhibitors such as papaverine, alpha-adrenergic receptor blockers such as phenoxybenzamine and prazosin and prostaglandin E_1 (PGE_1) agents such as alprostadil. There is some evidence that early treatment (starting 1 month after radical prostatectomy) with intracavernosal alprostadil injection results in an improved potency

---

Intracavernosal injection of prostaglandin E₁

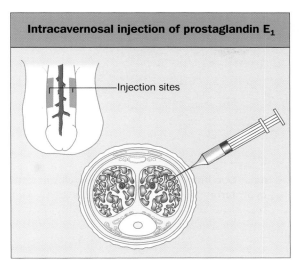

Injection sites

15.4 Intracavernosal injection of prostaglandin E₁.

rate³⁰. It is thought that PGE₁ maintains cavernous oxygenation and avoids hypoxia-induced damage to erectile tissue, which can subsequently impair erectile function. Intracavernosal injection of alprostadil will produce an erectile response in 75% or more of men who suffer from erectile dysfunction following prostate surgery (**15.4**). Transurethral alprostadil therapy with the *medicated urethral system for erection (MUSE)* is well tolerated with few side effects. In one study of 384 radical prostatectomy patients who had erectile dysfunction 70.3% of men were able to achieve an erection sufficient for sexual intercourse with MUSE therapy³¹ (**15.5**). Similar results have been reported with

---

Intraurethral therapy with PGE₁

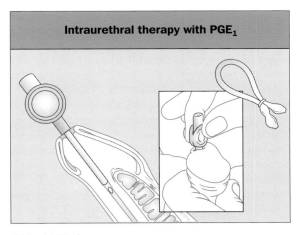

15.5 MUSE therapy.

Mechanism of action of sildenafil

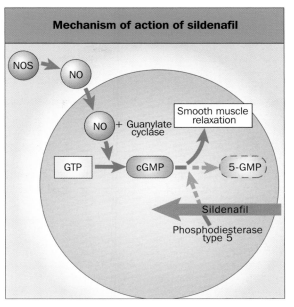

15.6 Mechanism of action of sildenafil. 5-GMP, 5-'guanosine monophosphate; cGMP, cyclic guanosine monophosphate; GTP, guanosine triphosphate; NO, nitric oxide; NOS, nitric oxide synthase.

the oral agent sildenafil citrate (Viagra™). In a study of 15 men who had erectile dysfunction following bilateral nerve-sparing radical prostatectomy 80% had a positive response to oral sildenafil citrate (**15.6**). Those in whom both the erectile nerves had been sacrificed had a poor response³².

In the future, other treatments for erectile dysfunction in prostate cancer are likely to become available. One possibility is intraoperative reconstruction of damaged cavernous nerves using a genitofemoral nerve interposition graft. This technique has been successfully used in rats to restore erectile function following surgical damage to the neurovascular bundle³³. Inhibitors of lipid peroxidation, which is probably an important mediator of cavernous nerve dysfunction following crushing injury, are also being investigated in the rat to determine whether prophylactic administration of these agents might have a useful role in preventing operative neural damage³⁴.

EJACULATORY DYSFUNCTION

Anatomy and Physiology of Normal Ejaculation

Erectile function, which has been comprehensively described above, is clearly an important issue when

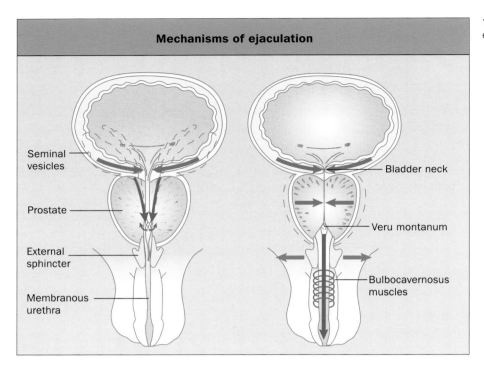

Mechanisms of ejaculation

Seminal vesicles

Prostate

External sphincter

Membranous urethra

Bladder neck

Veru montanum

Bulbocavernosus muscles

15.7 Mechanisms of ejaculations.

considering ejaculatory dysfunction. However, the neural pathways subserving ejaculation are to a large extent separate from those leading to erection. Ejaculation or antegrade emission of spermatic fluid is brought about by stimulation via the sympathetic nervous system leading to contraction of smooth muscle of the bladder neck, prostate, seminal vesicles, urethra and vas deferens (**15.7**).

Anorgasmia or loss of ejaculation rarely occurs as a congenital problem or can arise secondary to drug treatments (particularly with alpha-adrenoceptor blockers), diabetic autonomic neuropathy or psychological problems. However, the commonest cause of loss of ejaculation is surgical damage at some step in the pathway. The general urologist is most aware of this phenomenon following TURP. However, open surgical procedures, particularly those within the retroperitoneum and pelvis may also lead to sympathetic nerve fibre damage. The sympathetic nerve fibres thought to be most important in stimulating ejaculation arise from the upper three or four lumbar sympathetic ganglia. The post-ganglionic fibres decussate anterior to the aorta and begin to merge just distal to the inferior mesenteric artery before passing distally to form the hypogastric nerve plexus just inferior to the bifurcation of the

aorta. The post-ganglionic fibres from the right side pass behind the inferior vena cava and emerge into the inter-aortocaval groove close to the left-sided lumbar veins before passing anteriorly over the aorta. In some cases the nerve fibres and ganglia, particularly L2/3, may appear to be merged together. From the hypogastric plexus nerve fibres pass distally to innervate the smooth muscle comprising the ejaculatory mechanism at the bladder neck, prostatic urethra, seminal vesicles and proximal vas deferens. At the time of orgasm and ejaculation the sympathetic nerve fibres stimulate contraction of smooth muscle within the ejaculatory apparatus and hence antegrade egress of seminal fluid.

Ejaculatory Dysfunction after Prostate Surgery

The most frequently encountered complication of prostatic surgery is disturbance of normal ejaculation. Patients should be pre-warned of this complication before surgery. Transurethral incision of the prostate leads to retrograde ejaculation in 38.8%, TURP causes retrograde ejaculation in 70.4% and open enucleative surgical procedures for benign prostatic hyperplasia is associated with retrograde ejaculation in 80.8% of men[20]. It is possible to retrieve sperm from the urine of patients who have retrograde ejaculation after prostatic surgery with a view for artificial insemination. After radical prostatectomy for prostate cancer normal ejaculation is not possible and all patients are rendered infertile. This should be explained to all patients pre-operatively because a small proportion may wish to store sperm. Ability to achieve orgasm is usually preserved and some men do notice emission of some fluid with orgasm – this is most likely to derive from bulbo-urethral glands. The quality of orgasm following radical prostatectomy has been less widely studied. In informal surveys, Geary and colleagues noted that only 10% of patients (regardless of potency) reported decreased orgasmic sensation[13]. This is important in that it makes these patients ideal candidates for intra-cavernosal injection therapy, MUSE therapy, sildenafil, vacuum devices or penile prostheses (**15.8**). However, in a study from the Netherlands, which was based on a semi-structured interview and a self-administered questionnaire, the majority of men experienced a change in orgasmic sensation after radical prostatectomy. From the patients interviewed 50% complained that orgasmic sensation was weakened and 64% suffered involuntary loss of urine at orgasm, but all but one were completely continent at other times. This caused half of these men to avoid sexual contact. Diminished

libido was also common[35]. The pathophysiology of these changes in orgasmic sensation is poorly understood, but may relate to the unavoidable excision of small nerve fibres surrounding the prostate and seminal vesicles.

Treatment of Ejaculatory Dysfunction

Loss of ejaculation after prostate surgery is of concern to some patients who worry that accumulation of spermatic fluid may lead to serious consequences. In the majority of cases simple reassurance is all that is needed. A number of treatments have been used in an attempt to correct post-TURP loss of ejaculation with variable success rates. Alpha-adrenoceptor agonists such as phenylpropanolamine hydrochloride and ephedrine sulphate have been used to stimulate bladder neck contraction. Electro-ejaculation, in which pulsed electrical current is applied to the periprostatic plexus, successfully induces ejaculation in 75% of patients. Sperm may be harvested from the specimens obtained for intrauterine insemination[36].

CONCLUSIONS

Greater understanding of the pelvic neuroanatomy has led to a reduction in the sexual morbidity of prostate surgery. Although eradication of prostate cancer remains of paramount importance, it is now possible to preserve sexual function in many patients without compromising disease control. Refinements in surgical technique have been matched by comparable improvements in the treatment of erectile dysfunction so that men now have a reasonable chance of either retaining or regaining potency after prostate surgery. In the treatment of advanced disease the use of antiandrogen monotherapy with Casodex™ 150 mg has been shown to preserve sexual interest and potency in a proportion of patients while still producing results equivalent to those of orchiectomy or luteinizing hormone-releasing hormone analogues. Loss of ejaculation and infertility is a less important issue in the age group of men who have prostate cancer. It is now possible to retrieve sperm using a variety of techniques, before or after surgery in the few men in this age group who wish to father children.

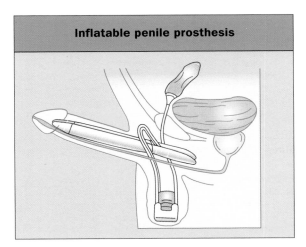

Inflatable penile prosthesis

15.8   Inflatable penile prosthesis.

REFERENCES

1 Garnick MB, Gittleman M, Steidle C, *et al*. Abarelix (PPI-149), a novel and potent GnRH antagonist, induces rapid and profound prostate gland volume reduction (PGVR) and androgen suppression before brachytherapy (BT) or radiation therapy (XRT). *J Urol* 1998;**159**:220.

2 Walsh PC, Donker PJ. Impotence following radical prostatectomy: insight into etiology and prevention. *J Urol* 1982;**128**:492–497.

3 Lepor H, Gregerman M, Crosby R, *et al*. Precise localization of the autonomic nerves from the pelvic plexus to the corpora-cavernosa: a detailed anatomical study of the adult male pelvis. *J Urol* 1985;**133**:207–212.

4 Walsh PC, Schlegel PN. Radical pelvic surgery with preservation of sexual function. *Ann Surg* 1988;**208**:391–400.

5 Breza J, Aboseif SR, Orvis BR, Lue TF, Tanagho EA. Detailed anatomy of penile neurovascular structures: surgical significance. *J Urol* 1989;**141**:437–443.

6 Schover LR. Sexual rehabilitation after treatment for prostate cancer. *Cancer* 1993;**71**:1024–1030.

7 Walsh PC, Lepor H, Egglestone JC. Radical prostatectomy with preservation of sexual function: anatomical and pathological considerations. *Prostate* 1983;**4**:473–485.

8 Walsh PC, Epstein JI, Lowe F. Potency following radical prostatectomy with wide unilateral excision of the neurovascular bundle. *J Urol* 1987;**138**:823–827.

9 Reiner WG, Walsh PC. An anatomical approach to the surgical management of the dorsal vein and Santorini's plexus during radical retropubic surgery. *J Urol* 1979;**121**:198–200.

10 Egglestone JC, Walsh PC. Radical prostatectomy with preservation of sexual function: pathological findings in the first 100 cases. *J Urol* 1985;**134**:1146–1148.

11 Catalona WJ, Dresner SM. Nerve-sparing radical prostatectomy: extraprostatic tumour extension and preservation of erectile function. *J Urol* 1985;**134**:1149–1151.

12 Wahle SM, Reznicek MJ, Fallon B, *et al*. Incidence of surgical margin involvement with various forms of radical prostatectomies. *Urology* 1990;**36**:23–26.

13 Geary ES, Dendinger TE, Freiha FS, Stamey TA. Nerve sparing radical prostatectomy: a different view. *J Urol* 1995;**154**:145–149.

14 Quinlan DM, Epstein JI, Carter BS, Walsh PC. Sexual function following radical prostatectomy: influence of preservation of neurovascular bundles. *J Urol* 1991;**145**:998–1002.

15 Catalona WJ, Basler JW. Return of erections and urinary continence following nerve sparing radical retropubic prostatectomy. *J Urol* 1993;**150**:905–907.

16 Drago JR, Badalement RA, York JP, *et al*. Radical prostatectomy: OSU and affiliated hospitals' experience 1985–1989. *Urology* 1992;**39**:44–47.

17 Bahnson RR, Catalona WJ. Papaverine testing of patients following nerve sparing radical prostatectomy. *J Urol* 1988;**139**:773–774.

18 Polascik TJ Walsh PC. Radical retropubic prostatectomy: the influence of accessory pudendal arteries on the recovery of sexual function. *J Urol* 1995;**153**:150–152.

19 Fowler FJ Jr, Barry MJ, Lu-Yao G, *et al*. Patient-reported complications and follow-up treatment after radical prostatectomy. The national Medicare experience: 1988–1990 (updated June 1993). *Urology* 1993;**42**:622–629.

20 Roehrborn C. Standard surgical interventions. In: *Textbook of Benign Prostatic Hyperplasia*. Oxford: Isis Medical Media; 1996:341–378.

21 Goldstein I, Feldman M, Deckers PJ, Krane RJ. Radiation associated impotence – a clinical study of its mechanism. *JAMA* 1984;**1251**:9031–9036.

22 Turner SL, Adams K, Bull CA, Berry MP. Sexual dysfunction after radical radiation therapy for prostate cancer. *Urology* 1999;**54**:124–129.

23 Roach MI, Chinn DM, Holland J, Clarke M. A pilot study of sexual function and quality of life following 3D conformal radiotherapy for clinically localised prostate cancer. *Int J Radiat Oncol Biol Phys* 1996;**35**:869–874.

24 Wallner KE, Roy J, Harrison L. Tumour control and morbidity following transperineal iodine 125 implantation for stage T1/T2 prostatic carcinoma. *Int J Radiat Oncol Biol Phys* 1996;**14**:449–453.

25 Zeitlin SI, Sherman J, Raboy A, Lederman G, Albert P. High dose combination radiotherapy for the treatment of localized prostate cancer. *J Urol* 1998;**160**:91–96.

26 Onik G, Cohen JK, Reyes GD, Rubinsky B, Change Z, Baust J. Trans-rectal ultrasound guided percutaneous radical cryosurgical ablation of the prostate. *Cancer* 1993;**72**:1291–9.

27 Abosief S, Shinohara K, Borirakchanyavat S, Deirmenjian J, Carroll PR. The effect of cryosurgical ablation of the prostate on erectile function. *Br J Urol* 1997;**80**:918–922.

28 DiSilverio F, Serio M, D'Erano G. Zoladex vs Zoladex plus cyproterone acetate in the treatment of advanced prostatic cancer. A multi-centre Italian study. *Eur Urol* 1990;**18**:54–61.

29 Mazur DJ, Hickman DH. Patient preferences. Survival versus quality of life considerations. *J Gen Int Med* 1993;**8**:374–377.

30 Montorsi F, Guazzoni G, Barbieri L, *et al*. Recovery of spontaneous erectile function after nerve sparing radical prostatectomy with and without early intracavernous injections of prostaglandin E_1: results of a prospective randomized trial. *J Urol* 1996;**155** (**Suppl**):468A.

31 Costabile RA, Spevak M, Fishman IJ, *et al*. Efficacy and safety of transurethral alprostadil in patients with erectile dysfunction following radical prostatectomy. *J Urol* 1998;**160**:1325–1328.

32 Zippe CD, Kedia AW, Kedia K, Nelson DR, Agarwal A. Treatment of erectile dysfunction after radical

prostatectomy with sildenafil citrate (Viagra). *Urology* 1998;**52**:963–966.

33 Quinlan DM, Nelson RJ, Walsh PC. Cavernous nerve grafts restore erectile function in denervated rats. *J Urol* 1991;**145**:380–383.

34 Karakiewicz PI, Bazinet M, Zvara P, *et al*. Inhibitors of lipid peroxidation may successfully reduce impotence following radical prostatectomy: a rat model. *J Urol* 1996;**155** (**Suppl**):617A.

35 Koeman M, van Driel MF, Schultz WC, Mensink HJ. Orgasm after radical prostatectomy. *Br J Urol* 1996;**77**:861–864.

36 Brindley GS. Electroejaculation: its technique, neurological implications and uses. *J Neurol Neurosurg Psychiatr* 1981;**44**:9–14.

Chapter 16

Reasons to be cheerful

Although at first sight some of the statistics may seem depressing, there are in fact many reasons to feel increasingly optimistic about the future prospects for sufferers of prostate cancer.

EARLIER DETECTION

Awareness about prostate cancer, among both the general public and health-care professionals, has risen steeply over the past few years: a 'Cinderella subject' up to the 1980s, prostatic diseases have recently become a favourite topic of conversation of men over 50 as well as their wives and families. In the USA and Europe, the media have developed an almost obsessive interest in the subject, and this fixation, which has already resulted in increased health-care seeking behaviour by men beyond middle age, is now being translated into earlier clinical detection in clinical practice – the 'stage migration' so frequently emphasized in previous chapters. However, while this potentially provides the means of achieving cure in many more patients, the possibility of over-treatment of men whose cancers were destined never to become clinically significant still remains a matter of some concern. These issues will only be resolved by randomized studies.

BETTER FUNDING FOR RESEARCH

New-found public interest in prostate cancer has also resulted in a recent increase in resources for clinical research, although this remains only a small proportion of the funds directed towards other major cancer killers, such as breast, lung and colonic carcinoma. The traditional explanation for the parsimony of governmental and research-body funding for prostate cancer has been the unimpressive number of average life years – around nine – lost due to the disease. However, as pointed out in Chapter 2, as the disease is so common, the cumulative loss of life years due to prostate cancer is third among all cancers; those nine twilight years at jeopardy in the later decades of life are also often considered *the* most precious by both the patients and their loved ones, and now the more elderly segment of society is becoming more vocal about its right to medical care.

The increased awareness surrounding the clinical aspects of prostate cancer has also resulted in an increase in funding for basic research which is now yielding significant rewards. The disease area has attracted the attention of experts other than urologists, and many more players have recently become involved – family practitioners, biostatisticians, epidemiologists, health economy and policy analysts all now contribute expertise and opinions. Although their views may sometimes be difficult to reconcile with those of urologists – the group who predominantly provide actual care to the patients – new perspectives on cost:benefit ratios of various treatment options and economic modelling can only enhance our understanding of the socio-economic impact of this very prevalent disease.

The trend towards detection of earlier stage prostate cancer in the USA has become most marked since 1987, the year when widespread prostate-specific antigen (PSA) testing became available. Since then, there has been a rapid rise in the number of transrectal biopsies undertaken (**16.1**), and therefore a rise in the number of potentially curable prostate cancers diagnosed, as well as the number of curative procedures performed (**16.2**), such as radical prostatectomies. The question remains open as to whether all of this activity will eventually translate into a reduction in the mortality of prostate cancer. Patients with metastatic disease are already reported to be becoming less often seen in everyday urological practice, at least in the USA, and prostate cancer mortality has recently declined by 7% in the States.

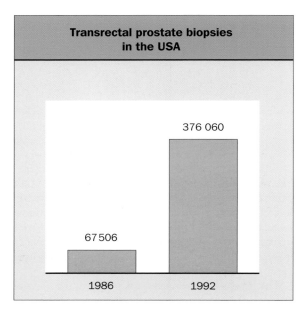

16.1 The rising number of TRUS-guided biopsies in the USA between 1986 and 1992. (Medicare data kindly supplied by L Holtgrewe.)

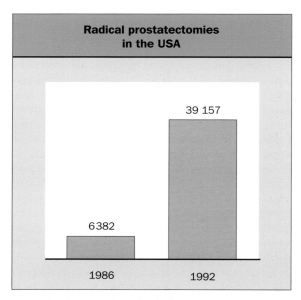

16.2 The rising number of radical prostatectomies performed in the USA. (Medicare data kindly supplied by L Holtgrewe.)

MORE ACCURATE DIAGNOSIS

While PSA testing carries indisputable potential for the earlier diagnosis of prostate cancer, it also carries the drawback of a significant incidence of false positive results. Since transrectal ultrasound imaging does not reliably identify every small focus of cancer, effectively every individual testing positive (PSA >4.0 ng/ml) is likely to require transrectal ultrasound-guided biopsy to rule out cancer. Around 15% of screened populations of men over 50 years test PSA-positive, but only 2–5% prove positive in fact on biopsy. Thus, between two-thirds and four-fifths of men will be worried that they *may* have cancer until the biopsy result is known (the psychological effects and sequelae of this period of anxiety are unknown), and perhaps 3% of those testing false positive and undergoing biopsy will suffer significant morbidity from the procedure (such as sepsis or bleeding). However, the near future holds the promise of more specific PSA tests. New assays based on differentiating free-PSA from complexed-PSA, significantly reduce the incidence of false positive testing[1].

Since serum PSA levels show a tendency to rise with age, a given individual screened by PSA testing will be more likely to test positive simply by virtue of being older. While the incidence of prostate cancer also rises steeply with age, it is probably more important to diagnose the disease in younger men because their greater life expectancy gives them more years 'at risk' of developing disease progression and metastases. These considerations have led Oesterling *et al.*[2] to advocate age-adjustment of PSA cut-offs (**Table 16.1**) based on the 95-percentile values for PSA in a population of men *without* prostate cancer.

Another promising avenue is the extra information available from sequential PSA determinations – or the so-called 'PSA slope'. Carter *et al.* compared serial PSA values in individuals with benign prostatic hyperplasia, prostate cancer and controls,

Table 16.1 Age-specific reference ranges for PSA as suggested by Oesterling	
Age (years)	**Upper limit of serum PSA (ng/ml)**
40–49	2.5
50–59	3.5
60–69	4.5
70–79	6.5

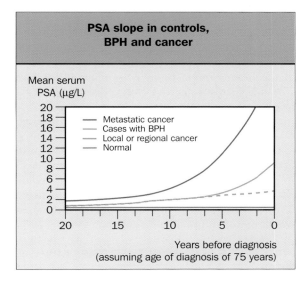

16.3 Annualized PSA rise in a small series of controls, patients with BPH and those with prostate cancer. (Reproduced with permission from Carter HB, *et al*. Longitudinal evaluation of prostate-specific antigen levels in men with and without prostate disease. *JAMA* 1992;**267**:2215–2220.)

and reported that an annualized PSA rise of more than 0.75 ng/ml was associated with a diagnosis of cancer (**16.3**). In his ongoing study of PSA screening, Brawer[3] reported a diagnosis of prostate cancer in 17% of those men whose PSA increased by more than 20% over one year. Other promising serum markers include human kallikrein 2 (Hk2) and insulin-like growth factor (IGF-2).

ENHANCED PROGNOSTIC INDICATORS

As previously emphasized, the central issue in prostate cancer management is deciding clinically which lesions should be managed conservatively, and which require more aggressive therapy. Although Gleason scoring and tumour-volume estimation give a reasonable indication of subsequent tumour behaviour, molecular biological markers seem to hold the promise of more accurate prognostic information. Already, E-cadherin estimation appears to correlate with subsequent metastatic potential[4], and a host of other markers (see Chapter 2) are currently being evaluated in this context. It appears to be only a matter of time before we will be in a position to prognosticate the future behaviour of a given prostate cancer much more accurately, and thereby balance the risks of tumour progression

against the probabilities of demise due to other comorbid conditions, before advising a specific form of therapy.

Evolving molecular biological techniques should also permit the identification of those individuals at particular risk of prostate cancer because of a familial tendency. Linkage analysis on the chromosomal configurations of groups of individuals with a strong family history of prostate cancer have already resulted in the identification of two 'prostate cancer genes', analogous to the 'breast cancer gene' already characterized[5] (see Chapter 4). Individuals carrying a susceptibility gene (or more plausibly suffering from a particular tumour-suppressor gene deletion) would be obvious candidates for close surveillance, early biopsy and therapy before extracapsular extension and metastatic progression occur.

Better Staging

One of the more potent arguments against the use of radical prostatectomy for the management of localized prostate cancer has been the historically high (30–40%) positive margin rate. These patients are at high risk of subsequent disease recurrence and would, in most cases, probably be better managed by alternative, less invasive, forms of therapy. New imaging technology, employing endorectal magnetic resonance imaging coils and gadolinium enhancement, microbubble technology and three-dimensional transrectal imaging, as well as developments such as radioisotopes attached to prostate cancer-seeking compounds, now hold the prospect of more accurate tumour volume estimation and staging information. This should eventually translate into more effective patient selection for curative procedures.

Identification of Micrometastases with Polymerase Chain Reaction Technology

Currently, one of the greatest drawbacks in accurately staging prostate cancer is the inability to detect the prevalence of systemic micrometastases. It is not until metastases reach a certain critical size that they can be identified with imaging such as radionuclide bone scanning. This being the case, a number of patients are treated for disease that is assumed to be localized at a stage when, in fact, micrometastases have occurred and more systemic forms of therapy are appropriate. The recent advent of polymerase chain reaction (PCR) technology may have provided the means whereby these micrometastases can be identified (**16.4**).

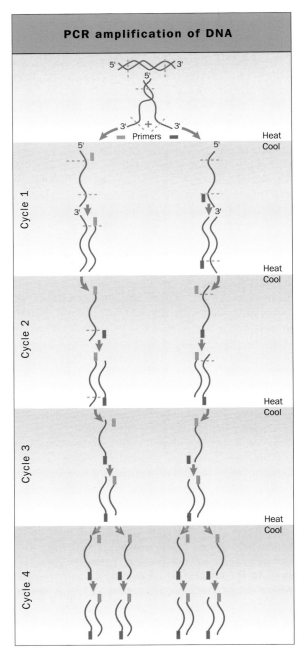

PCR amplification of DNA

Cycle 1 · Cycle 2 · Cycle 3 · Cycle 4

Primers — Heat/Cool

16.4 Polymerase chain reaction (PCR) amplification of a DNA segment can be used to detect PSA producing cells outside the prostate.

PCR technology allows the amplification of tiny amounts of either DNA or RNA. In the normal individual, transcription of the portion of the DNA that encodes prostate specific antigen for messenger RNA, and subsequently PSA, should be confined to epithelial cells of the prostate. The finding, therefore, of tiny amounts of mRNA for PSA either in the blood stream or in bone marrow aspirate would be highly suggestive of the presence of micrometastases of prostate-cancer tumour cells.

As mentioned in the earlier chapter on staging, early studies were very promising[7,8].

Unfortunately, other workers have to date not been able to reproduce these preliminary findings[9]. In particular PCR testing for PSA did not correlate with subsequent PSA relapse after radical prostatectomy[10]. More work is currently ongoing is this area which has obvious clinical potential.

PROSPECTS FOR IMPROVED THERAPY

The treatment options for patients with prostate cancer will undoubtedly continue to expand and improve. In expert hands, the incontinence rate within 6 months of radical prostatectomy should now be less than 3%, potency may be preserved in many younger men, and post-operative mortality should be exceedingly uncommon. Technical improvements in surgical technique – for example, with the development of an automatic anastomotic 'gun' or laparoscopic prostatectomy – could conceivably reduce the incontinence rate to virtually zero. A recent series of 3170 radical prostatectomies from the Mayo Clinic reported a mortality rate of only 0.3%[11].

Radiotherapy for prostate cancer is also likely to become more effective. Conformal techniques already permit better localization of tumoricidal doses to the prostate, thus reducing morbidity due to the involvement of adjacent structures (**16.5**)[12]. Early reports suggest that development of new modalities of radiation therapy, such as fast-neutron treatment generated using cyclotron technology, may enhance tumoricidal activity without significantly increasing side-effects[13]. Brachytherapy has already been discussed in detail in Chapter 11.

Pharmacotherapy

Many of the potential therapeutic advances that offer the best prospects for future sufferers of prostate cancer are pharmacological. As already discussed, maximal androgen blockade seems, at least in a subset of patients, to hold a small but significant advantage over monotherapy with luteinizing hormone-releasing hormone (LHRH) analogues.

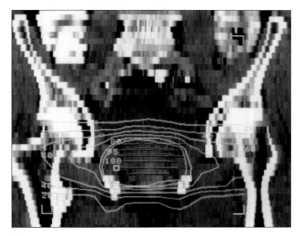

a

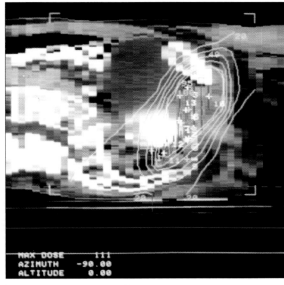

b

16.5 Conformal imaging of the prostate prior to cyclotron treatment using accelerated neutrons. **a.** AP view. **b.** Lateral view. (Reproduced from Austin-Seymour M, Caplan R, Russell K, *et al*. Impact of a multileaf collimator on treatment morbidity in localized carcinoma of the prostate. *Int J Radiat Oncol Biol Phys* 1994:**30**;1065–71 © 1994 with permission Elsevier Science.)

The recent data relating to Casodex™, an antiandrogen, confirm that this compound, when administered orally at a dose of 150 mg once per day, may be at least as efficacious as conventional therapy, at least in patients who do not have bone metastases, but without the quality of life impairment due to adverse effects on sexual function. There may also be a role for antiandrogen therapy in earlier stage, localized disease, especially in older patients, but this needs to be confirmed by long-term, randomized studies.

A new modality, gonadotropin-releasing hormone (GnRH) antagonists, are under development. The most advanced is abarelix which blocks production of GnRH and inhibits production of luteinizing hormone (LH) and follicle-stimulating hormone (FSH)[14]. These actions cause immediate suppression of testosterone and dihydrotestosterone (DHT) to castrate levels. Abarelix also causes an immediate decrease in FSH[15] (see 13.10) in contrast to LHRH agonists. Unlike LHRH agonists, abarelix does not cause an initial stimulation of LH, FSH, testosterone or DHT. This lack of testosterone surge prevents temporary worsening of the condition. Serum concentrations of PSA were also found to be decreased as were those of testosterone. After cessation of treatment with abarelix, PSA levels remained low whereas testosterone concentrations recovered to greater than castrate levels in 4–5 weeks for most patients[16]. In a comparative study with leuperorelin and goserelin (all groups, with or without antiandrogen), abarelix showed chemical castration in 76% of patients by day eight as opposed to 0% in the leuperorelin and goserelin groups. Testosterone surge was absent in the abarelix group but occurred in all patients treated with leuperorelin or goserelin[17].

Other new approaches include angiogenesis inhibition, inhibition of DNA topoisomerase and tyrosine kinase inhibitors. Phase II studies in all these and other areas are in progress.

Chemoprevention

Chemoprevention can be defined as the administration of drugs with the aim of interfering with carcinogenesis, cancer growth or tumour progression. In the context of carcinoma of the prostate, where latent microscopic cancer is so common, the most likely target for chemoprevention would probably be the inhibition of steps that are critical to cancer progression. Men between 40 and 70 years of age might be suitable for such intervention if it were to become available. If the toxicity of the interventional drug were minimal, potentially it could be offered to all men older than 40 years in areas where prostate cancer is common. Alternatively, if the drug toxicity was relatively minor, but still present, and if better markers of prostate cancer progression were developed, the middle-aged

Table 16.2 Potential chemopreventive agents
Difluoromethylornithine (DFMO)
Fenretinide (N-4-hydroxyphenyl retinamide) and other retinoids
Finasteride (5 alpha-reductase inhibitor)
Vitamin D analogues
Vitamin E
Selenium

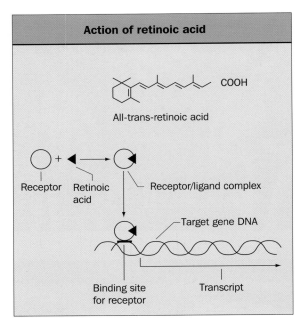

Action of retinoic acid

16.6 Mechanism of action of retinoids in modulating gene expression.

population could be screened with a view to inclusion only of those at high risk of cancer development and progression. Chemoprevention is clearly likely to be of little or no benefit in men older than 70 years of age.

Characteristics of available chemopreventive drugs

The list of potential chemopreventive agents is long. It appears that, based on pre-clinical studies as well as on chemoprevention studies in other human tumours, four categories of drugs might be considered for prostate cancer chemoprevention (**Table 16.2**).

Difluoromethylornithine (DFMO)

DFMO is an effective chemopreventive agent in a variety of animal tumours by virtue of its activity as an irreversible inhibitor of ornithine decarboxylase, the enzyme responsible for the first and rate-limiting step in mammalian polyamine synthesis. Polyamines are normal cell constituents that are important for the regulation of cell proliferation and cell differentiation; the mammalian prostate contains some of the highest concentrations of polyamines anywhere in the body. The administration of DFMO to immature animals prevents normal prostatic development. It has been shown that DFMO inhibits ornithine decarboxylase activity in the Dunning R3327 rat prostatic carcinoma, and also inhibits the growth of this tumour both *in vitro* and *in vivo*. In animal studies, a cyclic regimen of administration involving low doses of the drug reduced toxicity while maintaining chemotherapeutic efficacy. As such, DFMO seems to deserve serious consideration in prostate cancer chemoprevention[18].

Retinoids

Vitamin A (retinol) and its natural analogues (retinoids) are important modulators of epithelial proliferation and differentiation (**16.6**). Retinoids appear to exert their activity by binding to specific nuclear receptors. Mice that had these receptors eliminated by sophisticated gene deletion techniques were born with a dysplastic or absent prostate gland, thus establishing an important potential role for retinoids in prostate development. Many studies have demonstrated the ability of retinoids to suppress carcinogenesis, both *in vitro* and *in vivo*, and synthetic retinoids were shown to inhibit the growth of a carcinogen-induced prostate cancer, perhaps by enhancing the expression of transforming growth factor beta (TGF beta)[19]. The synthetic retinoid, fenretinide, when added to the diet, reduced the incidence and slowed the progression of oncogene-induced prostate cancer in mice[20]. Whereas epidemiological studies attempting to correlate dietary retinoids with a risk of developing prostate cancer have usually been equivocal, evidence that low serum retinol levels correlate with an increased risk of prostate cancer is somewhat stronger[21,22].

The natural retinoids, although effective in inhibiting carcinogenesis, display significant toxicities which preclude their use as general chemopreventive agents. Synthetic retinoid analogues that retain their biological activity and possess a favourable toxicity profile are, however, currently available. The best known, and most extensively studied, is fenretinide.

The safety of fenretinide has been demonstrated in a large breast-cancer chemoprevention trial in Europe, which involved the administration of a daily dose of 200 mg, with a three-day period each month when the drug was not given[23]. Several groups in the USA are currently planning chemoprevention prostate cancer studies using this compound.

Finasteride

The prostate is dependent upon dihydrotestosterone (DHT) for its development and subsequent function. The ability of drugs like finasteride to suppress DHT levels without significantly altering testosterone-dependent functions like muscle strength and libido, has prompted the US National Cancer Institute to propose a large chemopreventive study using this agent. This study has now completed accrual and enrolled 1800 healthy men between 55 and 70 years of age who have been randomized into treatment groups receiving either 5 mg of oral finasteride each day or placebo. Both groups have been biopsied at the end of 7 years and followed for an overall period of at least 10 years. The study's design will allow detection of a 25% decrease in new tumours or local progression with a roughly 90% statistical certainty. Newer dual inhibitors of 5 alpha-reductase such as dufasteride are in development and may also have a chemopreventative role in prostate cancer.

Vitamin D

Recently, Schwartz and his colleagues proposed that low levels of vitamin D could increase the risk of clinical prostate cancer, and they presented some epidemiological evidence to support this theory[24]. Experimental evidence also suggests that vitamin D does possess tumour-inhibitory properties. The human prostate and prostate cancer cell lines contain vitamin D receptors and, furthermore, vitamin D can promote differentiation of prostate cancer lines *in vitro*. Administration of high doses of vitamin D maybe, however, associated with toxicity including hypercalcaemia. Analogues of vitamin D that do not induce hypercalcaemia have now been synthesized, and should be considered for evaluation in prostate cancer chemoprevention.

Potential for Gene Therapy

Recently there has been tremendous enthusiasm in the concept of gene therapy for many neoplastic and non-neoplastic disease areas, and some of these developments may have special application to pro-

state cancer. Gene therapy involves the transference of new genetic material into the cells of a patient in the prospect of therapeutic benefit, hopefully with the induction of few concomitant side effects. In order for gene therapy to work it will of course be necessary to select a gene which encodes the desired therapeutic effect and secondly to develop effective vectors for gene delivery[25,26]. In essence, gene therapy offers three potential mechanisms by which patients with prostatic cancer may be helped:

- Restoration of normal controls over cell division. This could be conceivably achieved by reintroducing deleted tumour suppressor genes or alternatively by insertion of functional homologues which inhibit prostate tumour oncogene expression.
- By enhancement of the natural host cytotoxic and immunostimulatory defence mechanisms against cancer[27].
- Either the delivery of toxic products specifically to cancer cells or the induction of sensitivity to toxic drugs which specifically kill prostate cancer cells.

Effector genes and their mechanisms

As discussed in Chapter 3, prostatic cell division is regulated by a delicate balance of growth promoting oncogenes and growth constraining tumour suppressor genes. Loss of tumour suppressor gene activity may remove a constraint on oncogene expression and thereby allow prostate cancer cells to proliferate. One potential for gene therapy therefore is to facilitate reinsertion of negative regulatory sequences. The genetic insertion of wild-type tumour suppressor genes could prevent neoplastic cell behaviour and restore normal growth patterns[28].

Cytokines

Among the most important elements of anti-tumour activity in normal individuals are naturally occurring cytokines. These substances are able to induce direct tumoricidal effects and they are also capable of initiating and maintaining natural immune surveillance against cancer. Cytokine genes could be transferred into either tumour cells or natural effector cells, thereby promoting an immune attack against neoplastic tissue and subsequent immune surveillance[29].

Cytoreductive therapy

Currently, much interest is focused on the transference of drug susceptibility by gene therapy. After transfer of a gene to cancer cells encoding an enzyme which converts a prodrug into a suicide substrate, the prodrug could be administered systemically thereby eliminating malignant target cells that have been genetically modified. This approach has been pioneered as brachytherapy in malignant brain tumours. One therapeutic combination is intravenous ganciclovir administration after herpes simplex virus thymidine kinase (HSV-tk) gene transfer. In this system, HSV-tk phosphorylation of ganciclovir (GCV) leads to the formation of ganciclovir tri-phosphate, a potent nucleotide competitor which interferes with DNA synthesis and thereby results in programmed cell death.

Gene Delivery Techniques

Integral to all forms of gene therapy is the vector used for gene transfer. Vectors are usually engineered DNA or RNA sequences which contain a site into which a therapeutic gene can be inserted. These vectors are then used to transfer the therapeutic gene into target cancer cells. The therapeutic gene in question is positioned in the vector adjacent to a promoter sequence for RNA polymerase which allows for the expression of messenger RNA of this gene after the vector enters the target for gene therapy. Promoter sequences control the expression of downstream genes and thus constitute a critical engineering component of most gene transfer vectors.

Retrovirus transduction

Genetic material in retroviruses occurs in the form of double-stranded RNA. Once an individual cell is infected with a retrovirus, the RNA genome is reverse transcribed into DNA which then stably integrates into the host DNA. Although retroviral vector mediated gene transfer can be durable, the decay of the viral titre when given intravenously will often impede their potential for direct intravenous *in vivo* gene transfer to disease cells. In fact, retroviruses appear far better suited for *in vitro* gene transfer into living cells that are subsequently returned to the patient (**16.7**). Unfortunately retroviral vectors require target cell proliferation for genomic integration; since gene transfer will only succeed in actively dividing cells. In addition, the possibility of pathogenic metagenesis during chromosomal insertion of the vector and the difficulty in isolating high enough titres for clinical use are further limitations associated with this vector system.

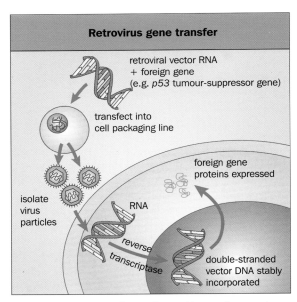

16.7 Retroviruses can be used to stably transfer genetic material into host cells.

Adenovirus transduction

Unlike retroviruses, adenoviruses are capable of infecting non-dividing cells and can also potentially carry large quantities of genetic material. They are therefore capable of mediating durable genetic transduction and are themselves sufficiently stable for potential direct *in vivo* gene transfer. However, integration of adenovirus genomes into target cell DNA has so far been associated with a greater tendency towards unwanted deletions and rearrangements during gene transfer.

An adenoviral vector nonetheless has been used to transfect prostate cancer cells with an efficacy as high as 65%[28]; the transfection is of only transient duration however and therefore repeated inoculations may be needed for continuous *in vivo* effective gene delivery. Nonetheless, expression appears to last for up to two weeks and this may be sufficient for adequate immunostimulation. Adeno-associated viruses (AAV) integrate into non dividing cells with a high efficiency but can only accept relatively small fragments of DNA. There is evidence that the AAV genome reproducibly integrates into a region of the human chromosome 19, which in itself has some advantages in terms of manipulation and exploitation. Adenovirus vectors have been chosen for the transmembrane regulatory gene transduction in cystic fibrosis gene therapy, partly because the virus particles are amenable to purification and concentration without significant loss of transduction activity.

However, the sophisticated mechanisms of pathogenicity of the parent viruses from which all of these vectors are derived do require equally sophisticated genetic engineering to render them clinically safe. Currently no single vector possesses all the desirable features for every therapeutic application. Desirable features include permanence of transduction, high efficiency of gene transfer, target tissue specificity and fidelity of gene expressions over time. When choosing a vector system for clinical application, the relative importance of each feature needs to be considered. In a related technique, liposomes can be complexed with effector gene DNA and then injected into the peripheral circulation. Liposomes with target cell membranes can thereby deliver DNA to their cytoplasm. A liposome–DNA complex containing interleukin-2 bearing adeno-associated virus (AAV) has been successfully used by Vieweg *et al* to transfect prostate cancer cells[30] with a roughly 50% efficacy and a stable expression for around 2 weeks duration.

Potential Approaches for Gene Therapy in Prostate Cancer

Restoration of normal growth regulation

As has already been discussed, oncogene activity via specific growth factors and their receptors may well be an important mechanism in the development of the various stages of prostate cancer. In theory, at least, gene therapy could be used to insert functional homologues into existing prostate cancer cells that might inhibit the deleterious effects of abnormal oncogene expression.

Mutations in the tumour suppression gene *p53* are known to be associated with uncontrolled proliferation of tumour cells and deletions involving this gene may well be involved in the development of androgen dependent and independent growth of prostate cancer.

In vitro tumour inhibition has been demonstrated in prostate cancer cells in culture by replacing *p53* suppressor gene activity which adds credence to the suggestion that mutation and deletion of the *p53* tumour suppressor gene may increase malignant potential in this disease[31].

Other tumour suppressor genes including the retinoblastoma (*RB* gene) may also be important

in the development of prostate cancer. Potentially, therefore, gene therapy could replace mutated *RB* genes. *In vitro* studies by Stiener *et al*[32] suggest that the replacement of the *RB* gene may increase the sensitivity of cells to transforming growth factor beta (TGF beta) and thereby slow tumour growth. Another approach may be to restore androgen receptor activity which potentially could result in the restoration of androgen sensitivity to tumour cells[33].

A number of further growth factors and cell adhesion molecules that can modulate prostate cancer cells have been identified, including fibroblast growth factor and transforming growth factors alpha and beta. Currently several groups are studying the oncogenic effects of these specific elements and the ways in which these can be manipulated to facilitate the development of gene therapy. As mentioned earlier in this book, an absence of E-cadherin may be important in the development of metastatic prostatic malignancy[4]; its restoration by gene therapy may potentially be beneficial. The way in which rapidly evolving knowledge in this field can be clinically utilized for the development of gene therapy for prostate cancer has yet to be fully established, but clearly the potential is enormous.

Cytoreductive Immunotherapy

The most extensively studied form of cytoreductive gene therapy involves augmentation of host immune responses against malignancy by vaccinating affected patients with genetically modified tumour cells. The goal of immunotherapy is to sensitize immune effector cells to tumour antigen, and thereby precipitate a cytotoxic response directed at the tumour with minimal associated systemic toxicity. Recent work in several centres has demonstrated that immunogenicity of neoplastic prostate tissue and its potential susceptibility to immunotherapy[28,34]. Current interest is focused on cytokines and the many growth factors which are involved in the proliferation of both neoplastic cells and cytotoxic cells directed against tumour antigens. A variety of cytokines that modulate antitumour immune response have been used in gene modified tumour vaccines for gene therapy. One of the first studies using this strategy showed induction of anti-tumour effect in nude mice by means of vaccination of tumour cells transduced to secrete interleukin-2 (IL-2). This study aimed to achieve nonspecific (T-cell independent) antitumour effect by producing significant systemic levels of IL-2. Subsequently other cytokines including IL-4, IL-6 and granulocyte-macrophage colony-stimulating factor (GM-CSF), were also shown to have the ability to eliminate microscopic tumour cell deposits when mouse tumour cells were transduced with the respective cytokine genes and when these cytokine-secreting tumours were reintroduced into the animals.

Tumour Vaccines

At present, most tumour vaccine protocols exploit the ability of cytokines to increase tumour cell immunogenicity thereby increasing host cell immune surveillance and tumour lysis. The need for individual patient cancer cell harvesting for cell culture and tumour burden reduction currently make urological surgery a necessary component. After removal of the patient's primary lesion, tumour cells can be cultured and transfected with cytokine genes *ex vivo*. These cells, with enhanced cytokine production potential, are then readministered to the patient

subcutaneously to stimulate an antitumour immune response. Although cytokine production will only occur at the implant site, the stimulated immune effector agents then diffuse throughout the host to pursue and destroy diffuse tumour foci (**16.8**). Studies in animals with subcutaneously innoculated vaccines demonstrate potent specific and long lasting anti-tumour immunity. A tumour vaccine has been recently created in the Dunning R3327-MatLyLu prostate tumour cell line. Vieweg *et al*[30] investigated an interleukin-2 secreting tumour vaccine which they found could cure animals with established tumour and induce immunological memory in the subjects protecting them from succeeding tumour challenge.

Transfer of Drug Susceptibility Genes

Another form of cytoreductive gene therapy under development involves the transfer of drug susceptibility genes. After transfer of a gene to cancer cells encoding an enzyme which converts a prodrug into a suicide substrain, the prodrug can be administered

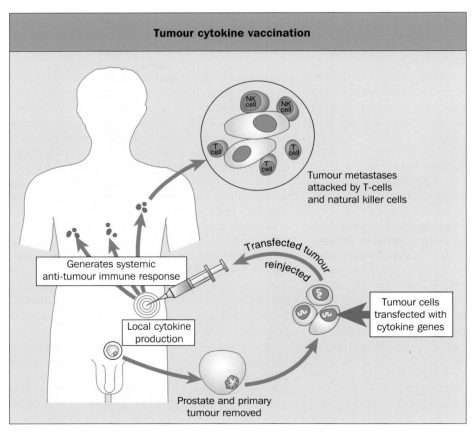

Tumour cytokine vaccination

Tumour metastases attacked by T-cells and natural killer cells

Generates systemic anti-tumour immune response

Transfected tumour reinjected

Local cytokine production

Tumour cells transfected with cytokine genes

Prostate and primary tumour removed

16.8 Vaccination therapy for prostate cancer may involve harvesting tumour cells, transfecting them with cytokine genes and reintroducing them where they may stimulate immune responses against tumour cells by T cells and natural killer (NK) cells.

systemically thereby eliminating malignant target cells that have been genetically modified. Eastham et al.[35] have used a recombinant adenovirus carrying the herpes simplex virus thymidine kinase (HSV-tk) gene to confer sensitivity to gangciclovir (GCV) to prostate cancer cells in culture.

The 'Bystander Effect'

An important new concept in gene therapy is that of the 'bystander effect'. This refers to the successful destruction of an entire tumour burden despite sub-total transfection of tumour cells with the target gene. This implies some mechanism whereby non-transduced cancer cells in the vicinity of a trans-duced cancer cell can also be killed after exposure to the drug. The pathways of cell death in the bystander effect still needs elucidation. Clearly there is a risk that this effect could also lead to toxicity related to the bystander effect harming local normal cells in the vicinity of the tumour.

The bystander effect is an important concept in terms of gene therapy for prostate cancer. Prostate tumour masses are known to consist of a very heterogeneous collection of cells, some of which are very immature. A sufficiently intense local immune response, however, may be enough to ensure that not only mature but also surrounding immature cancer cells will also be destroyed.

Other new approaches include targeting the bcl-2 gene to delay androgen-independent progres-sion and enhance chomosensitivity using antisense bcl-2 oligodeoxynucleotides[36].

Target Tissue Specific Gene Delivery

Vectors are currently being constructed that contain tissue specific promoters which restrict expression of a transferred cytotoxic gene. Prostate cancer is potentially an optimal target for such approaches. By designing a construct with a gene of interest whose expression is controlled by the PSA promoter and regulatory sequences, only cells which normally express PSA will express the transferred therapeutic gene product. Pilot studies have examined this approach by evaluating expression of luciferase (a reporter gene which encodes a readily assayed gene product) transcribed downstream from the human PSA promoter sequence after transfection with pro-state cancer cells in vitro[29]. Peng et al[37] have con-firmed the specificity to prostate derived tissue with this approach and increased the activity fourfold by combining the PSA promoter with an upstream cytomegalovirus (CMV) promoter sequence.

In conclusion, the prospects for gene therapy in prostate cancer seem promising. For further information the reader is directed to the excellent review by Sanda and Simmonds[34] together with that of Sokolov and Belldegrun[38].

CONCLUSION

Some may find the many uncertainties associated with prostate cancer, perhaps one of the most enigmatic of cancers, unsettling. But, as we have tried to convey throughout this book, there are currently numerous grounds for optimism. Although prostate cancer research has lagged behind that of breast cancer – its endocrine-related equivalent in females – this balance is now beginning to be redressed; many of the fundamental issues are currently being tackled in well designed, long-term, randomized studies.

Chemoprevention, screening, staging and optimal therapy for both localized and metastatic disease are all currently under intense scrutiny. Commercial considerations related to the demographic shift and the rising prevalence of prostate cancer will ensure that the already considerable investment in new pharmacological, molecular, biological and techno-logical therapy continues apace. Many of the contro-versies surrounding prostate cancer will be resolved only when the results of long-term, randomized studies are available, but in the meantime it falls to us as clinicians to work together in partnership and communicate clearly and sympathetically to our patients and their families the range of diagnostic and treatment options available, together with their various merits and demerits.

As in many other areas of medicine, there are few absolute rights and wrongs in the treatment of prostate cancer; the selection of therapy is some-times more of an art than a science. Until definitive data are available, we must continue to do the very best we can for our patients, even if we do not know all of the answers for sure. It should be remembered that communication with a caring sympathetic professional, conversant with the very latest infor-mation, can often do as much for the quality of life of the patient as the actual treatment employed. We hope that the second edition of this book will promote this informed communication.

REFERENCES

1 Christensson A, Bjork T, Nilsson O, *et al*. Serum prostate-specific antigen complexed to alpha-1-antichymotrypsin as an indicator of prostate cancer. *J Urol* 1993;**150**:100–105.

2 Oesterling JE, Jacobsen SJ, Chute CG, *et al*. The establishment of age-specific reference ranges for prostate-specific antigen. *J Urol* 1993;**149**:510A.

3 Brawer MK, Beatie J, Wener MH, *et al*. Screening for prostatic carcinoma with prostate-specific antigen: results of the second year. *J Urol* 1993;**150**:106–109.

4 Umbas R, Schalken JA, Aalders TW, *et al*. Expression of cellular adhesion molecule E-cadherin is reduced or absent in high-grade prostate cancer. *Canc Res* 1992;**52**:5104–5109.

5 Black DM, Nicolai H, Borrow J, *et al*. A somatic cell hybrid map of the long arm of human chromosome 17, containing the familial breast cancer locus (BRCA1). *Am J Hum Genet* 1993;**52**(4):702–710.

6 Roth MS, Antin JH, Ashe R. Prognostic significance of Philadelphia chromosome positive cells detected by the polymerase chain reaction after allogeneic bone marrow transplant for chronic myelogenous leukaemia. *Blood* 1992;**79**:276–282.

7 Wood DP, Banks ER, Humphreys S, *et al*. Sensitivity of immunohistochemistry and polymerase chain reaction in deleting prostate cancer cells in bone marrow. *J Histochem Cytochem* 1994;**42**:505–511.

8 Cama C, Olsson CA, Raffo AJ, *et al*. Molecular staging of prostate cancer II. A comparison of the application of an enhanced reverse transcriptase polymerase chain reaction assay for prostate-specific antigen versus prostate specific membrane antigen. *J Urol* 1995;**153**:1373–1378.

9 Ellis WV, Vessella RL, Corey E, *et al*. The value of reverse transcriptase PCR testing in preoperative staging and follow up of prostate cancer. *J Urol* 1998;**159**:1134.

10 Oefelein MG, Ignatoff JM, Clomens JQ, Watkin W, Kaul K. Clinical and molecular follow up after radical prostatectomy. *J Urol* 1999;**162**:307–311.

11 Zincke H, Oesterling JE, Blute ML, *et al*. Long term (15 years) results after radical prostatectomy for clinically localized (Stage T2c or lower) prostate cancer. *J. Urol* 1994;**152**: 1850–1857.

12 Leihel SA, Zelefsky MJ, Kutcher GJ, *et al*. Three dimensional conformal radiation therapy in localized carcinoma of the prostate: interim report of phase 1 dose-escalation study. *J Urol* 1994;**152**:1792–1978.

13 Russell KJ, Caplan RJ, Laramore GE, *et al*. Photon versus fast neutron external beam radiotherapy in the treatment of locally advanced prostate cancer: results of randomized prospective trials. *Int J Radiation Oncology Biol Phys* 1993;**28**:47–54.

14 Molineaux CJ, Sluss PM, Bree BS, Gefter ML, Sullivan BS, Garnick MB. Suppression of plasma gonadotrophins by abarelix: a potent new LHRH antagonist. *Molecular Urology* 1998;**2**:265–268.

15 Garnick MB, Campion M, Abarelix Depot Study Group. Abarelix depot, a GnRH antagonist V. LHRH superagonists in prostate cancer: differential effects on follicle-stimulating hormone. *Mol Urol* 2000;**4**:275.

16 Garnick MB, Gittleman M, Steidle C, *et al*. Abarelix (PPI-149), a novel and potent GnRH antagonist, induces rapid and profound prostate gland volume reduction (PGVR) and androgen suppression before brachytheray (BT) or radiation therapy (XRT). *J Urol* 1998;**159**:220.

17 Garnick MB, Tomera K, Campion M, Kuca MA. Abarelix-depot (A-D). A sustained-release (SR) formulation of a potent GnRH pure agonist in patients (pts) with prostate cancer (PrCa): Phase II clinical results and endocrine comparison with superagonists Lupron (L) and Zoladex (Z). *J Urol* 1999;**161**:340.

18 Kadmon D. Chemoprevention in prostate cancer: The role of difluoromethylornithine (DFMO). *J Cell Biochem* 1992; **16H(Suppl)**:122–127.

19 Sporn MB. Chemoprevention of Cancer. *Lancet* 1993;**342**: 1211–1213.

20 Slawin K, *et al*. Dietary fenretinide, a synthetic retinoid, decreases the tumour incidence and the tumour mass of ras + myc-induced carcinomas in the mouse prostate reconstitution model system. *Cancer Res* 1993;**53**:4461–4465.

21 Hayes RB, *et al*. Serum retinol and prostate cancer. *Cancer* 1988;**62**:2021–2026.

22 Reichman ME, *et al*. Serum vitamin A and subsequent development of prostate cancer in the first National Health and Nutrition Examination Survey Epidemiologic Follow-up Study. *Cancer Res* 1990;**50**:2311–2315.

23 Rotmensz N, *et al*. Long-term tolerability of fenretinoid (4-HPR) in breast cancer patients. *Eur J Cancer* 1991;**27**: 1127–1131.

24 Hanchette CL, Schwartz GG. Geographic patterns of prostate cancer mortality: Evidence for a protective effect of ultraviolet radiation. *Cancer* 1992;**70**(12):2861–2869.

25 Morgan RA, Anderson WF. Human gene therapy. *Ann Rev Biochem* 1993;**62**:191–217.

26 Mulligan RC. The basic science of gene therapy. *Science* 1993;**260**(5110):926–932.

27 Hill ADK, *et al*. Cytokines in tumour therapy. *Br J Surg* 1992;**79**(10):990–997.

28 Sanda MG, Ayyagari SR, Jattee EM, *et al*. Demonstration of a rational strategy for human prostate cancer gene therapy. *J Urol* 1994;**151**: 622–628.

29 Taneja SS, Belldegrun A, de Kernion JB, *et al*. Adenoviral vector mediated high efficiency gene transfer in prostate cancer cell lines [abstract]. *J Urol* 1994;**151**(5):253A.

30 Vieweg J, Heston WDW, Fair WR, *et al*. Use of cytokine gene-modified prostatic tumor cells for the treatment of advanced prostate cancer. *J Urol* 1994;**151**(5):492A.

31 Isaacs WB, Carter BS, Ewing CM. Wild-type p53 suppresses growth of human prostate cancer cells

containing mutant p53 allele. *Cancer Res* 1992;**51**(17):4716–4720.

32 Steiner MS, Anthony CT, Case T, *et al.* Retinoblastoma (RB) gene replacement in advanced human prostate cancer increases transforming growth factor beta-1 sensitivity and slows tumor growth. *J Urol* 1995;**153**:306A.

33 Yuan S, Trachtenberg J, Mills GB, *et al.* Androgen-induced inhibition of cell proliferation in an androgen-insensitive prostate cancer cell line (PC3) transfected with a human androgen receptor complementary DNA. *Canc Res* 1993;**53**:1304–1311.

34 Sanda MG, Simons JW. Gene therapy for urologic cancer. *Urology* 1994;**44**:617–624.

35 Eastham JA, Chen SH, Sehgal I, *et al.* Prostate cancer gene therapy: HSV-tk gene transduction followed by ganciclovin in the mouse prostate reconstitution model. *J Urol* 1995;**153**:307A.

36 Gleave ME, Miayake H, Goldie J, *et al.* Targeting bcl-2 gene to delay androgen-independent progression and enhance chemosensitivity in prostate cancer using antisense oligodeoxynucleotides. *Urology* 1999;**54**:36–46.

37 Peng S, Sokoloff M, Teneja S. Prostate tissue-specific gene therapy utilizing a unique prostate-specific antigen cytomegalovirus (PSA–CMV) promotor. *J Urol* 1995;**151**:307A.

38 Sokoloff M, Belldegrun A. Gene therapy for prostate cancer *Prospectives* 1995;**5**:1–8.

Index

225